Foot and ankle in rheumatoid arthritis

Springer
Paris
Berlin
Heidelberg
New York
Hong Kong
Londres
Milan
Tokyo

Maurice Bouysset, Yves Tourné and Karl Tillmann

Foot and ankle in rheumatoid arthritis

Springer

Maurice Bouysset
126, rue Philippe-Héron
69400 Villefranche-sur-Saône
France

Yves Tourné
Groupe Chirurgical République
15, rue de la République
38000 Grenoble
France

Karl Tillmann
Arzt-für Orthopaëdie Rheumaklinik
24572 Bad Bramstedt Holst.
Germany

ISBN-10 : 2-287-59757-3 Springer Paris Berlin Heidelberg New York
ISBN-13 : 978-2-287-59757-2 Springer Paris Berlin Heidelberg New York

SPIN: 10864155

Cover Design: Nadia OUDDANE

List of authors

Dr Bonnin Michel	Clinique Sainte-Anne-Lumière, 85, cours Albert-Thomas, 69003 Lyon (France)
Dr Bouysset Maurice	126, rue Philippe-Héron, 69400 Villefranche-sur-Saône (France)
Dr Caro W.	Universitätsklinik Regensburg, im BRK Rheuma-Zentrum Kaiser-Karl V – allee 3, 93077 Bad Abbach (Germany)
Dr Colombier Jean-Alain	Clinique de l'Union Boulevard Ratalens 31240 Saint-Jean (France)
Dr Crevoisier Xavier	FMH chirurgie orthopédique, hôpital orthopédique de la Suisse romande, Pierre-Decker 4, 1005 Lausanne (switzerland)
Pr Fink B.	Klinik und Polichlinik für Orthopädie, Universität Hazmburg-Eppendorf Martinistr. 52, D-20246 Hamburg (Germany)
Dr Gintz Bruno	CHU Albert-Michallon, BP 217, 38043 Grenoble Cedex 09 (France)
Pr Grifka Joachim	Orthopädische Universitätsklinik Regensburg, im BRK Rheuma-Zentrum Kaiser-Karl V – Allee 3, 93077 Bad Abbach (Germany)
Dr Guaydier-Souquières Gennevième	Centre hospitalier universitaire de Caen 14033 Caen Cedex (France)
Dr Heers G.	Orthopädische Universitätsklinik Regensburg, im BRK Rheuma-Zentrum Kaiser-Karl V – Allee 3, 93077 Bad Abbach (Germany)

Dr Hugueny Pascale	126, rue Philippe Heron 69400 Villefranche-sur-Saône (France)
Dr Jalby Jocelyne	126, rue Philippe-Héron, 69400 Villefranche-sur-Saône (France)
Dr Judet Thierry	Hôpital Tenon 4, rue de la Chine 75020 Paris (France)
Dr Koeck F.X.	Orthopädische Universitätsklinik Regensburg, im BRK Rheuma-Zentrum Kaiser-Karl V – Allee 3, 93077 Bad Abbach (Germany)
Pr Kofoed Hakon	30 Norasvej DK 2920, Charlottenlund (Denmark)
Dr Lapeyre Françoise	Centre de grand appareillage, 53, rue de Créqui, 69006 Lyon (France)
Dr Leemrijse Thibaut	Cliniques Universitaires Saint-Luc Avenue Hippocrate, 10 1200 Bruxelles (Belgium)
Pr Miossec Pierre	Hôpital Edouard-Herriot, pavillon F, Service de rhumatologie et de pathologie osseuse 5, place d'Arsonval, 69437 Lyon Cedex 03 (France)
Dr Noël Eric	Clinique Sainte-Anne Lumière 85, cours Albert Thomas 69003 Lyon (France)
Pr Souter W.A.	Surgical Arthritis Unit, Princess Margaret Rose Orthopaedic Hospital, Edinburgh (Grait Britain)
Dr Siguier Thierry	Clinique Jouvenet 6, square Jouvenet 75016 Paris (France)
Dr Tavernier Thierry	Clinique de la Sauvegarde, av. Ben-Gourion, service de radiologie, 69009 Lyon (France)
Pr Tebib Jacques	Centre hospitalier Lyon-Sud, service de rhumatologie, 69310 Pierre-Bénite (France)
Dr Thabe Heiner	Diakonie-Anstalten Ringstrasse 58-60, D 55 543 Bad Kreuznach (Germany)
Pr Tillmann Karl	Arzt für Orthopaëdie Rheumaklinik, 24572 Bad Bramstedt Holst (Germany)
Dr Tourné Yves	Groupe Chirurgical République 15, rue de la République 38000 Grenoble (France)
Dr Valtin Bernard	Clinique des Lilas CEPIM, 41-49, avenue du Maréchal-Juin, 93260 Les Lilas (France)

Aknowledgements

With specific aknowledgements to professor J. Tebib without his help this book would not have been possible.

And for their help a special gratitude to doctor Michel Bonnin, who read several translations of surgical chapter, and Corinne Gauthier, the secretary of the book.

The following people are aslo thanked for their direct or indirect participation in the making of this book: Véronique Belin, Jean-Luc Besse, Maurice Bouvier, Jean-François Brantus, Roland Chapard, Jeanne Charrin, Frédéric Colson, Nina Crowte, P.-D. Delmas, Laurence Denoual, Stéphanie van Duin, Jean-Pierre Duivon, Roger Elkaim, Joachim Grifka, Sophie Guillemot, Pascale Hugueny, Nathalie Huilleret, Jocelyne Jalby, Catherine Jolly, Jean-Paul Larbre, Patrick Lavault, Guy Lorca, P.-J. Meunier, Pierre Miossec, Chantal Nemoz, Eric Noël, Annie-Claude Ortiz, Jean-Claude Vianey, Eric Vignon.

Foreword

One of the earliest signs of rheumatoid arthritis may be pain in the foot. However, this part of the body is very often neglected during clinical assessment of the illness in favour of the articulations of the upper limbs, knees and hips.

Nevertheless, it appears evident that a detailed clinical examination of the forefoot, ankle and heel could be useful in order to get closer to a rheumatological diagnosis.

Thanks to blood tests and conventional imaging, completed with a scanner or MRI if needed, every doctor should be in a position to detect the beginning of rheumatoid arthritis in the foot or ankle.

As well as its diagnostic contribution, this book broaches the theme of the most recent medicinal treatments, that of orthoses, made-to-measure shoes (the prescription of which practitioners and the rheumatologists often hand over to the orthopaedic surgeons), and finally that of local injections. These elements constitute the main treatment of the rheumatoid foot.

Taking care of the ill subject does not necessarily stop there and a surgeon may need to operate on the forefoot, which is more common, or on the mid-foot or the ankle. One of the strong points of this book is that a large part of it covers the diverse surgical possibilities that are now available. These measures need to be carefully thought about beforehand with regards to their usefulness for each patient, if possible with an exchange between rheumatologists and orthopaedists. The complementary nature of the surgical and conservative clinical approach appears clearly in the structure of this book.

The credit of this book is due to A.M. Bouysset, Y. Tourné and K. Tillmann. With the « Pied en rhumatologie » published in 1998 and « Pathologie ostéo-articulaire du pied et de la cheville » published in 2000, Maurice Bouysset has already given us a foretaste of the perfection he achieves in the books he inspires and whose publications he directs.

Pr Jean-Charles Gerster
CHU Vaudois
Hôpital Nestlé
Avenue Pierre Decker 5
CH 1010 Lausanne
Switzerland

Preface

We all have a great and ever increasing interest in the international efforts of describing, understanding and solving foot and ankle problems. More and more orthopaedic surgeons are going to specialize in the treatment of disorders of the foot. The European Foot and Ankle Society - EFAS, aiming to promote the development of foot and ankle surgery and to advance education, study and research in this speciality observes a popular interest and demand for instructional courses and for specialized literature.

It is essential to collect the experience and the expertise of more than one specialist to provide a substantial contribution to a subject. This book is certain to be a substantial contribution. Twenty percent of rheumatoid arthritis starts in the foot and ankle area. Not only specialists should know the pathomechanism and the spectrum of the conservative and operative treatment but also master later stages and to be able to soothe the suffering.

It is not an easy task to write comprehensible texts for all levels of rheumatologists, foot surgeons and professional groups engaged in foot treatment. In my view, all participating authors of this book have done just that, respecting the multiple layers of this chronic inflammatory disease. They share their great experience and their knowledge, respecting biomechanical features, giving a clear description of the current state of the art concerning operative treatment and conservative therapeutic and aftercare measures. Specialists and editors have succeeded in composing a unique textbook, reflecting the high level of the authors' experience. All fundamental information is well illustrated and arranged in a enjoyable didactical way.

Rheumatologists such as Maurice Bouysset and orthopaedists such as Yves Tourné and Karl Tillmann as editors and most of the participating authors of this are highly experienced in the treatment of inflammatory and post-inflammatory residual disorders of the human joints, and it was them who set the pace in many directions of research and development concerning the foot. This book provides us with an insight to the European rheumatologists' skills, being an enrichment for everybody's library.

Pr Hans Heino Kuster
Professor of orthopaedic surgery
Director orthopaedic Department
Sankt-Elisabeth Hospital
Stadtring Kattensroth 130
33332 Gütersloh-Germany

Contents

Diagnosis of rheumatoid arthritis at an early stage

P. Miossec and J. Tebib

Definition

Rheumatoid arthritis (RA) is the most frequent chronic inflammatory arthritis. It affects about 0.5% of the population, four times more often women. It can start at any age but more frequently between 35 and 55 years.

Its severity is the consequence of a chronic inflammation of the synovial membrane of joints and tendons. This inflammation leads gradually to a destruction of bone and cartilage, responsible for loss of function.

RA is also a systemic disease with extra-articular manifestations, some of which can have lethal consequences. RA is a significant health problem because 50% of the patients stop their professional activity less than 5 years after the beginning of their disease. Furthermore life expectancy of these patients is on average reduced from 5 to 10 years. Finally, costs due to this disease are high, more because of an exclusion from the active economic system than because of high medical and pharmaceutical costs.

Pathophysiology

RA is a disorder and its precise origin is not known. However, RA has been classified as an autoimmune disease because of the presence of signs of auto-reactivity.

Several inducing factors have been identified:

- *hormonal:* with a clear female association and a better control during pregnancy;
- *genetic:* there is an incomplete association with HLA DR4 and DR1 alleles, particularly with the DRB1 0401, 0404 and 0101 subtypes. More recently was identified the positive or negative contribution of cytokine gene polymorphisms with opposite effects from pro- and anti-inflammatory cytokines. It is important to note, however, that concordance for RA in homozygous twin sisters is only 17.5%.
- *environmental:* various candidates have been suspected including bacterial (mycobacterial heat shock proteins) or viral (exogenous or endogenous retrovirus, Epstein Barr virus, parvovirus) agents.

The consequences of synovial membrane inflammation are now better understood. This has led to several therapeutic applications to control the action of proinflammatory cytokines such as interleukin 1 and tumour necrosis factor alpha.

Chronic inflammation of the synovial membrane leads to a chronic synovitis characterized by interactions between mononuclear cells migrating from blood, which, after extra-vascular emigration, come into contact with mesenchymal cells in joints (fibroblasts/synoviocytes).

The development of RA synovitis induces a pannus formation, the chronicity of which leads to bone and cartilage destruction. At an early stage, there is a hyperplasia with proliferation of lining cells next to the articular cavity, an intense new blood vessel formation, which favours the migration of lymphocytes, especially of the CD4 memory phenotype, that accumulate as perivascular lymphoid nodules.

These T lymphocytes express markers of activation and contribute to the secretion of cytokines of the Th1 type (Interferon γ, interleukin 17) (9). In addition, these lymphocytes, directly and through their soluble factors, activate resident cells in combination with an effect on the secretion of proinflammatory cytokines such as interleukin 1 and tumour necrosis factor alpha. These cytokines activate mesenchymal cells, which release enzymes, namely metalloproteases, responsible for the degradation of the extra-cellular matrix.

In contrast, there is a local defect in the production of cytokines of the Th2 type, which have an anti-inflammatory effect, such as interleukin 4 and interleukin 10.

This local cell activation induces an intense cell accumulation, which results from an increased proliferation not compensated by the elimination by programmed cell death or apoptosis, which is globally deficient.

Prolonged local inflammation is susceptible to lead to molecular changes very similar to those found in tumour cells. The presence of activation, even alteration, of some oncogenes such as p53 may explain the limitations of controlling these abnormalities at a late disease stage (6). This concept is a strong argument for an early therapeutic control not only of inflammatory features but more so of local factors, which control cell proliferation.

The specific control of these targets has made a significant step in the right direction. Today, inhibition of TNFα with a monoclonal antibody or with a soluble receptor is part of the current RA treatment. However, the efficiency of these new approaches will not be able to compensate for the need for early treatment.

Clinical diagnosis

Diagnosis of RA must indeed be made as soon as possible, in particular before articular destruction occurs. It is at this stage that a treatment may have a chance to be effective. Two totally opposite pictures of the disease can be defined:
- at an early stage, diagnosis is difficult to establish and differential diagnoses are numerous;
- at a late stage, diagnosis is obvious but treatment is difficult.

Early diagnosis of RA is difficult, above all based on clinical examination. At this stage the goal is to find enough arguments to suggest and not necessarily to establish such diagnosis. It is often difficult to establish a diagnosis of RA after the first visit and there are other differential diagnoses. Biologic data are often not useful. At this stage diagnosis of RA must be suggested and only a symptomatic treatment without steroids given. It is critical to see the patient again for a follow-up to search for more chronic signs.

Different clinical presentations can be observed:

Distal oligo-arthritis

This is the most frequent mode of initiation. This presentation is suggestive by:
- the location: affecting wrists, metacarpo-phalangeal joints (especially 2nd and 3rd) and forefeet;
- the expression: bilateral and relatively symmetric;
- type of pain: inflammatory, at night, maximal in the morning, with articular morning stiffness, decreasing after joint exercise;
- clinical manifestations are still limited, more obvious in the morning with joint stiffness, sometimes swelling;
- the most suggestive sign is hand finger flexor tenosynovitis, with often a carpal tunnel syndrome, and extensor tenosynovitis.

It is necessary to underline the importance of the chronic character of these manifestations. The association of stiffness of both hands, forefoot pain and synovitis of finger flexor tenosynovitis is practically pathognomonic of RA.

Intermittent polyarthralgias

This is also a common mode of disease initiation. There is a contrast between the functional signs described by the patient: arthralgias with an inflammatory mode, fatigue, occasional episodes of synovitis, and negative or poor examination. These intermittent and migratory manifestations were previously described in the context of palindromic rheumatism. The intermittent character implies that very often examination is normal, in particular without arguments for chronic synovitis. There are incomplete forms where articular signs are part of self-limited synovitis on average with a good prognosis.

These manifestations are also signs of Sjögren's syndrome: defined by sicca syndrome with kerato-conjunctivitis (xerophtalmia) with the sensation of sand in eyes, linked to a reduced lachrymal secretion (measured by the Schirmer's test) and salivary gland secretion (xerostomia). Sjögren's syndrome is defined as secondary when associated to another disease, often RA. Diagnosis is made on the basis of a salivary gland biopsy showing a dense lymphoid infiltrate.

Tenosynovitis with compression syndromes

Tenosynovitis represents a major sign of synovial inflammation. Almost constant, they can lead eventually to tendon ruptures. They affect tendons of various muscles: extensors and flexors of fingers with carpal tunnel syndrome or nodular tenosynovitis responsible for episodes of flexion blockade.

The involvement of the synovial membrane with hypertrophy around tendons is not always painful, but becomes noticeable through the consequences of local compression.

Compression of the median nerve at the carpal tunnel is often an early isolated sign. The presence of a synovitis of the tendons of finger flexor muscles increases compression. At this stage, especially if some clinical signs question the common character of the carpal tunnel syndrome, it makes sense to propose a surgical access. Magnetic resonance imaging with gadolinium injection is useful to better clarify the anatomical situation by showing the contribution of the synovial hypertrophy to the compression. In addition to treatment, surgical access allows a biopsy. In this context, it remains logical to prefer an open surgical access to a simple section of the ligament under arthroscopy.

Inaugural foot involvement

Foot symptoms can represent the first manifestations of numerous inflammatory arthritis. The involvement of the forefoot is the most usual presentation in RA. This induces pain when walking but morning pain during the first steps is particularly suggestive. Examination can notice pain following pressure across the forefoot and on the 5th metatarso-phalangeal joint.

Sometimes the patient will complain of changes in pain first associated with more common deformities. Often there is already a common hallux valgus deformity with triangular forefoot, which becomes more painful.

The involvement of the Achilles tendon is more suggestive of spondylarthropathies, especially when the inflammatory character is present with morning pain. During RA, the involvement of this tendon is mostly secondary to changes in foot pressure, which results from forefoot involvement.

The very inflammatory, isolated or asymmetric involvement of one toe is more suggestive of psoriatic arthritis, reactive arthritis and spondylarthropathies.

Rarer forms of early manifestations

An inflammatory involvement of proximal joints is more common after sixty years of age, associated with important systemic changes with fever, pain and stiffness in hips and shoulders and myalgias. Differential diagnosis between RA with proximal manifestations and polymyalgia rheumatica is very difficult. This later diagnosis is often used in excess. Sometimes only follow-up will clarify the diagnosis, in particular with difficulties to decrease steroids and the appearance of more distal articular signs.

In aged individuals, crystal arthritis can be misleading. However an association with RA is always possible especially for chondrocalcinosis. Synovial fluid examination can be a simple way to clarify.

A subacute or chronic mono-arthritis implies first to eliminate infectious arthritis. This can be clarified with a biopsy of the synovial membrane. The optimal use of the more modern molecular tools should reduce the percentage of arthritis, which remains of unknown aetiology. Inflammatory diseases such as RA will become a possibility only when infection has been ruled out.

Systemic symptoms with extra-articular signs (vasculitis, rheumatoid lung) with fever are rarely found early. They are rather characteristic of the expression of adult Still disease.

Contribution of additional investigations

At this stage, they often do not provide specific enough arguments and diagnosis remains above all clinical. They will serve as reference for follow-up.

Morphological tests

X-ray films of hands and feet are normal or show a simple osteoporosis band of the metacarpo-phalangeal joints. In the foot, the most specific lesion is that of the 5th metatarso-phalangeal joint. Changes are delayed by several months with regard to clinical signs. The presence of erosions is a turn in disease evolution because it demonstrates its destructive character. Certainly it allows diagnosis clarification. It is necessary, however, to realize that the progress in disease control will be significant only if active treatments are used early when that diagnosis is only a possibility and before the stage of erosions.

Quantification of radiological lesions can be performed using different radiographic methods (Steinbrocker, Sharp, Larsen). Today the Sharp's method modified by Van der Hedge is often selected in drug trials (12).

The contribution of the other morphological tools remains to be better defined before they can be used routinely on all patients. Magnetic resonance imaging allows an appreciation of soft tissues. With such an approach with synovitis, its contribution to nerve compression can be better analysed (8). Ultrasound imaging goals are similar with more simple means. The use of this tool during ambulatory clinic may give such information directly as a supplement to the clinical examination (7). The training experience of the examiner is however critical for valid conclusions. Bone absorptiometry of sites at risk of bone degradation, essentially wrists and hands, is susceptible to quantify early bone loss before X-ray damage appears. Progress has been made in hardware and software (4). When examining wrists and hands, one problem associated with reproducibility is related to the difficulty in finding the exact same position for each measurement.

Biological and immunological tests

The presence of a biologic inflammatory syndrome is almost constant but has no diagnostic specificity. Its presence and magnitude will be useful for follow-up under treatment. It is difficult to justify a choice between sedimentation rate and C reactive protein measurements.

The degree of anemia is variable. Its mechanism is mostly inflammatory with a high ferritine level; or mixed with a low ferritine level, mostly from gastro-intestinal bleeding.

When looking at autoantibodies, the test for rheumatoid factors remains the routine reference. These autoantibodies are directed against the Fc part of IgG. Only agglutinating rheumatoid factors of the IgM class are detected by the Waaler-Rose and latex agglutination tests. ELISA tests, which are more sensitive but also less specific, allow the detection of the other immunoglobulin classes.

Agglutination tests are positive only several months after the beginning of the disease. Their sensitivity is from 60 to 80%, lower for the Waaler-Rose test. When tests for rheumatoid factors are negative, RA is classified as sero-negative. Rheumatoid factors are not RA specific since they can be detected in patients with connective tissue diseases, especially Sjögren's syndrome, infectious diseases (endocarditis), lung and hepatic disorders, and mixed cryoglobulinemia, even in elderly normal subjects.

Antikeratin and antiperinuclear antibodies can represent an interesting tool for an early diagnosis. They are directed against a skin protein, fillagrine, which is citrulinated (11). Both specificities are combined as anti-fillagrine antibodies. Their detection by the classical immunofluorescence test with esophagus sections remains difficult. ELISA assays with anti-citrullin peptides (cc), which are now commercially available, should give a better access to this test, which is very specific for RA (10).

Antinuclear antibodies detected by indirect immunofluorescence are sometimes present usually at low titers, rarely with the presence of anti-native DNA antibodies. The other specificities are often found in associations with Sjögren's syndrome for anti-SSA antibodies.

Genetic markers are not yet with major interest for diagnosis. They have a better prognostic value but results have been obtained on populations of patients and not on individual cases. An association with a more severe prognosis has been described for HLA DR4 subtypes 0401 and 0404 (3). Other markers have been associated with a severe or benign prognosis (pro- and anti-inflammatory cytokines) (2). For the future, the goal is to be able to predict response to treatment through the use of pharmaco-genomic evaluation.

Pathology findings

The study of synovial fluid, even of a synovial biopsy, is more useful to eliminate other diagnoses. RA synovial fluid is inflammatory, sterile, and rich in cells, especially polymorphonuclear cells with low synovial complement levels (C4).

Synovial biopsy shows mostly signs of a non-specific subacute synovitis. Some aspects are suggestive of RA diagnosis, such as a hyperplasia of the lining layer, an increased neovascularisation and a lymphocytic infiltrate with perivascular nodules.

Evolution

RA is a very heterogeneous disease and its severity may be variable from one patient to another. It is important to remember when discussing treatment that most of the articular destruction will be already achieved after the first two years.

Differential diagnosis is difficult at an early stage and depends on the mode of disease presentation. The American College of Rheumatology (ACR) proposed criteria for the classification of RA (1). They are often of limited value in the presence of incomplete or atypical forms. Often only follow-up will allow clarification of the exact diagnosis. It is important to see the patient again and to use at this stage only symptomatic treatment. To use of high dose steroids from the beginning is to risk modifying symptoms, no longer allowing differentiating RA from another steroid-sensitive disease.

Follow-up is made:

- on clinical data: degree of disease activity (number of painful and swollen joints, Ritchie index disease activity score (DAS) 28), of joint function (Lee's index), morning stiffness duration, and level of pain;
- on biologic data: level of inflammation;
- on radiographic data: speed of degradation measured by different indices;
- on the level of response to treatments quantified by indices of ACR 20, 50 and 70 response (5).

Markers of poor prognosis have been identified, such as a high inflammatory syndrome, high rheumatoid factor levels, a polyarticular initial presentation, the presence of HLA DR4, early radiological erosions and a poor response to the first slow acting drug treatment.

General principles of RA treatment

RA treatment must be established as soon possible and combines four important aspects:

- patient information (sessions of patient information, information brochures, psychological support, social and occupational therapy);
- systemic and local drug treatments;
- rehabilitation;
- surgical treatment.

Although we are still waiting for the preventive or final curative treatment of RA, it is doubtless that an early use of these aspects by a multi-member team constitutes at present the best therapeutic approach of this disease. Therapeutic progress obtained recently with cytokine inhibitors further supports the need for early and correct definition of the prognostic.

References

1. Arnett, F. C., S. M. Edworthy, D. A. Bloch, D. J. McShane, J. F. Pries, N. S. Cooper, L. A. Healey, S. R. Kaplan, M. H. Liang, H. S. Luthra, T. A. Medsger, D. M. Mitchell, D. H. Nenstadt, R. S. Pinals, J. G. Schaller, J. T. Sharp, R. L. Wilder and G. C. Hunder (1988). "The American Rheumatism Association 1987 revised criteria for the classification of rheumatoid arthritis." Arthritis Rheum. 31: 315-324.
2. Buchs, N., F. S. di Giovine, E. Vannier, G. W. Duff and P. Miossec (2001). "IL-1B and IL-1Ra gene polymorphims and disease severity in trheumatoid arthritis: Interaction with their plasma levels." Genes Immunity 2: 222-228.
3. Combe, B., J. F. Eliaou, J. P. Daures, O. Meyer, J. Clot and J. Sany (1995). "Prognostic factors in rheumatoid arthritis. Comparative study of two subsets of patients according to severity of articular damage." Br J Rheumatol. 34 (6): 529-34.
4. Deodhar, A. A., J. Brabyn, P. W. Jones, M. J. Davis and A. D. Woolf (1995). "Longitudinal study of hand bone densitometry in rheumatoid arthritis." Arthritis Rheum 38 (9): 1204-10.
5. Felson, D. T., J. J. Anderson, M. Boers, C. Bombardier, D. Furst, C. Goldsmith, L. M. Katz, R. Lightfoot, Jr., H. Paulus, V. Strand and *et al.* (1995). "American College of Rheumatology. Preliminary definition of improvement in rheumatoid arthritis." Arthritis Rheum 38 (6): 727-35.
6. Firestein, G. S., F. Echeverri, M. Yeo, N. J. Zvaifler and D. R. Green (1997). "Somatic mutations in the p53 tumor suppressor gene in rheumatoid arthritis synovium." Proc Natl Acad Sci USA 94: 10895-10900.
7. Karim, Z., R. J. Wakefield, P. G. Conaghan, C. A. Lawson, E. Goh, M. A. Quinn, P. Astin, P. O'Connor, W. W. Gibbon and P. Emery (2001). "The impact of ultrasonography on diagnosis and management of patients with musculoskeletal conditions." Arthritis Rheum 44 (12): 2932-3.
8. McGonagle, D., P. G. Conaghan, R. Wakefield and P. Emery (2001). "Imaging the joints in early rheumatoid arthritis." Best Pract Res Clin Rheumatol 15 (1): 91-104.
9. Miossec, P. and W. van den Berg (1997). "Th1/Th2 cytokine balance in arthritis." Arthritis Rheum 40 (12): 2105-15.
10. Nogueira, L., M. Sebbag, C. Vincent, M. Arnaud, B. Fournie, A. Cantagrel, M. Jolivet and G. Serre (2001). "Performance of two ELISAs for antifilaggrin autoantibodies, using either affinity purified or deiminated recombinant human filaggrin, in the diagnosis of rheumatoid arthritis." Ann Rheum Dis 60 (9): 882-7.
11. Sebbag, M., M. Simon, C. Vincent, C. Masson-Bessiere, E. Girbal, J. J. Durieux and G. Serre (1995). "The antiperinuclear factor and the so-called antikeratin antibodies are the same rheumatoid arthritis-specific autoantibodies." J Clin Invest 95 (6): 2672-9.
12. Van der Heijde, D., P. Van Riel, M. Van Leeuween, M. Van't Hof, M. Van Rijswijk and L. Van de Putte (1992). "Prognostic factors for radiographic damage and physical disability in early rheumatoid arthritis. A prospective follow-up study of 147 patients." Br J Rheumatol 31: 519-528.

The rheumatoid foot. Pathomechanics, clinical and radiological features. Therapeutic conditions

M. Bouysset and P. Hugueny

General remarks

The incidence of rheumatoid arthritis in the general population is 0.5%. This progressive disease affects 3 times more women than men and occurs at any age, but especially between 40 and 60 years. Initially, it may remain localized to the foot and ankle for a long time. During its progress, the foot is affected in 90% or more of cases (1, 19, 78, 82, 97, 104, 109).

Despite progress in therapeutics, rheumatoid arthritis often remains a serious disorder with severe morbidity (3, 98). Disability related to the foot in rheumatoid arthritis has not been objectively assessed but the frequency of foot surgery enables us to give an estimate: it occurs in approximately 20 to 30% of cases (96, 106, 107). This high incidence is an argument for optimal management of the foot in rheumatoid arthritis.

Pathomechanics

Biomechanical factors account for the main deformities of the rheumatoid foot; the great variety of factors involved is evidenced by the numerous atypical forms. It is impossible to summarize the pathophysiology of the foot in rheumatoid arthritis in a few lines but the following schema may be suggested.

Inflammatory synovitis predominates and is the initial factor. It leads to weakening of the structures which support the foot: joint capsules, ligaments, tendons and certain muscles. Its consequences appear more in the metatarsal area, on the subtalar joint complex and on the tendon of the tibialis posterior muscle. Some authors make a comparison with the hyperlaxity of Ehler-Danlos disease (99).

At a later stage there is osteoarticular destruction with subsequent dislocation (or, in certain cases, ankylosis). In some lesions, the healing process with postinflammatory contracture plays a part in causing deformities (2, 86, 105).

In this weakened setting, mechanical stresses, which are common, appear as factors predisposing to deformity. These are anatomic or functional factors of congenital or acquired origin. They are situated not only in the feet (morphotype of the forefoot, more or less marked pronation of the hindfoot), but also at the hips and knees (genu valgum, fixed flexion of the knee) (2, 86, 105).

Other factors promote and aggravate the deformities. The footwear may either stress the foot or fail to support it (wearing of slippers or worn-out shoes) (109). Weight-bearing is particularly harmful during inflammatory crises.

The causes cited increase muscular imbalance, between the flexor and extensor muscles and between the abductor and adductor muscles. Not only are the intrinsic muscles affected (lumbricals, interossei, extensor digitorum brevis) but also the extrinsic muscles, whose eccentric action gives rise to deformity (105, 112). Ordinary movements, particularly intense activity, accentuate the imbalance of forces. Some authors minimize the role of this muscular imbalance which is difficult to study during walking (85). Thus, inflammatory rheumatism make certain deformations appear, or worsen them when previously these deformities had been prevented by healthy supporting structures. The mechanism of deformation, if understood, enables us to envisage treatment programmes better.

Hindfoot deformities

Pes planovalgus is the commonest deformity of the rheumatoid hindfoot. Its causes are varied and complex. Even the minimal calcaneal valgus, which is present beforehand and which is usual in the general population, is a predisposing factor in the great majority of cases. The inflammatory disease impairs the structures which stabilize the subtalar joint complex and the valgus deformity appears as a result of lesions of the supporting soft tissues (63, 105, 108, 109). Other causes exist but are often more difficult to distinguish (see below).

Several disease sites promote this tendency: the tarsus and especially the medial articular chain of the foot; the talonavicular and subtalar joints, which are more subject to mechanical stress, are the most frequently affected (14, 24, 109). Tillmann emphasizes the role of tarsometatarsal arthritis which is also frequently observed by Resnick (87, 105). The increased susceptibility to torque accentuates the tendency to valgus deformity (or sometimes varus, if there was prior varus) (1, 96, 99, 102, 109, 111). On the whole, the flat-foot is initially flexible, and then becomes rigid. This secondary rigidity of the deformity is due to the consequences of tarsal arthritis

(106, 108, 109). Some authors state that the rigid flat-foot is caused by spasm of the fibular muscles, which may be provoked by any cause of stiffening or ankylosis of the tarsus. The principal muscle concerned is the fibularis brevis (2). The two deforming processes – weakening of the supporting structures of the foot and spasm of the fibular muscles – can combine to lead to pes planovalgus (108).

The importance of retromalleolar tenosynovitis in the development of pes planovalgus is generally undervalued (11, 17, 33, 34, 54, 95). The tendon of the tibialis posterior muscle is of primary importance as it plays a major role in maintaining the dynamic stability of the foot. All lesions of this tendon, simple stretching of inflammatory origin or even rupture, may explain the flattening of the midfoot and the valgus deviation of the hindfoot. Loss of function of the fibular tendons does not have such repercussions on the structure of the foot. The tendons of other muscles can be affected, in particular those of the flexor hallucis longus and flexor digitorum longus muscles (17, 33, 54, 95, 105). The respective roles of tenosynovitis and arthritis in the appearance of pes planovalgus are debatable (34, 54, 59, 95).

Ankle arthritis appears later (14, 60, 95, 105, 109). The lateral talocrural narrowing, which is more frequent, promotes valgus deformation (105) or may itself be caused by preexisting calcaneal valgus.

Other factors may be involved in the appearance of pes planovalgus: abnormal gait and/or antalgic positions. Arthritis of the first metatarsophalangeal joint prevents the patient from standing on this painful joint and causes supination of the forefoot. If, after the inflammatory crisis, the forefoot resumes its initial position, the compensatory deformation of the hindfoot into pronation, relative to the forefoot, may remain fixed and thus cause planovalgus (105, 109). This clinical sequence may explain the varus of the forefoot observed by Vavahnen (105, 108) and corresponds to Hohmann's description of " pes postice pronatus, antice supinatus " (105).

Deformities of the other joints of the lower limb also play a part: a varus knee may sometimes give rise to a valgus hindfoot. If there is a calcaneal valgus and then a valgus knee develops, the latter worsens the valgus hindfoot, though it may sometimes bring about a varus hindfoot (105). Likewise, a large angle of gait while walking stresses the mid-hindfoot and favours the tendency of the hindfoot to pronate. Numerous other factors may be involved in the development of the rheumatoid valgus flat foot (2, 105).

The frequency of **cavus foot** varies according to the authors: 4% for Potter (86), higher for others (19). Among other causes, sclero-inflammatory contracture of the soft parts may be responsible (2, 19). It can be in a valgus or varus position. An initial hindfoot varus seems to ensure relative protection from the development of hindfoot deformities.

Stiffness in flexion of the **hip or knee** may make the pathology of the foot more pronounced and provoke functional imbalance (2, 26); abnormal gait or an antalgic position can have the same effect. Thus, contracture of the triceps surae muscle following fixed flexion of the hip or knee causes plantarflexion and inversion of the foot with dorsiflexion of the proximal phalanges and plantarflexion of the distal phalanges. Persistence of this position may lead to secondary cavus deformity (modern knee and hip replacements have certainly reduced the frequency of these conditions). For some authors, cavus foot is due to spasm of the fibularis longus muscle, which causes a valgus cavus foot with heightening of the longitudinal arch, forefoot abduction and calcaneal valgus (2).

Forefoot deformities

Forefoot and hindfoot deformities, whether of mechanical or inflammatory origin, are interrelated, with each influencing the other (105, 107).

Hallux valgus and metatarsus varus of the first ray are examples of deformities of both mechanical and inflammatory origin (105). Hallux valgus is logically correlated with other deformities and articular lesions of the forefoot and mid-hindfoot, but the relation between flattening of the arch and metatarsus varus of the first ray is direct; above all, it does not depend on the duration of the disease (18). Habitual mechanical causes of hallux valgus are metatarsus varus of the first ray, deviation into pronation of the hallux by the tendon of the long flexor and extensor muscles, but an inflammatory component worsens the consequences of the mechanical stresses. The latter favour the appearance of hallux valgus and are diverse:

- prior static disorders, particularly the common marked valgus of the hindfoot (65, 86, 105);
- inadequate footwear and abnormal weight-bearing, especially during an inflammatory period, increased by obesity, over-exertion, too heavy bed covers and any external mechanical constraint on the foot;
- certain torsional or flexion abnormalities of the lower limb in the foot (forefoot varus, equines hindfoot) or in the hips and knees (2);
- gait abnormalities which may or may not be secondary to the preceding causes;
- other general conditions with a weakening effect (articular laxity) (65).

When there is inflammation, the reciprocal influences between the forefoot and hindfoot are exacerbated. Rheumatoid hallux valgus can cause a hindfoot deformity which will then augment the hallux valgus, the reverse order of events may also occur (25, 63, 105).

Other lesions can arise in the development of rheumatoid hallux valgus (105). Tarsometatarsal arthritis can play a part in the splaying of the forefoot; the tendon of the abductor hallucis muscle, which is inserted between two inflammatory sites (superficial bursitis and deep articular synovitis), can be damaged and weakened; lateral displacement of the extensor hallucis longus tendon is also involved more in rheumatoid arthritis (as with the other extensors), due to synovitis of the first metatarso-phalangeal joint.

Sometimes the first ray is unaffected. There is often a favourable morphotype of the forefoot with an intact metatarsophalangeal joint in patients who wear adequate footwear (1, 111). This respect of the first ray is often the case in male patients (110), stressing the fact that certain deforming factors are more frequent in women (narrow shoes, postmenopausal flat-foot).

Splaying of the forefoot

The periarticular edema and intermetatarsal bursitis displace the metatarsal heads (1, 33). The extra mobility of the first and fifth metatarsals particularly favours their deviation and therefore their role in the spreading of the metatarsal bones (46).

Tarsometatarsal arthritis certainly arises in this process (105) and also stretching of the intermetatarsal ligaments (2). The influence of these different lesions is combined and determines the appearance of the deformity (97, 99).

Deformities of the toes

Deformities of the lesser toes depends on mechanical factors (fig. 1): the flattening of the medial arch and spreading of the forefoot increase the tension of the short flexor tendons, which passively flex the proximal interphalangeal joints. The proximal phalanx is not subject to the action of the flexor muscles and the balancing action of the interosseous and lumbrical muscles is lacking, so that the extensor muscles exert a great force on the proximal phalanges (105).

In rheumatoid arthritis, the tendency to deformity worsens as the muscular involvement particulary affects the interosseous and lumbrical muscles. These muscles are active in 40% of the gait cycle (68) and their reduced efficiency, of inflammatory origin, becomes evident during this cycle. At the end of stance, the metatarsal heads tend to be placed under the proximal phalanges (2, 105, 111). The other articular support structures (capsules, ligaments) are also weakened and subluxation of the first phalanx is accentuated. The cartilaginous and bony destruction worsens the deformity and healing with secondary fibrosis can make it become fixed (1, 105).

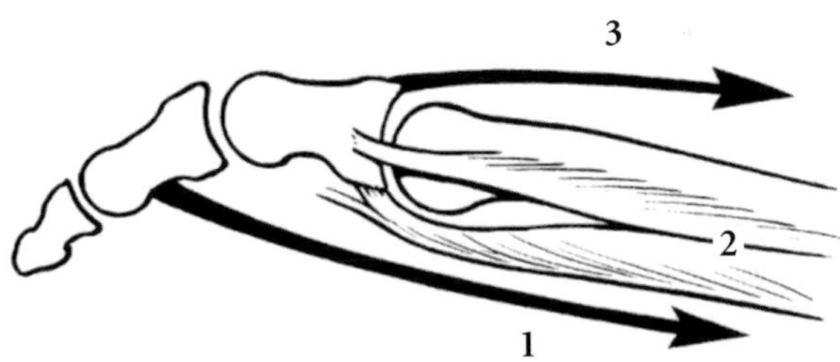

Fig. 1 - Clawed toes and tendency to subluxation of the proximal phalanges (toes 2, 3, 4). **1** short flexor tendons; **2** interosseous and lumbrical muscles; **3** extensor tendons.

Other causes also play a part in this dorsal subluxation of the proximal phalanx, with flexion of the interphalangeal joint: tenosynovitis of the flexor (2) or extensor muscles (105); inflammatory lesions of the plantar aponeurosis which is situated between the deep articular pannus and the more superficial plantar bursitis (105); and inflammation of the tarso-metatarsal joints. At a late stage interdigital displacement of the flexor tendons also plays a part (1, 105).

The lateral deviation of the toes is largely due to the role of the extensor digitorum brevis muscle (fig. 2). Flattening of the medial arch and abduction of the forefoot deviate the axis of traction of this muscle outwards and upwards; lateral deviation of the toes occurs in this way. On the other hand, the varus of the first metatarsal increases the tension of the extensor hallucis brevis tendon and favours valgus deformation of the hallux in addition to the other causes of hallux valgus. The metatarso-phalangeal joint capsules are weakened early on by the inflammation, facilitating this process, which also affects the long extensor tendons of the toes (1, 105). It has been suggested that the deviated hallux may displace the lateral toes (1, 55).

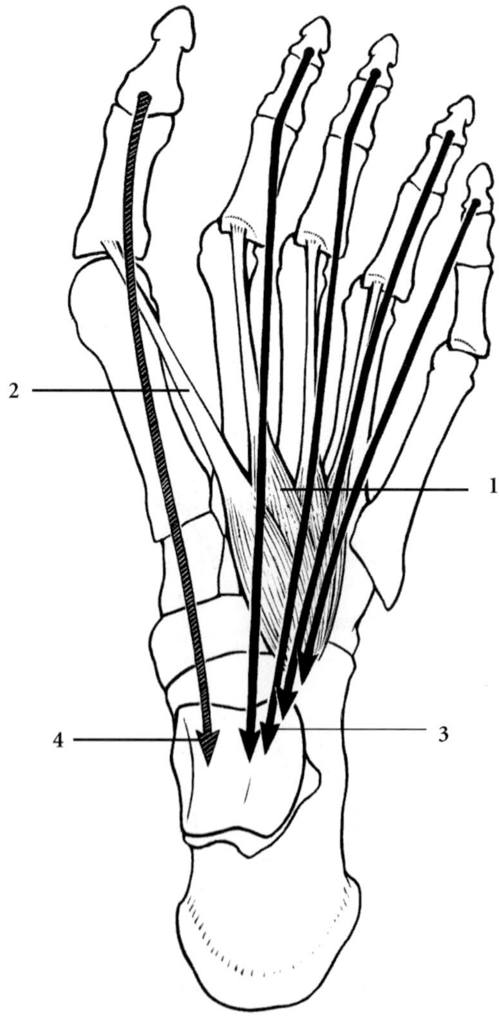

Fig. 2 - Lateral deviation of toes 2, 3, 4. **1.** Extensor digitorum brevis muscle; **2.** Extensor hallucis brevis tendon: **3.** -Extensor digitorum longus tendon; **4.** Extensor hallucis longus tendon. (from K TILLMANN).

The fifth toe is not subject to the action of the extensor digitorum brevis muscle but (like the hallux) is particularly subject to footwear constraints. Other influences exist (105) (fig. 3): inflammation of the tarsometatarsal joints accentuates the abduction of the fifth metatarsal, stretching the tendon of the abductor digiti minimi muscle; the fifth toe can then deviate into adduction. Moreover, the flattening of the anterior arch favours pronation of the fifth metatarsal and in consequence the insertion of the long extensor tendon of the fifth toe becomes medial and the pull of this tendon takes a medial direction. Finally, lateral displacement of the tendon of the flexor digitorum longus to the fifth toe displaces the fifth metatarsal head outwards, just as the former is displaced inwards.

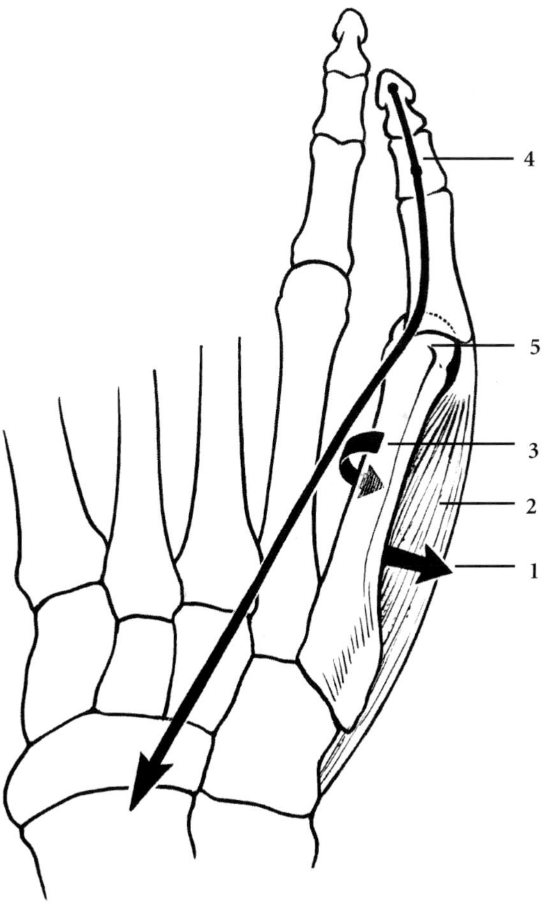

Fig. 3 - Specifics of the fifth toe. **1.** Abduction of the fifth metatarsal; **2.** Stretched abductor digiti minimi tendon; 3. Pronation of fifth metatarsal bone; 4. Insertion of the long extensor tendon of fifth toe becomes medial; 5. The fifth metatarsal head displaces outwards because there is a lateral displacement of the tendon of the flexor digitorum longus (from K. TILLMANN).

The congenital morphotype of the forefoot influences the deformities. Viladot distinguishes two types of rheumatoid forefoot (111):

- the triangular forefoot, caused by combined hallux valgus and varus of the fifth toe. This deformity, which Morton called the atonic foot, is characterized by the weakened intrinsic musculature of the first and fifth rays and shortness of the first metatarsal, with consequent spreading of the metatarsal bones. This results in a predominance of the extrinsic musculature. The long flexor and extensor tendons of the first and fifth rays deviate outwards the first and the fifth metatarsals and the corresponding toes inwards, resulting in the typical triangular forefoot deformity;
- the forefoot with lateral deviation of the toes is characterized by a long first metatarsal and a predominating intrinsic musculature. The reflex contracture of the tendons of the abductors hallucis and flexor hallucis brevis muscles, due to inflammatory involvement, deviates this hallux into valgus. This favours the lateral deviation of the median toes. The extensor digitorum brevis, as we have seen, accentuates this deviation except at the fifth toe, which is unaffected by the deviation.

These deformities often occur with a long hallux, which, as it is subject to more mechanical strain, becomes deformed more easily. A short hallux is less sensitive to the pressure of the shoe and becomes deformed less frequently. Needless to say, these rules do not apply uniformly. Other factors influence the deformities, as we have already seen, and account for the numerous atypical forms when they are not correlated with any particular metatarsal or digital morphotype.

Clinical features

At the onset

In the great majority of cases there is a forefoot involvement. The first signs are an inflammatory and symmetric involvement of the metatarsophalangeal joints (19, 33, 61) which is also often present at the metacarpophalangeal joints. These two localisations dominate the pathology of rheumatoid arthritis at the onset, even if their relation frequency varies (33, 41, 73, 104). Radioclinical involvement of the forefoot may be the inaugural manifestation of rheumatoid arthritis in 10 to 25% of cases (1, 19, 20, 24, 82, 87, 96, 100). The initial symptoms are sometimes asymmetric (68, 93).

Clinically, the lateral metatarsophalangeal joints are those most affected in the initial stage (33). Actually the pain is due to joints but also to intercapito-metatarsal bursae. Braun particularly emphasizes the prime localisation at the fifth metatarsal head; this is a lesion which must be searched for clinically as it is not always painful spontaneously (19). First metatarsophalangeal joint involvement appears less frequently. Nevertheless, some patients who have generalized rheumatoid arthritis, and who have undergone a recent operation for hallux valgus, suggest that the pain was caused by the arthritis and was not of mechanical origin (33).

The examination shows swelling of the metatarsophalangeal region with oedema on the dorsal side of the forefoot and global widening of the forefoot. This inflammatory involvement may be detected early on by pain on lateral compression of the metatarsal bones, which is not painful in a normal foot (33). Selective pressure between the thumb and index on each metatarsophalangeal joint highlights those most affected and the radiologic detection of early bony erosion may confirm the examination (19, 33). At its maximum, when the forefoot is enlarged by the periarticular oedema, the toes are separated (" daylight sign ") (33).

Radiography at this early stage of the disease is often characteristic enough to permit the detection of other signs which are not specific at this time (19, 73). Regional demineralisation is frequent at the inflamed joints and is initially juxta-articular (19, 41, 73). Oedema of the soft tissues with articular synovitis, effusion and periarticular oedema can be detected at the metatarsophalangeal joints. Radiographic evidence of cysts is common at this stage (19) but metatarsal bony erosion (fig. 4) predominates in the initial radiographic findings (19, 112). In the forefoot, it precedes joint narrowing.

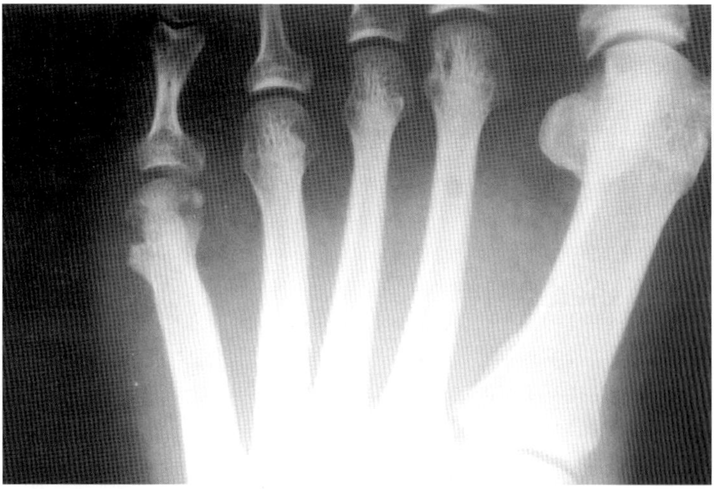

Fig. 4 - Metatarsal bony erosion predominates in the initial radiographic findings.

Being the first sign whose observation is uniformly interpreted on the radiograph, erosion is sometimes the prime feature of inflammatory rheumatism (19, 112). The earliest signs of erosion correspond to the bony areas at the sides of the joint, which are not covered by articular cartilage. These erosions are normally detected on the medial side of the metatarsal heads, apart from the fifth, where the initial erosion is normally found on the lateral side and sometimes on the medial side. As the disease progresses the plantar aspect of the metatarsal head is eroded (rarely it is involved at the beginning) (41, 73, 90). Generally speaking, there is erosion of the interphalangeal joint of the hallux which is affected more often and earlier on. Though bony erosion often precedes the clinical onset of the disease or occurs soon afterwards (19, 75, 104), it sometimes appears only after six months or more (73). The observation of osseous erosions is the witness of destructive disease and has to be taken in consideration for therapeutics (cf corresponding chapters). The joint narrowing is always uniform and is difficult to assess in standard views of the metatarso-phalangeal joints (73).

Other manifestations at the initial phase of foot involvement are possible; involvement of a single metatarsophalangeal joint (113); tarsitis (33, 37, 92) or retromalleolar tenosynovitis (11, 33); pain, swelling or widening of the intermetatarsal spaces (the second and third are the most cited but sometimes the fourth). The initial diagnosis is often Morton's metatarsalgia (7, 76, 81) but sometimes the symptoms are those of an ordinary bursitis without neurologic compression (32, 76, 93, 52).

The symptoms of inflammatory rheumatism advance at different joints. If it were not the case before, the lesions become bilateral and symmetric and then in the majority of cases the clinical course, generally progressing with acute inflammatory episodes, is the same with some small variants; the oedema of the soft parts, synovitis and articular effusion appear more clearly; the phase of advanced destruction and deformation develops progressively.

The criteria for RA diagnosis include ACR criteria (86). Recently other criteria have been proposed (112) (cf. chapter: "Management of the patient with rheumatoïd arthrites").

The established state

Generally speaking, the clinical manifestations predominate clearly over either the forefoot or hindfoot but rarely at both sites at the same time, except for cases of severe and very progressive diseases (4, 33). The physical examination specifies the possible reversible character of any deformity. Probably the biological treatments will modify the course.

The forefoot

The pain provokes a disability which increases the need of the patient for more care. Thin feminime shoes, high heels and too supple a sole of the shoe increase mechanical stresses on the metatarsal area and consequently increase pain. Valgus hindfoot deformity increases the pressure on the forefoot (102). The incidence of involvement and seriousness of lesions increase with disease duration.

Clinical features

There is typically deformation with a **triangular-shaped forefoot** and lateral deviation of the toes 1, 2, 3, 4 (111). Hallux valgus, the most frequent deformity of the rheumatoid forefoot, appears or is accentuated if it existed before (50, 99, 109) (figs. 5, 6). The first metatarsal bone presents a major varus deformation. The incidence of hallux valgus increases with the duration of the disease (99, 109). In men, the deformity occurs especially in cases of advanced inflammatory lesions of the first metatarso-phalangeal joint (110). The bony hypertrophy which is characteristic of non-rheumatoid hallux valgus is uncommon (61).

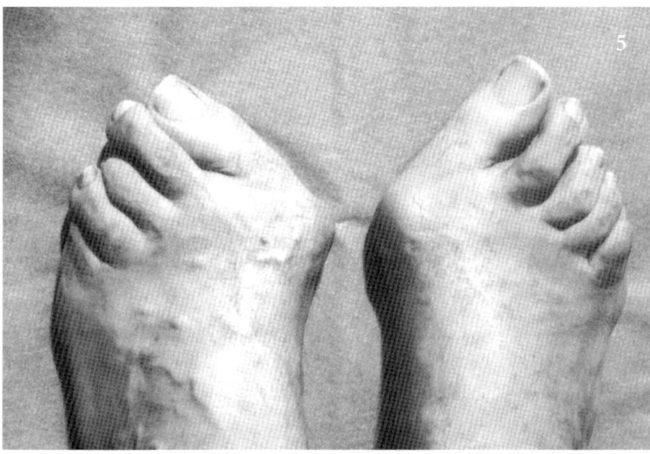

Fig. 5 - Rheumatoid forefoot: hallux valgus deformity, lateral deviation of toes, except the fifth toe (left foot).

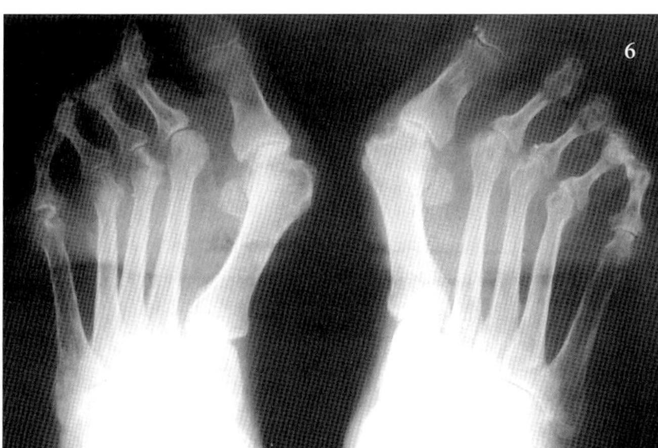

Fig. 6 - X-ray: Rheumatoid forefoot. Hallux valgus, subluxation of metatarso-phalangeal joints 2, 3 and 4; lateral deviation of toes 2, 3, 4 and the fifth toe remains in the axis of fifth metatarsal bone.

The spreading of the forefoot occurs at the same time as the deviation of the first ray and is accompanied by a plantar depression of the metatarsal heads. It also affects the fifth ray and may even start there (109).

Clawed toes and subluxation of the metatarsophalangeal joints complete this clinical picture. Deformation of the metatarsophalangeal joints 2, 3, 4 and 5 increases in frequency with disease duration (99) and after ten years almost all patients seem to be affected (109). All types of toe deformities can be variously associated (clawed toes, hammer-toes, swan-neck). The deformity, which is initially flexible, rapidly becomes fixed (109). The metatarsophalangeal joints become partially subluxed and the toes lose their role in walking, which accounts for the formation of corns, callosities and sometimes bursitis. Malalignment of the metatarsophalangeal joints is typical at a later stage, with lateral deviation of toes 1, 2, 3 and 4 and quintus varus, thus defining the triangular forefoot deformity (1, 19, 105, 111). Classically, the deviation of the toes decreases from the first toe of the fourth.

Apart from this commonest clinical form of triangular forefoot there are **numerous variants of rheumatoid forefoot deformities** (19, 111). First, there is the forefoot with outward deviation of all the toes. This deviation decreases from the hallux to the fifth toe, which may remain centred. Next come numerous atypical forms which include: rare monarticular forms (111, 113) affecting a single metatarsophalangeal joint (in the great majority of cases at the onset of the disease); forms where the hallux remains centred with outward deviation of the other toes; anarchic deformities which defy description (19); tibial deviation of the toes which is more characteristic of rheumatoid arthritis according to Dixon (33).

The hallux may present other lesions such as hallux rigidus; its frequency is variable. Usually there is absent or reduced dorsiflexion of the first metatarsophalangeal joint secondary to fibrous (or, much more rarely, bony ankylosis) (61, 99, 105, 109). Other deformities of the hallux seem even rarer (hallux flexus, hallux malleus) (61).

Radiography

Radiography defines the osteo-articular destruction clearly and shows the malalignment of the axes. In rheumatoid arthritis, foot involvement is, exceptionally, monarticular (73) and the radiographic signs generally increase in frequency with disease duration (14, 104, 109).

Standard radiographic views must include lateral and frontal views of the foot and ankle with and without weight-bearing. Others may prove useful: 3/4 obliques, axial sesamoid views (33, 40) or others (62).

Erosive features

In the forefoot, the most affected metatarsal head is the fifth (19, 104) and the first is the least affected from a radiographic viewpoint (104). When the disease is chronic, the number of involved metatarsal heads increases (approximately 80% of cases after 10 years of disease duration) and the severity of the lesions become more pronounced (fig. 7). Likewise, advanced radiographic changes go hand-in-hand with more symmetric lesions and a more frequent positive latex test (104). Radiographic signs of rheumatoid arthritis may be observed even when there is no history of clinical symptoms (15% of cases for Thould and Simon) (19, 104) but if there has not been any foot pain the number of affected metatarsal heads is minimal (104).

The initial image of erosion increases; progressive destruction of the metatarsal head occurs and often tends to prevail at plantar level under the metatarsal head (41) (fig. 8). In rare cases, complete destruction of one or more metatarsal heads occurs (19, 33, 73) (fig. 7). Both sesamoids, embedded in the articular capsule, may be affected by these lesions (41, 73, 88, 105, 109). Tangential radiography of the forefoot specifies their state, but also spike-erosions of the metatarsal heads, thinning of the fibrofatty cushion and inversion of the transverse arch (33, 40). Lastly, as the destructions worsen, generalized and progressive demineralisation of the foot occurs.

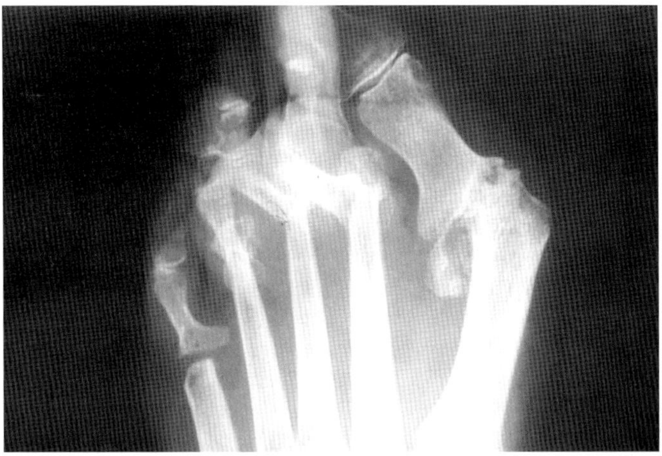

Fig. 7 - Advanced rheumatoid forefoot, subluxation of median metatarso-phalangeal joints, complete destruction of fifth metatarsal head.

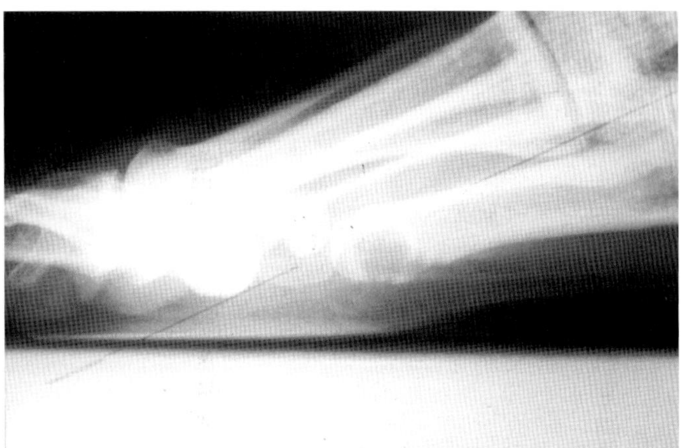

Fig. 8 - Plantar erosion of fifth metatarsal head.

Radiography of the forefoot helps to identify the patients who have erosive arthropathy and whose prognosis is poor. In this context, X-rays of the feet and hands every six months during the first two years of the disease can be useful in identifying the patients who risk having severe articular lesions (20).

The midhinfoot and the ankle

Clinical symptoms

Joint pathology

The involvement is quite frequent (14, 37, 86, 108, 109) and almost always associated with metatarsophalangeal involvement (87, 78). The lesions, which are less characteristic than those of the forefoot, appear more asymmetrically (100, 103, 108, 109). In the majority of cases, midtarsal pain is described by the patient as ankle pain. When there is subtalar involvement, walking on uneven ground is painful and the valgus hindfoot deformity must be looked for. On the whole, the feet with eroded metatarsal heads and flattened feet appear during the same period of the duration of the disease and have a shorter duration of the disease than feet with tarsitis (16). This observation emphasizes the importance of the earliest clinical features of tarsitis in order to attempt to control the deformation at the beginning.

A weight-bearing and non-weight-bearing examination considers the lower limb in its entirety and observes walking. It studies the passive movements of each joint. Active movements against resistance are useful to determine the integrity of the tendons. With clinical assessment it is possible to detect symptoms early, which allows the timely institution of medical treatment more adapted to mid-hindfoot involvement. When there is midtarsal involvement, the dorsum of the midtarsus is warm to palpation and pronation and supination are painful; localized redness is rarer.

Subtalar involvement often presents swelling behind the medial and lateral malleoli and the beginning of valgus hindfoot deformity (fig. 9); at the latter side

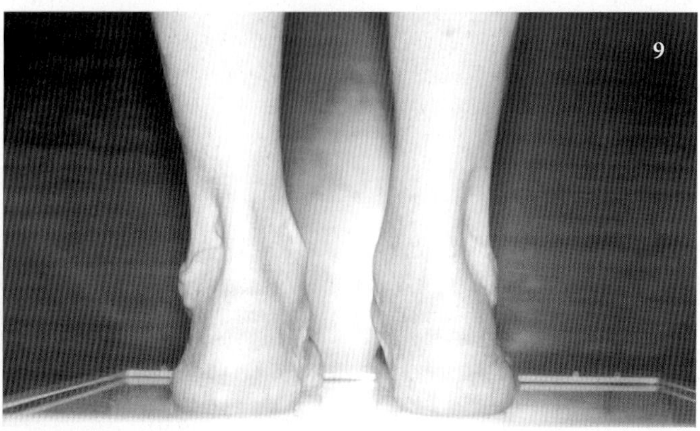

Fig. 9 - Subtalar arthritis (right foot): swelling behind medial and lateral malleoli and beginning of valgus hindfoot deformity.

there is a palpable swelling which must also be searched for at the lateral orifice of the sinus tarsi or at the calcaneo-cuboïd joint. Midtarsal and subtalar movements are studied, with particular attention to the presence of subtalar laxity and calcaneal valgus; the deformities of the hindfoot must be assessed in weight-bearing, and especially during walking (fig. 10). It must be kept in mind that all the valgus

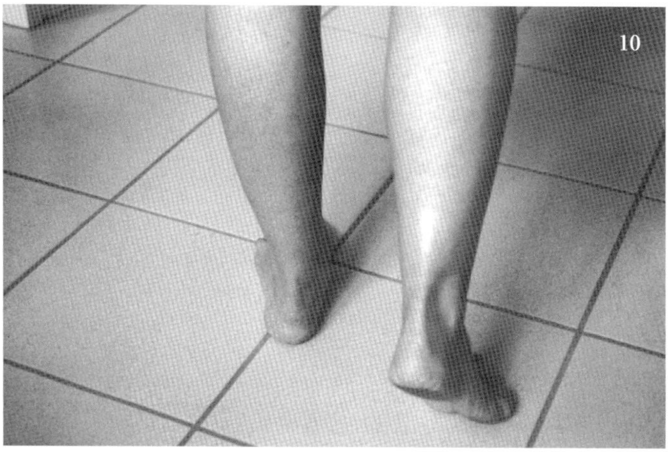

Fig. 10 - The deformity of the hindfoot must be assessed in weight-bearing rather during walking.

hindfoot deformities are not due to RA. This clinical assessment will indicate whether a tarsal ankylosis appears to be in an acceptable position from the functional viewpoint. All the rheumatoid hindfeet do not have hindfoot valgus deformity, and varus hindfoot deformity may be observed (fig. 11).

The ankle itself is often spared until a late stage of the disease (14, 33, 60, 109). The examination may identify an increase in local warmth or anterior joint swelling (fig. 12). However, the detection of an effusion or a proliferative synovitis generally proves difficult due to inflammatory involvement of the neighbouring soft parts. Finally, a decrease in talocrural movements may be noted; dorsiflexion is limited in a quarter of the cases (99).

Tendinous involvement (79)

In addition to articular involvement, tendinous lesions must be systematically studied and any swelling in the course of the tendons noted. The tibialis posterior tendon which maintains the medial longitudinal arch is of particular importance (48, 89). Previous degenerative chronic tenosynovitis and also very often a rheumatoid tenosynovitis weaken the tendon. Repeated corticosteroid infiltrations are harmful. The examination searches for local oedema or a swelling under the medial malleolus (fig. 13) and seems to be obvious only when the effusion inside the sheath is important (figs. 14, 15, 16) (17, 19), but also evaluates the loss or decrease

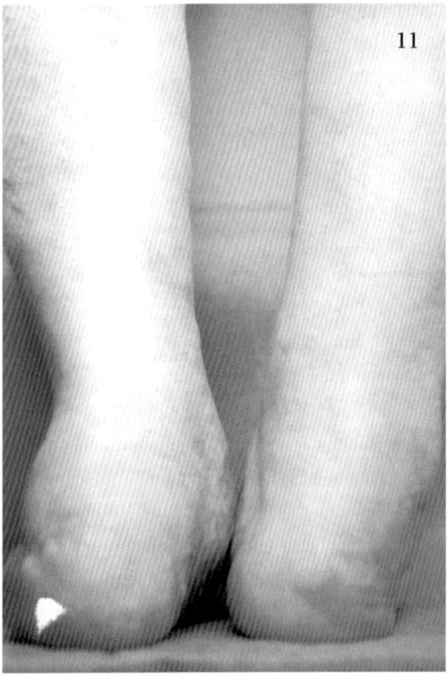

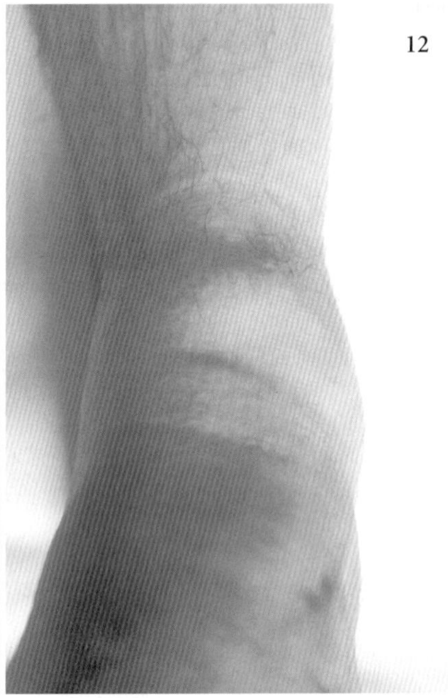

Fig. 11 - Right foot: varus hindfoot deformity must be observed.

Fig. 12 - Effusion and proliferative synovitis of the ankle.

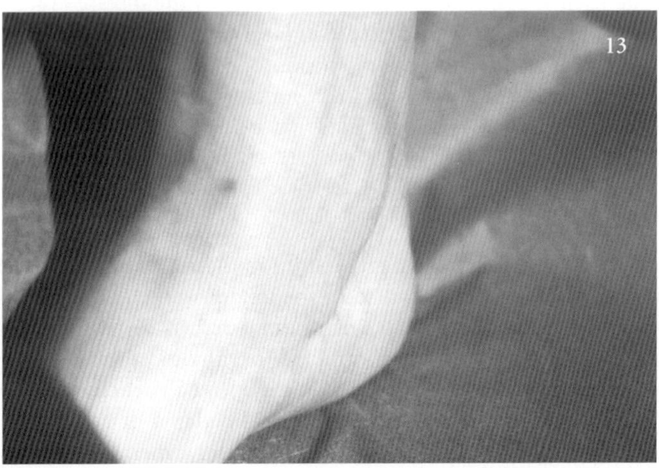

Fig. 13 - Tenosynovitis of the tendon of the tibialis posterior muscle.

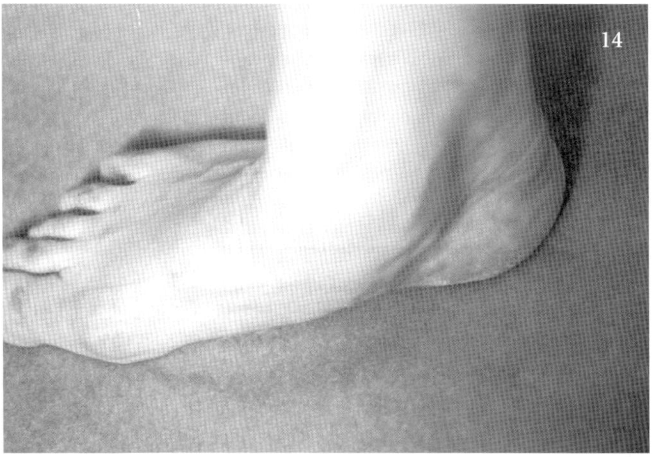

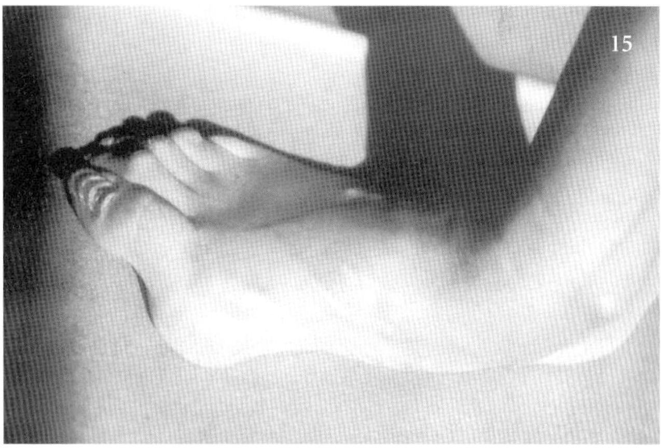

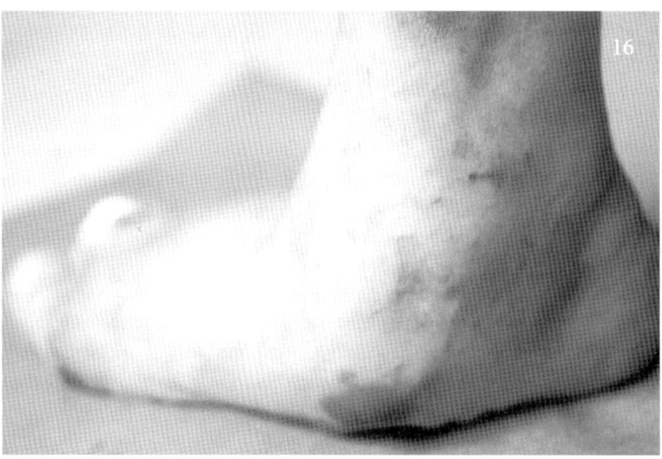

Figs. 14, 15, 16 - Progressive flattening of the medial arch. On figs. 14 and 15 tenosynovitis of the tendon of the tibialis posterior muscle may be observed.

of active inversion against resistance. The tibialis posterior tendon is not palpated during this test if it is completely ruptured (34, 95). The function of this tendon may also be assessed by examining the heel from the rear in order to check if hindfoot inversion is satisfactory when the patient is on tiptoe (fig. 17). These difficulties in clinical examination may make us underestimate lesions of the tendon, whose rupture generally goes unrecognised in its early stage (17, 34). The features must be systematically looked for (19, 36). Other tenosynovial structures in the foot may be affected by inflammatory involvement (4, 11, 62, 105, 109). Their functional repercussions are less evident than those of the tibialis posterior tendon and here again, clinical examination appears difficult in the case of rheumatoid arthritis, chiefly during inflammatory crises. In fibular tenosynovitis, there is a typical swelling of the tendinous tract on the lateral side of the heel, localized tenderness and possible weakening or loss of foot abduction. The possibility of rupture of the calcaneal tendon is reported but it may be uncertain whether this is of mechanical or inflammatory origin, or both.

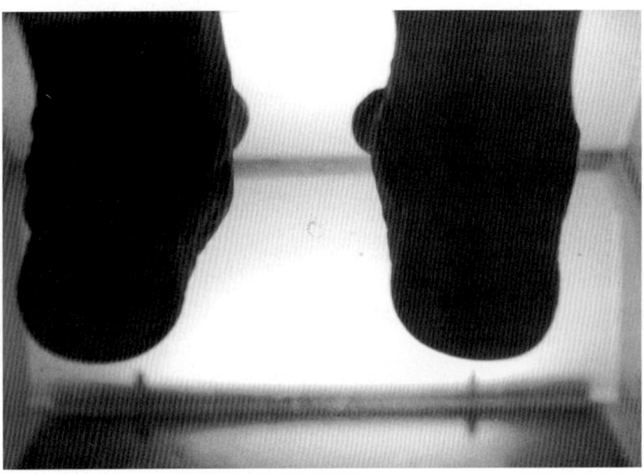

Fig. 17 - Posterior tibial tendon insufficiency: when standing on tiptoe the left foot does not invert.

Evolution

Frequently, the disease evolves towards a pes plano-valgus which is initially flexible. Sometimes the articular laxity worsens, but normally pronation and supination lessen and the flat-foot becomes rigid; consequently the maximum frequency of flexible flat-foot is in the initial period of foot involvement, this then decreases as a rigid flat-foot increases with prolonged disease. However, some mobile flat-feet which arise during inflammatory crises can be cured by suitable treatment, which leads to a normally shaped, stable foot (109).

Radiography

Bone and joint involvement

In the hindfoot and midfoot (and ankle too), radiographic signs are often delayed (14, 103) and are more asymmetric than those in the forefoot. Swelling of the soft parts due to joint effusion, synovial pannus and periarticular oedema is common (62). Articular space narrowing, sometimes with osteosclerosis, is almost always present; it is the first lesion which can be uniformly interpreted at this level and it is irreversible (73). Unlike the forefoot, erosions are not frequent in the midfoot (99, 100) or are of small size (87).

The joints of the subtalar joint complex, subtalar and talo-calcaneo-navicular, are affected earlier and more frequently (14, 108, 109) (fig. 18). Joint involvement increases in frequency with disease duration to reach or exceed 50% of cases after 10 years (14, 92, 108, 109). All the tarsal joints may be involved, including tarso-metatarsal joints (fig. 19), with different degrees of severity, exhibiting joint-narrowing with variable bone destruction, sometimes very marked. Sometimes during the course a dislocation of the tarsus is observed (fig. 20) (19, 24, 33, 102). In rare cases talonavicular subluxation is observed. Fibrous or osseous ankylosis of the tarsus may be observed (fig. 21), exceptionally it concerns all the tarsus (fig. 22) (15, 87, 105, 109). Sometimes during the course a dislocation of the tarsus is observed (19, 24, 33, 102). Some rheumatoid feet with inflammatory clinical signs of tarsitis are protected from the appearance of valgus hindfoot deformity it is particularly the case for the calcaneal varus feet (fig. 23).

Arthrosis signs on the midfoot may be observed, sometimes they appear before the inflammatory rheumatism (19, 20).

Finally, it must be kept in mind that clinical features of the tarsus may be due to septic arthritides (fig. 24) or due to stress fractures (cf later).

Deformations

Radiography also clearly shows the malalignment of the axes.
Hallux valgus, splayed forefoot and marked calcaneal valgus increase in frequency with disease duration. Metatarsus varus of the first ray only is correlated with midfoot lesions, tarsitis and flattening of the medial arch, and is independent of disease duration. These last findings confirm the interrelation between mid-hindfoot and forefoot involvement (6, 60, 105, 107, 108, 109). The incidence of flat-foot is higher in feet affected by tarsitis and generally there is a relation between tarsal arthritis, disease duration and flat-foot (14).

Inflammatory involvement can also affect the accessory bones; the structures of the foot are weakened, especially if the os tibiale is concerned, whose involvement is often followed by a pes planovalgus (109). The trigonal and fibular accessory bones can also be affected (109).

Talocrural arthritis

Talocrural arthritis occurs later, rarely without tarsal involvement, and may represent 14% of cases after ten years of the disease. The joint narrowing rather concerns the lateral side of the joint. The observation of a tibial cyst is not rare (fig. 25). Complete destruction of the joint (fig. 26) or bony ankylosis is possible.

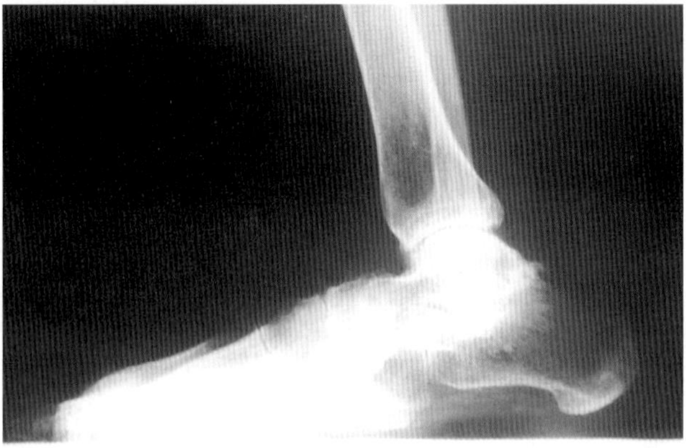

Fig. 18 - Subtalar and talo-navicular joints seem to be affected earlier and more frequently.

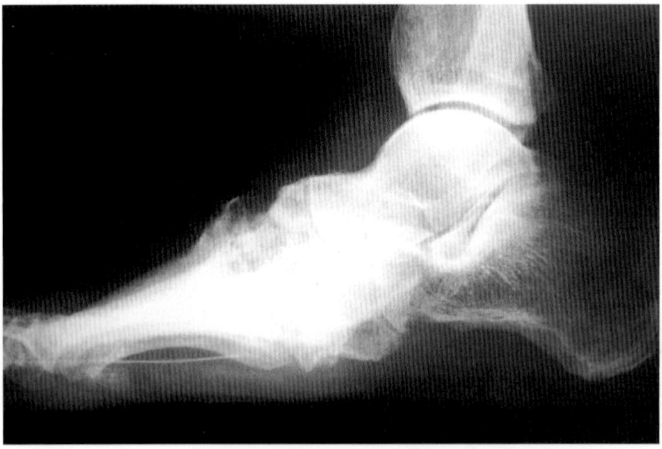

Fig. 19 - All the joints of the tarsus may be involved in rheumatoid arthritis including tarso-metatarsal joint which may be predominantly involved.

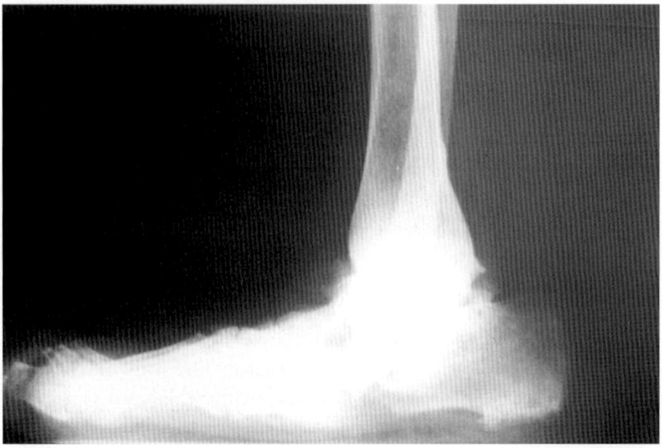

Fig. 20 - During the course a dislocation of the tarsus may be observed.

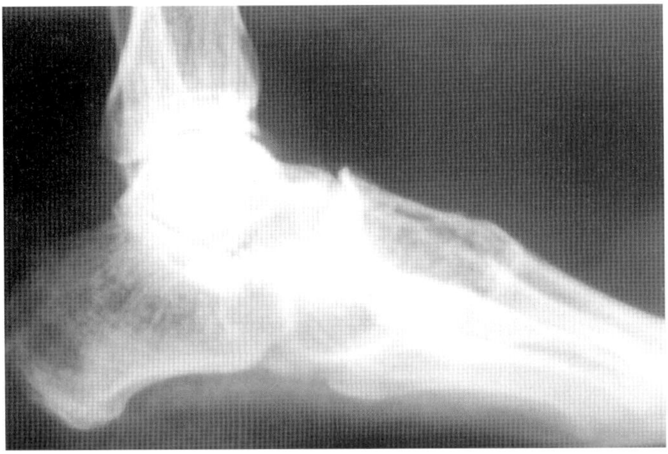

Fig. 21 - Osseous ankylosis of the anterior tarsus and fibrous ankylosis of the posterior tarsus.

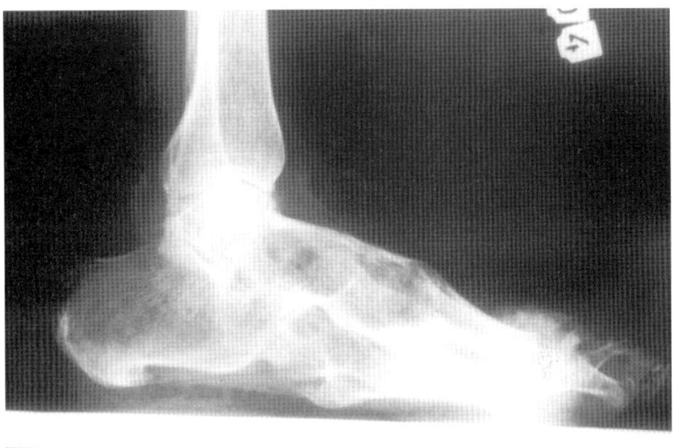

Fig. 22 - Global spontaneous ankylosis of the tarsus.

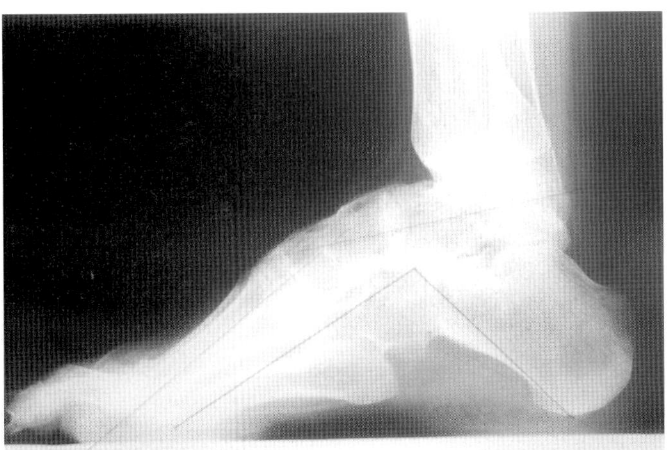

Fig. 23 - Some rheumatoid feet with important inflammatory involvement of the tarsus are protected from the appearance of valgus hindfoot deformity: cavus varus foot.

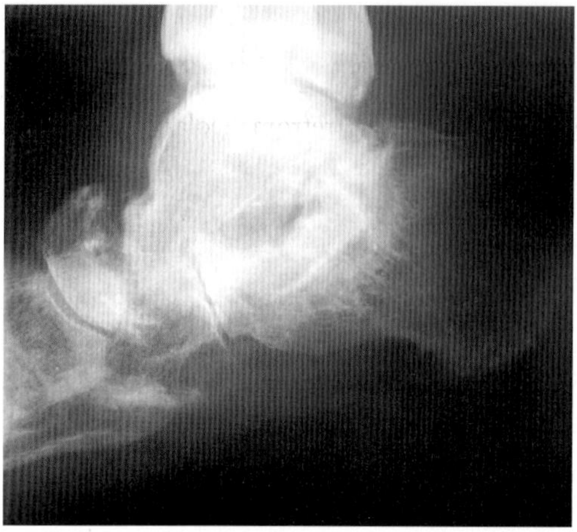

Fig. 24 - The possible presence of septic arthritis must not be forgotten.

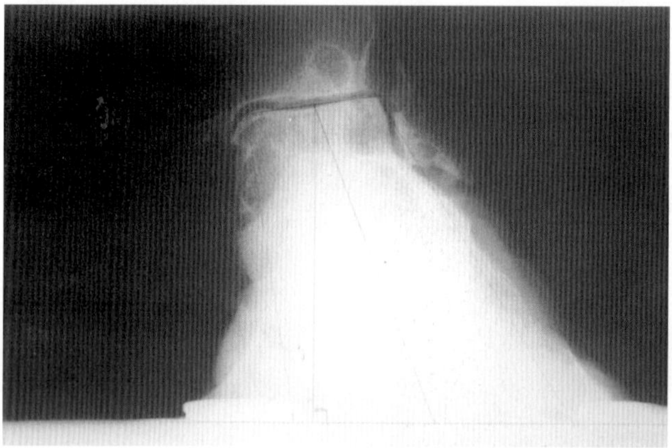

Fig. 25 - Lateral talo-talar narrowing and presence of cyst of tibia.

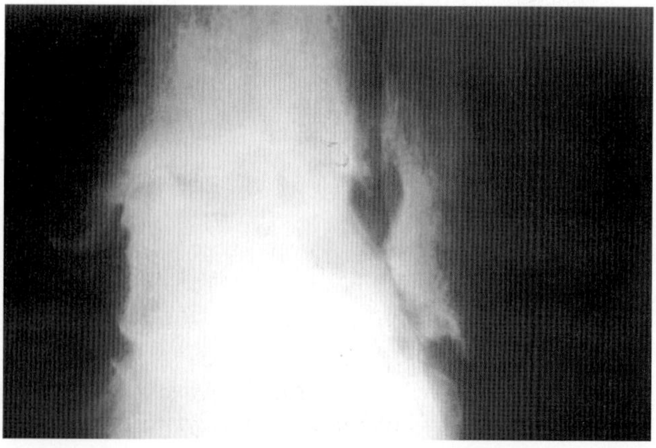

Fig. 26 - Destruction of talo-crural joint due to arthritis.

If there is a diffuse swelling of the midfoot, hindfoot and ankle, it becomes difficult to make a distinction between different articular and extra-articular rheumatoid pathologies; moreover, one of these lesions is often predominant (62, 73). Thus, when there is posteromedial pain, a medial retromalleolar tendinopathy can be suspected, and when there is lateral pain a posterolateral tendinopathy or an impingement syndrome may be suggested, and the possibility of a stress fracture should be remembered. The possible presence of ankle septic arthritis must not be forgotten (fig. 27). The pains normally have mechanical associations and paresthesiae or dysesthesiae of non mechanical nature must prompt a search for a tarsal tunnel syndrome or a peripheral neuropathy. Again, any weakening of the lower limbs must make us consider extra-articular etiologies such as a cervical myelopathy (62).

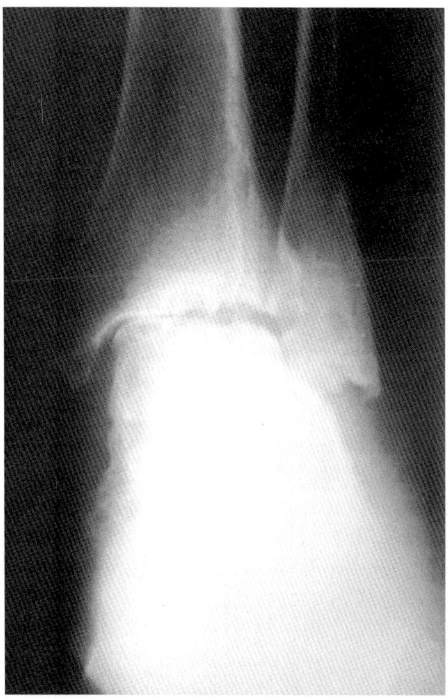

Fig. 27 - The possible presence of septic arthritis of the ankle must not be forgotten in rheumatoid arthritis.

Additional imaging techniques (cf corresponding chapter)

The X-ray assessment may be supplemented, when necessary, depending on the results of the clinical assessment, by CT, MRI with a gadolinium injection, or arthrography with CT (17, 34, 95). The gadolinium injection during the procedure helps to specify the inflammatory involvement. CT displays the bone and joint involvement better. MRI with a gadolinium injection detects soft part lesions better and chiefly of the tendons (tenosynovitis, rupture) (17) as well as the degree of synovial proliferation. However, it must be kept in mind that the information supplied by additional imaging, whatever its quality, must not be interpreted without comparison with the clinical findings.

The X-ray assessment may be completed after clinical interpretation by computed tomography (CT) or MRI with a gadolinium injection or CT with tenography. This last procedure has the inconvenience of being an invasive one (17, 34, 95). CT rather concerns observation of cortical bone. MRI rather concerns soft parts, tendinous lesions (tenosynovites, ruptures) (17), synovitis and spongy bone. The gadolinium injection during the procedure helps to observe the inflammatory lesions. The consequences of synovitis may be foreseen when this synovitis invades some anatomical structures (tendon of the tibialis posterior muscle, sinus tarsi).

Tenosynovitis may be observed on all the tendons of the foot but the tendon of the tibialis posterior muscle (ptt) is the most frequently involved (17, 54), and several grades of lesion are noted with a classification following the classification of Rosenberg (91). Stage 1, tendon thickening with longitudinal splitting; stage 2, hourglass of the tendon at the level of the lesion; stage 3, complete rupture. It is also possible to assess other anatomical lesions which have an important role in the maintaining of the shape of the rheumatoid hindfoot: destroyed inter-osseous talo-calcaneal ligament, possible involvement of the spring ligament.

A tendinous lesion of the tendon of the the ptt when there is an important stiffening of the subtalar joint complex does not incite to a surgical indication when the functional capacity has a good level. On the other hand, concerning tendinous lesions, the functional efficiency of the muscle or of other muscles which have the same ability (temporary replacement of activity instead of the concerned muscle) when clinically assessed of good quality must be taken in mind when compared with sectional imaging data.

A rheumatoid calcaneal tendinopathy was described on MRI (inflammatory involvement of retro-calcaneal bursa, no thickening of the tendon and observation of intrat-tendinous involvement) (101).

Finally, MRI may be useful to evaluate the prognosis of the disease (observation of an important synovial pannus around the ptt? in sinus tarsi? destruction of these anatomical elements?) and help to decide some earlier surgical forefoot indications after comparison with clinical data too (38). Ultrasonography may be a useful procedure for the assessment of tendinous involvement but must prove its value in the observation of the earliest eroded bone (114).

Other rheumatoid features

Plantar rheumatoid heel pain seems to be rare (2-3% of cases) and is perhaps no commoner than in the general population; posterior talalgia is less frequent (15, 22, 109). These heel pains appear more often on clinical examination (39) and are often mechanical in origin (15, 19, 22, 39). In the rheumatoid foot, as in the general population, there is no relation between talalgia and the presence of a plantar or posterior spur (17), or between talalgia and inflammatory involvement of the tarsus (15, 39).

Calcaneal spurs seem to be more common in rheumatoid arthritis than in the general population (9, 15). Age and perhaps disease duration play a part in their incidence. The inflammatory involvement certainly causes a modification in a preexisting spur or leads to its development (15, 22). Typically, an inflammatory exostosis is large and rounded-off, rarely, a periosteal reaction gives it a fluffy appearance (22, 39). The common mechanical exostosis is often small, well defined and generally sharp-pointed (22). There are numerous intermediate aspects between these typical forms (15) and these radiographic observations are not characteristic of the rheumatoid process as they are also found in spondylarthropathies (15, 87). The mechanical tension of the plantar aponeurosis, secondary to midfoot flattening, certainly explains the frequency of the plantar spur in flat-foot (111) but local inflammation also plays a part (15, 22, 109).

Retrocalcaneal bursitis is not painful or only slightly (15, 22, 109) and a local swelling is rarely noted. Bony posterosuperior erosion of the calcaneus appears in 5 to 8% of cases in lateral radiographs (15, 19, 39, 110). Its evolution is as follows: inflammatory bursitis is the first stage; then the underlying bone has a dimineralized and sometimes cavitary aspect; finally, an erosion appears just above the insertion of the calcaneal tendon. The cortical bone on the upper and posterior part of the calcaneus often remains intact (fig. 28) and rarely appears to be burnt out by the rheumatoid process (19, 22). A subchondral sclerosis may emphasize the bony erosion (15, 22). Hypertrophic modifications are rarely observed among elderly patients; they give the posterosuperior part of the calcaneus an irregular appearance

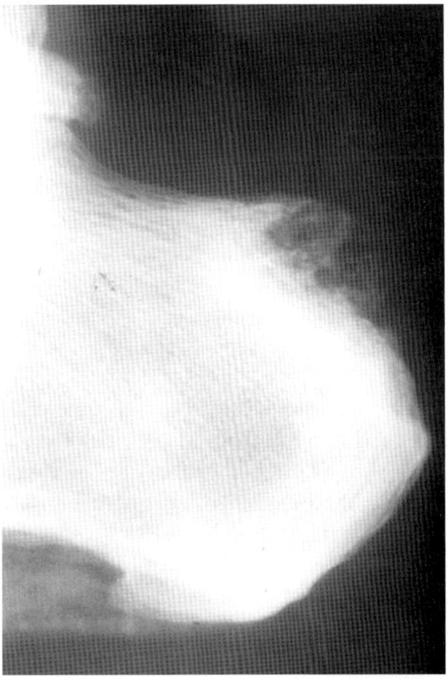

Fig. 28 - Postero-superior calcaneitis.

and can be caused by rubbing of the counter of the shoe against the posterosuperior region of the calcaneus (19, 109). In the majority of cases, this posterosuperior bursitis heals spontaneously (22, 39). On the radiography, when the thickening of the soft tissues decreases, remineralisation may occur, sometimes giving a surface of roughened appearance (22). The bony erosion often persists as a witness of burnt-out inflammation (22, 109). Histological changes are no different from those noted in the joints in rheumatoid arthritis. This also applies to plantar calcaneitis, which is much rarer (1 to 2% of cases) and which exceptionally erodes the bone to a depth of 1 cm (15, 19, 22, 109) (fig. 29). Rheumatoid calcaneitis increases in frequency with disease duration (15) and almost always appears associated with tarsal arthritis or metatarsophalangeal involvement (87); it is therefore and indicator of an advanced stage of the disease (110). A rupture of calcaneal tendon was described in RA with histologic evidence of enthesitis (75).

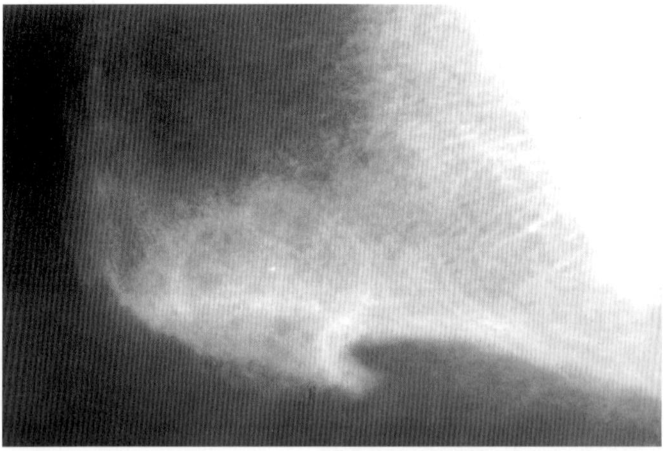

Fig. 29 - Plantar calcaneitis.

The tarsal tunnel syndrome can arise at any stage of the disease and in some cases is inaugural (23). It is very rare in ordinary practice in rheumatoid arthritis (33) but some systematic electromyographic studies show a higher proportion of cases, though often subclinical (43, 66). Paresthesia of the toes, often nocturnal, are sometimes accompanied by pain (11, 23, 62). Local infiltration is sometimes effective (23, 66). The pathology of the compression of the peripheral nerves of the foot is varied. This irritation of the posterior tibial nerve must of course be differentiated from the peripheral neuropathies observed in some advanced and chronic cases of rheumatoid arthritis (33, 66).

Nodules and bursitis between the metatarsal heads are sometimes noted, with certain symptoms reminiscent of Morton's metatarsalgia (7, 32, 52, 70, 76, 81, 84, 109). The local anatomic configuration explains the symptoms (12, 13). Pain caused by the nodule or by the bursitis, and widening of the intermetatarsal space and interdigital spaces are sometimes the only features, particularly at the second space (2, 4, 70, 93).

Subcutaneous nodules can appear at the calcaneal tendon (19, 33) or at points of hyperpressure due to footwear or weight-bearing (35, 82). Their specific treatment must be avoided unless there are local complications (erosions, infection, pain due to hyperpressure) (35).

Circulatory abnormalities may be observed: usually banal disorders of the venous circulation which can lead to ulcers (33, 62, 82). Foot and ankle oedema is frequent, often due to the almost permanent seated position of the patients (33). Raynaud's syndrome and some signs of vasculitis may be noted, especially in severe cases (33, 62, 82). These circulatory abnormalities increase the risk of sepsis, particularly after a surgical operation in the rheumatoid patient.

As the disease progresses *atrophy of the soft parts* develops. The thickness of the plantar subcutaneous tissues lessens and cutaneous abnormalities are customary; the skin becomes thin and fragile. The plantar skin, which is subject to hyperpressure, hypertrophies into painful callosities with corns. These can also occur at the toes. Plantar bursitis, which is sometimes very painful, is frequent.

During the course of the disease the *gait* becomes characteristic with shuffling movements. There is no longer an impact of the heel in walking; the foot is placed flat on the ground with the knee and hip maintained in slight flexion. Elevation of the forefoot is absent and the foot slides forwards. The two stages of swing and stance are short as the gait cycle is shortened. These abnormalities of gait are more obvious when the valgus hindfoot increases. Antalgic abnormalities of gait become common and the patient avoids standing on the painful parts of the foot (33, 72, 82).

Stress fractures seem to be rare (33, 60, 105) and are generally masked by the usual symptoms of rheumatoid arthritis. They must be suspected when there is severe and unexplained pain of sudden onset. Localisation at the lateral malleolus is typical (60, 105): hyperpressure due to calcaneal valgus produces painful fibulo-calcaneal contact (impingement syndrome) which may become complicated by a stress fracture of the fibula (figs. 30, 31). In fact, any of the standard sites of such fractures may be affected in these often osteoporotic patients. Deformities of the knee, ankle and subtalar joint are probably predisposing factors.

Course

The disease progresses with crises of variable length and intensity. Any articular and tenosynovial structure may be affected. Generally speaking, the forefoot involvement worsens, then midfoot and hindfoot lesions occur gradually and often insidiously. The symptoms progress and worsen as disease duration increases (14, 33, 99, 109). At a late stage, the metatarsophalangeal synovitis is less severe but more diffuse (99); the deformities become fixed by tendinous and muscular contracture. This highlights the importance of early supervision.

Whatever forefoot deformity there is, triangular-shaped forefoot or outward deviation of the toes, the stresses due to the wearing of the shoes becomes more

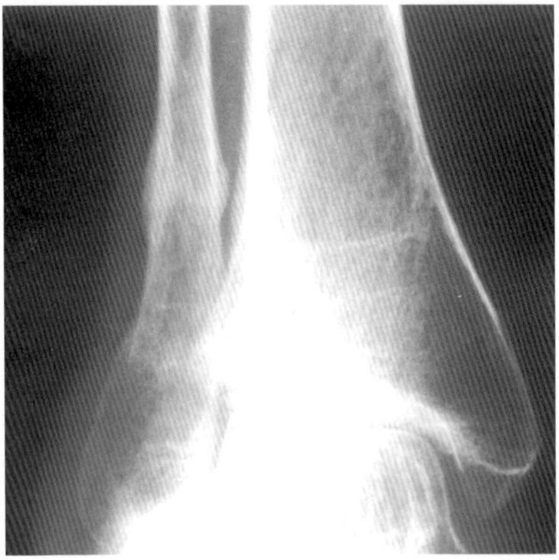

Fig. 30 - X-ray: stress fracture of the fibula.

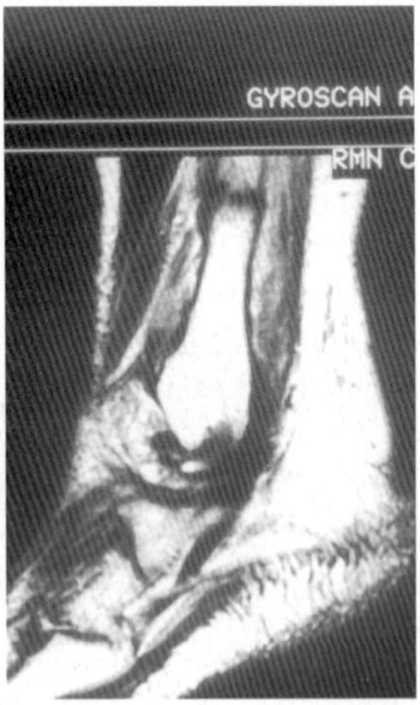

Fig. 31 - MRI: stress fracture of the fibula, before misdiagnosed on X-ray.

important during the course (figs. 33, 34). However, on the whole, rheumatoid forefoot deformities are not correlated with disability, while rheumatoid flat foot is (18). The knowledge of the probability of different possibilities of evolution and systematic observation of the rheumatoid foot allow an earlier care of the local involvement of the foot.

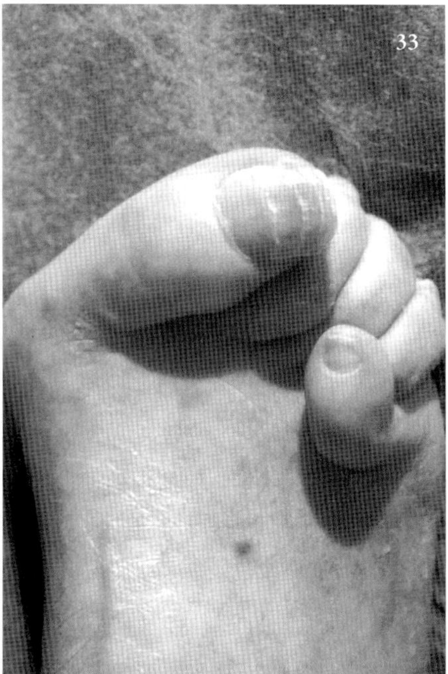

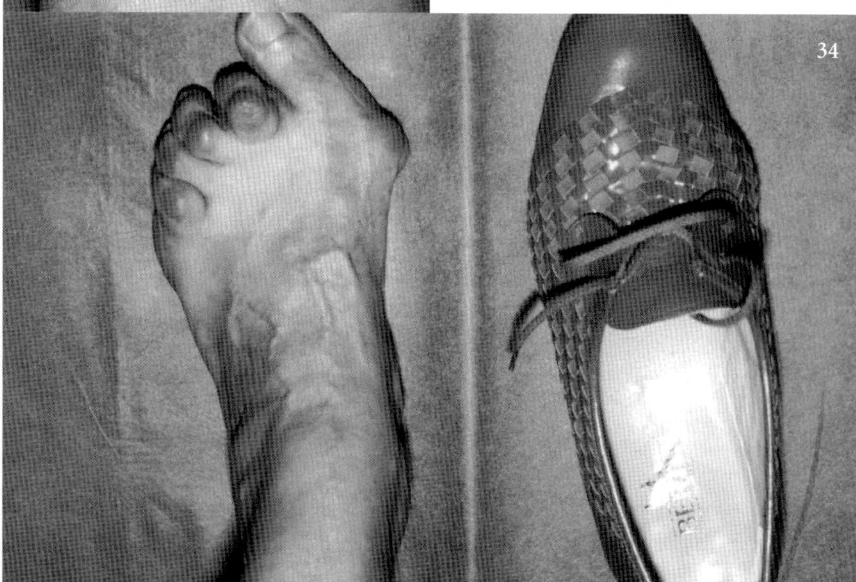

Fig. 33 - Advanced triangular rheumatoid forefoot deformity.

Fig. 34 - Advanced rheumatoid forefoot, clawed toes and stresses due to the wearing of the shoes.

Therapeutic indications

Now there is a tendency to make the earliest medical treatment of RA, with the most possible efficiency, before the appearance of bone erosions (cf corresponding chapters).

Invalidity caused by the lower limbs has decreased due to prostheses, and foot pathology is comparatively more striking. Often, unfortunately, in the treatment of the rheumatoid foot, the indications remain purely symptomatic; steroid infiltrations or radioactive injections for pain; suitable plantar ortheses for flattening: made-to-measure shoes when there is severe destruction. Finally, if arthritis does not respond to conservative treatment, we resort to arthrodesis. However, therapeutic indications vary widely among different schools of thought. Within two similar establishments which treat inflammatory rheumatism, the rate of foot surgery may be very different; at Bad Bramstedt in Germany and at Heinola in Finland (106) for example. The indications of treatment depend on the stage of seriousness (pain and deformity) but also depend on the evolutivity of the disease on the foot and ankle and on the other joints (particularly on the knee and the hip). The risk of evolution towards a disabling deformation of the foot and ankle must be particularly considered (42). For the quality it is better off the results that practitioners are experienced with RA.

The results of the medical treatment are discussed when there are serious deformities of the rheumatoid forefoot (71). Some authors underline the benefit of an adequate footwear (8); for other authors, conservative and surgical treatment have the same rate of good results on the rheumatoid forefoot (31). Probably the discussion of the best therapeutic indication is not solely a choice between conservative treatment and surgery. The question is rather: which conservative treatment or which surgical treatment for each case?

Some general notions must be stressed as regards treatment.
In this progressive disease the immediate treatment must not compromise future function. Here are a few examples:

- a plantar orthosis with an empty spot in the middle of the forefoot relieves the inflammatory forefoot but favours deformation into a rigid flattened forefoot which will present its own complications later;
- intra-articular corticosteroid injections permit a spectacular improvement but one wonders, especially if they are repeated, whether they further weaken an already weak joint and accelerate subluxation of the lateral toes.

When a surgical operation is planned:

- the lower limb must be observed on the whole: it is risky to do a subtalar arthrodesis to stabilize the hindfoot and subsequently to modify the axis of the limb by an operation on the knee. The same remarks may be made for the rheumatoid forefoot;
- one must be cautious about operations limited to the tendons; the fragile development of the supporting structures in the disease is well known. If one tendon is involved, the others will generally be involved too (17, 54);

- with the same idea, before practice of median metatarsal osteotomies, the probability of appearance of metatarsal head lesions or the risk of increasing these lesions must be considered. The important lesions of metatarso-phalangeal joints which appear later make the indication of a second forefoot surgery possible.

One must try to control the deforming tendencies in order to keep the foot in acceptable functional conditions: malalignment of the axes must be compensated in a vertical plane between the axis of the leg and hindfoot, but also in a horizontal plane between the hindfoot and forefoot (particularly at the first ray) (cf chapter "Footwear") (4, 107).

Ankle involvement generally occurs later, but its structure and function must be preserved as much as possible. This joint helps the correct progress of the patient's gait and must preserve a good range of movement, especially in dorsiflexion. Ankylosis of the ankle harms the mid-tarsal and subtalar joints. The difficulties increase when the first metatarsophalangeal joint is rigid.

General indications

The patient's contribution and a proper medical follow-up make it easier to implement measures of treatment.

The initial treatment remains medical. It is adapted to each case and acts upon the deforming factors: in general and if necessary by using local anti-inflammatory treatment (steroid or radioactive injections) and to the greatest possible extent, other local measures which present few secondary risks. In the first place, adequate footwear (cf corresponding chapter) and appropriate plantar orthoses maintain the foot in a good position. Likewise, relatively non-weight-bearing positions, cast immobilisation and a healthy life are recommended from the onset of inflammatory involvement of the foot. Finally, plantar or toe orthoses, chiropodal care and discerning rehabilitation prove useful aids.

The **nonoperative treatment**, apart from *general drugs*, first uses all different *means of articular protection*; the temporary non-weight-bearing position during an inflammatory crisis remains an indispensable measure and should be recommended untiringly (24, 86). The lessening of overloading helps to relieve the weakened joints (99). Devices which immobilize or protect the foot are certainly not used enough; they prevent or delay articular deformation. A support at the bottom of the bed avoids bed-cover pressure and prevents equines or hallux valgus. Appliances made of thermomodeled material immobilize the joints in a functional position; they are applied in the evening on going to bed and intermittently during the day. For example, a cast maintains the ankle at right angles or corrects a reducible hindfoot valgus. The hallux remains centered by a wedge between the first and second toes (4, 24, 62).

Concerning *ergotherapy*, the patient needs to be properly trained in order to respect a certain healthy life, adapted to each case (4). By carrying out a complete physical assessment of the patient's daily and professional life, the possible economy of weight-bearing can be evaluated. In the first place, the articular constraints encountered in everyday life must be reduced, e.g., the frequent use of the sitting position in household and professional activities. Standing strains must be reduced by using aids when carrying heavy objects (tea trolleys) and by using appropriate walking aids (sticks). Functional capacity can be greatly improved by the efficient use of such aids (4). Occupational therapy is used in some centres; it completes the rehabilitation and respects the same cautionary rules (24).

Toe orthoses are small devices which are molded on to one or several toes. They can correct a reversible deformity and slow down its course or even relieve a zone of hyperpressure. Their palliative role proves very useful when there is non-operable fixed clawing. They fill in the gap between the ground and the plantar side of the toes and in this way relieve the metatarsal heads (4, 24, 115). *Chiropodal* care makes a valuable contribution and alleviates lesions due to pressure and hyperkeratoses by nail care and the excision of corns. It sometimes abolishes the pain in a forefoot, even a very deformed one (4, 24, 33). Local hygiene is supplementary in patients who have difficulty in maintaining the hygiene of their feet. The fragile skin cover needs attention by trying to avoid maceration, and by the wearing of cotton socks. Adhesive epidermal protectors relieve the hyperpressure zones (24, 115).

Massages, rehabilitation and physical treatment are contraindicated when there is an acute inflammatory crisis or irreversible deformity. Rehabilitation must be carried out with caution and be related to the stage of the disease. Patient must also be trained to mobilize their joints. Passive mobilisation, if not painful, maintains the remaining range. Manual stretching combats contractures of muscles and ligaments (24).

All these methods, when properly used, bring relief which enables the practitioner to avoid the use of more aggressive care. They are all the more efficient if they are used early. In this way, improvement in the function of the foot is possible and also saves time, which is useful if surgical operations are scheduled for joints other than those of the foot.

These different types of care can have a preventive aim, particularly when there are static disorders. In this respect the appearance for a metatarsal or even a metacarpal bony erosion is a therapeutic indication for the prescription of adapted plantar ortheses.

Consequently, a *systematic clinical examination* searches for any involvement which is potentially destructive, especially tarsitis or tenosynovitis of the tendon of the tibialis posterior muscle. In this way, treatment can be prescribed early and in the light of the foreseeable evolution of the disease; when deformities have already appeared, care is essentially palliative in nature.

This treatment aims to prevent dislocation of the tarsus or its ankylosis in a bad position. To obtain such a result, the causes of the deformity must be controlled as much as possible. Nevertheless, certain feet will dislocate whatever happens, whereas other feet will present fibrous or bony ankylosis. Finally, the best possible solution seems to be to obtain a tarsal ankylosis in an acceptable position from a functional point of view (105); all means which permit this to happen are thus beneficial. In this perspective, the ankle itself must of course retain sufficient mobility. The difficulty in treatment is to act in this way for the feet whose disease state is intermediate (fig. 32). The forefoot may be rendered fit for walking by wearing appropriate footwear or by a surgical operation, depending on the stage of the disease.

Surgery is indicated for pain, deformity and functional incapacity and therefore depends on the efficiency of the maintenance treatment (44, 105) (fig. 35). It must

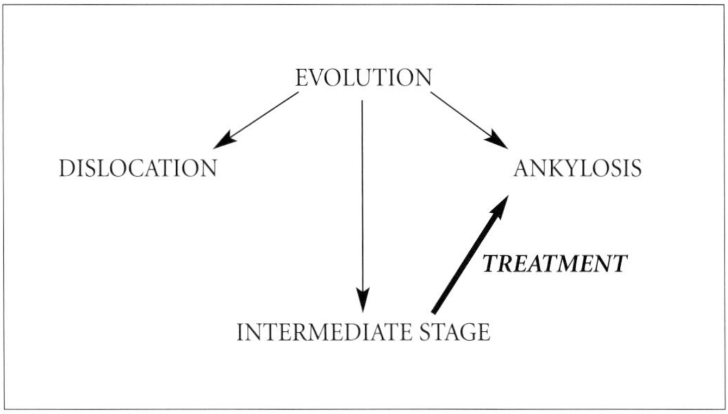

Fig. 32 - Some feet will dislocate whatever happens, others will develop fibrous or bony ankylosis in good positions. The difficulty in treatment is to act for the best for the feet at an intermediate stage of the disease.

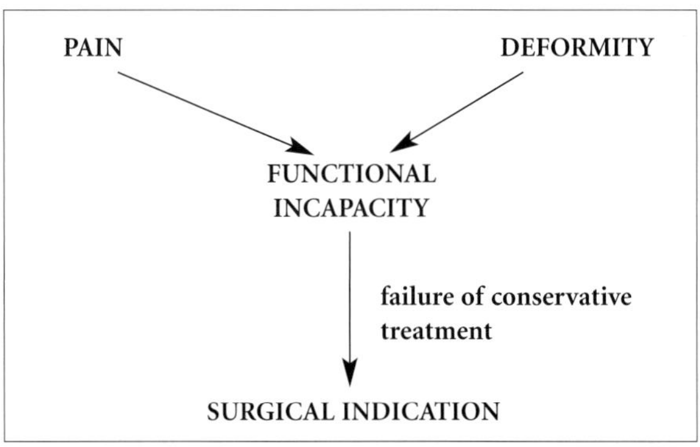

Fig. 35 - The surgical indications include pain, deformity and functional incapacity, and therefore depends on the efficrency of the conservative treatment.

also take into account the deforming potential of certain situations. The patient must be considered on the whole since RA is a systemic disease, is progressive and involves many joints. Carefulness is necessary: observation of the general state of the patient, planning of the next surgical operations on other joints. Long and recurred post-surgical convalescence periods may weaken the whole physical ability of the patient and must be evaluated in the long term (85). The surgical operation must be made at the good time and must rather use a procedure which avoids recurrent surgery if possible. On the other hand; it must be kept in mind that on the whole patients with RA have less demands than others about functional ability (85).

In patients whose disease is not very destructive, and who present localized involvement, simple early surgical treatment is sometimes indicated to maintain the correct functional conditions of the foot: talonavicular arthrodesis (6, 36, 58) or synovectomy of the tendon of the posterior tibialis muscle. On the contrary, if the arthritis is very painful and very destructive, surgery (arthrodesis) will be more radical at an earlier stage to prevent the dislocation of the tarsus (28, 44, 80, 105, 108).

Conclusion

Generally speaking, forefoot involvement appears earlier and is more obvious, while the tarsal lesion is later, often more insidious and often clinically mistaken for ankle involvement. The talocrural joint must be spared as much as possible. The metatarso-phalangeal bone erosion is the witness of the destructive character of RA, this erosion appears during the same period as the flattening of the midfoot and must incite the earliest preventive treatment.

When medical treatment fails, forefoot involvement, which is more frequent and disabling earlier, leads to surgical treatment, generally including arthrodesis of the first metatarsophalangeal joint. Then (or sometimes simultaneously) arthrodesis of the subtalar and midtarsal joints is performed in some cases.

Advanced talocrural disease can lead to the performance of an ankle arthrodesis or to the insertion of a prosthesis.

Finally, other factors must be taken into account now. In particular, the longevity of the rheumatoid patients is increasing and the new immunologic treatments should modify the destructive evolution of the disease.

All these considerations underline the importance of a global overview of the progressive nature of the disease. Consequently, the treatment of foot involvement must be carried out in the context of treatment of the rheumatoid arthritis as a whole.

References

1. Allieu Y, Claustre J, Simon L (1977) Étude anatomo-clinique et genèse des déformations du pied dans la polyarthrite rhumatoïde. In: Le pied inflammatoire. Maloine, Paris, pp 15-33
2. Amico (d') JC (1976) The pathomechanics of adult rheumatoid arthritis affecting the foot. J Am Podiatr Assco 66: 227-36
3. Amor B, Herson D, Cherot A, *et al.* (1981) Polyarthrites rhumatoïdes évoluant depuis plus de dix ans (1966-1978). An Med Interne (Paris) 132: 168-73
4. Anderson EG (1990) The rheumatoid foot: a sideways look. Ann Rheum Dis 4: 851-7
5. Arangio GA, Phillippy DC, Xiao D, *et al.* (2000) Subtalar pronation – relationship to the medial longitudinal arch loading in the normal foot. Foot and Ankle International 21, n° 3, 216-20

6. Asencio G, Bertin R, Megy B, *et al.* (1991) Intrication de l'arrière-pied dans la chirurgie de l'avant-pied rhumatoïde. Médecine et Chirurgie du Pied 7: 185-191
7. Awerbuch MS, Shepard E, Vernon-Roberts B (1982) Morton's metatarsalgia due to intermetatarso-phalangeal bursitis as an early manifestation of rheumatoid arthritis. Clin Orthop 167: 214-21
8. Barrett JP Jr (1976) Plantar pressure measurements: rational shoewear in patients with rheumatoid arthritis. JAMA: 235: 1138-9
9. Bassiouni M. (1965) Incidence of calcaneal spurs in osteoarthrosis and rheumatoid arthritis and in control patients. Ann Rheum Dis 24: 490-3
10. Benson GM, Johnson EW Jr (1971) Management of the foot in rheumatoid arthritis. Orthop Clin North Am 2: 733-44
11. Blotman F, Claustre J, Allieu Y, *et al.* (1977) Ténosynovites et syndromes canalaires du pied rhumatoïde. In: Le pied inflammatoire. Paris, Maloine p 35
12. Bonnel F, Farenc C, Claustre J, *et al.* (1989) Etude biométrique et radiographique du pied. Médecine et Chirurgie du Pied 5: 105-11
13. Bossley CJ, Cairney PC (1980) The intermetatarsophalangeal bursa: its significance in Morton's metatarsalgia. J Bone Joint Surg 62B: 184
14. Bouysset M, Bonvoisin B, Lejeune E, *et al.* (1987) Flattening of the rheumatoid foot in tarsal arthritis on X-ray. Scand J Rheumatol 16: 127-33
15. Bouysset M, Tebib J, Weil E, *et al.* (1989) The rheumatoid heel: its relationship to other disorders in the rheumatoid foot. Clin Rheumatol 8: 208-214
16. Bouysset M, Tebib J, Noël E, *et al.* (1993) When should orthopaedic treatment be prescribed to avoid the flattening of the rheumatoid foot? Clin rheumatol vol 12, n° 1
17. Bouysset M, Tavernier T, Tebib J, *et al.* (1995) CT and MRI evaluation or tenosynovitis of the rheumatoid hindfoot. Clin Rheumatol 14: 303-7
18. Bouysset M, Tebib J, Noël E, *et al.* (2002) Rheumatoid flatfoot and deformity of the first ray. J Rheumatol, 29: 903-5
19. Braun S (1975) Le pied dans les grands rhumatismes inflammatoires chroniques. Rhumatologie 27: 47-56
20. Brook A, Corbett M. (1977) Radiographic changes in early rheumatoid disease. Ann Rheum Dis 36: 71-73
21. Budiman-Mak K, Conrad K, Roach J, *et al.* (1993) Can foot orthoses prevent deformity in rheumatoid arthritis? American College of Rheumatology, San Antonio nov 7-11
22. Bywaters EGL (1953) Hell lesions of rheumatoid arthritis. Ann Rheum Dis 13: 42-50
23. Chatter EH (1970) Tarsal tunnel syndrome in rheumatoid arthritis (letter to the editor). Br Med J (Clin Res) 3: 406
24. Claustre J (1979) Le pied rhumatoïde. Problèmes podologiques pratiques. Rev Rhum 46: 673-8
25. Clayton ML (1960) Surgery of the forefoot in rheumatoid arthritis. Clin Orthop 16: 136
26. Clayton ML (1967) Surgical treatment of the rheumatoid foot. In: Giannestras NJ (ed) Foot and Disorders. Medical and Surgical Management. Lea and Febiger, Philadelphia
27. Clayton ML (1963) Surgery of the lower extremity in rheumatoid arthritis. J Bone Joint Surg (AM) 45: 1517-36
28. Coughlin MJ (1988) The rheumatoid foot. In: Chapman MW (ed). Operative Orthopedics, Philadelphia, JB Lippincott vol 3, pp 1845-55

29. Cracchiolo A (1997) Rheumatoid arthritis. Hindfoot Disease. Clin Orthop 340: 58-68
30. Cracchiolo AC III (1984) Surgery for rheumatoid disease. Part I: foot abnormalities in rheumatoid arthritis. In American Academy of Orthopedic Surgeons. Instructional Course Lectures. Vol 33. St Louis, Mosby-Year Book 386-404
31. Craxford AD, Stevens J, Park C (1982) Management of the deformed rheumatoid forefoot: a comparison of conservative and surgical methods. Clin Ortho 166: 121-6
32. Dedrick DK, Mc Cune J, Smith WS (1990) Rheumatoid arthritis presenting as spreading of the toes. J Bone Joint Surg 72A: 463
33. Dixon ASJ (1971) The rheumatoid foot. Mod Trands Rheumatol 2: 158-73
34. Downey DJ, Simkin PA, Mack LA, *et al.* (1988) Tibialis posterior tendon rupture: a cause of rheumatoid flat foot. Arthritis Rheum 31: 441-6
35. Duncan GS (1990) Recurrent rheumatoid nodule of the foot. J Am Podiatr Med Assoc 80, number 10: 552-5
36. Elbaor JE, Thomas WH, Weinfeld MS, *et al.* (1976) Talonavicular arthrodesis for rheumatoid arthritis of the hindfoot. Orthop Clin North Am 7: 821
37. Enjalbert M, Claustre J, Herisson C, Simon L (1989) Synovites du médio-tarse révélatrices d'un rhumatisme inflammatoire chronique. In: Claustre J, Simon L (ed). Le médio-pied. Paris, Masson 191-7
38. Forslind K, Larsson EM, Johansson A, *et al.* (1997) Detection of joint pathology by magnetic resonance imaging in patients with early rheumatoid arthritis. Br J Rheumatol 36(6): 683-8
39. Gerster JC, Wichert L, Bennami A, *et al.* (1977) The painful heel. Ann Rheum Dis 36: 343-8
40. Gheith and Dixon (1973) Tangential X-ray of the forefoot in rheumatoid arthritis. Ann Rheum Dis 32: 92-3
41. Gold RH, Basset LW (1982) Radiologic evaluation of the arthritis foot. Foot and Ankle, 2: 332-41
42. Gould JS (1982) Conservative management of the hypersensitive foot in rheumatoid arthritis. Foot Ankle, 2: 224-9
43. Grabois M, Puentes J, Lidsky M. (1981) Tarsal tunnel syndrome in rheumatoid arthritis. Arch Phys Med Rehabil 62: 401
44. Gracchiolo A III, Kitaoka HB, Pearson S (1988) Treatment of the painful, arthritic hindfoot (abstract). Orthop Transactions 12: 765
45. Grifka JK (1997) Shoes and insoles for patients with rheumatoid foot disease. Clin Orthop 340: 18-25
46. Haines RW, Mac Dougall A (1954) The anatomy of hallux valgus. J Bone Joint Surg 36-B: 272
47. Hamalainen M, Raunio P (1997) Long term follow-up of rheumatoid forefoot surgery. Clinical Orthopaedics and Related Research. 340: 34-8
48. Huber-Levernieux C (1993) La rupture du tendon du jambier postérieur. Synoviale 20: 10-7
49. Inman VT (1976) The joints of the Ankle. Baltimore, Williams and Wilkins
50. Jacoby RK et al. (1976) The great toe as a clinical problem in rheumatoid arthritis. Rheumatol Rehabil 15: 143-7
51. Jakubowski (1959) Early synovectomy in rheumatoid arthritis. Excerpta Medica Foundation: 149

52. Jan C, Delagoutte JP, Lobeuille D, *et al.* (1995) Polyarthrite rhumatoïde et kyste synovial: une localisation inhabituelle. Méd Chir Pied 11: 45-8
53. Janisse DJ, Ped C (1998) Prescription footwear for arthritis of the Foot and Ankle. Clin Orthop 349: 100-7
54. Jernberg ET, Simkin P, Kravette M, et al. (1999) The posterior tibial tendon and the tarsal sinus in rheumatoid flat foot: magnetic resonance imaging of 40 feet. J Rheumatol 26 (2): 289-93
55. Jörgensen G (1953) Uber die laterale abduction der zehen. Zbl Chir 78: 849
56. Keenan MAE, Peabody TD, Gronley JK, *et al.* (1991) Valgus deformities of the feet and characteristics of gait in patients who have rheumatoid arthritis. 73A, 2: 237-47
57. Kerschbaumer F, Von-Salomon D, Lehr F (1996) Der rheumatische Vorfuss. Der Orthopädie. 25 (4): 354-61
58. Kindsfater K, Wilson MG, Thomas WH (1997) Management of the rheumatoid hindfoot with special reference to talonavicular arthrodesis. Clin Orthop 340: 69-74
59. Kirkham BW, Gibson T (1988) Letter: comment on the article by Downey *et al.* Arthritis Rheum 31: 3
60. Kirkup Jr (1974) Ankle and tarsal joints in rheumatoid arthritis. Scand J Rheumatol 3: 50-2
61. Kirkup JR, Vidigal E, Jacob RK (1977) The hallux and rheumatoid arthritis. Acta Orthop Scand 48: 527-44
62. Kitaoka HB (1989) Rheumatoid hindfoot. Orthop Clin North Am 20: 593-604
63. Klenerman L (1995) The Foot and Ankle in Rheumatoid Arthritis. British Journal of Rheumatology 34: 443-8
64. Lapeyre-Gros F (1996) Le chaussage du pied rhumatoïde. Méd chir pied 12: 196-201
65. Mac Carthy DJ (1983) Surgical anatomy of the first ray. J Am Podiatr Assoc 73: 244-55
66. Mac Guigan L, Burke D, Fleming A (1983) Tarsal tunnel syndrome and peripheral neuropathy in rheumatoid disease. Ann Rheum Dis 42: 128
67. Mac Master PE (1933) Tendon and muscle ruptures: clinical and experimental studies of the causes and location of subcutaneous ruptures. J Bone Joint Surg 15: 705-22
68. Mann R, Inman VT (1964) Phasic activity of intrinsic muscles of the foot. J Bone Joint Surg 46A: 469
69. Mann RA, Schakel ME (1995) Surgical correction of rheumatoid forefoot deformities. Foot Ankle Int 16: 1-6
70. Manzi JA, Goldman F (1983) Rheumatoid nodule, an unusual variant. J Am. Podiatr Assoc 73: 205-8
71. Marmor L (1975) Resection of the forefoot in rheumatoid arthritis. Clin Orthop; 108: 223-7
72. Marshall RN, Myers DB, Palmer D (1980) Disturbance of gait due to rheumatoid disease. J Rheumatol 7: 617-23
73. Martel W (1970) Acute and Chronic Arthritis of the foot. Semin Roentgenol 5: 391-406
74. Matsuda Y, Yamanaka H, Higami K, *et al.* (1998) Time lag between active joint inflammation and radiological progression in patients with early rheumatoid arthritis. The Journal of Rheumatology 25(3): 427-32
75. Matsumoto K, Hukuda S, Nishioka J, Asajima S (1992) Rupture of the Achilles Tendon in Rheumatoid Arthritis with Histological Evidence of Enthesitis. A case report. Clin Orthop and Rel Res 235-40

76. Meachim G, Abberton MJ (1971) Histological findings in Morton's metatarsalgia. J Pathol 103: 209
77. Mereday C, Dolan C, Lusskin MD (1972) Evaluation of the University of California biomechanics laboratory shoe insert in " flexible " pes planus. Clin Orthop 82: 45-58
78. Michelson J, Easley M, Wigley FM, *et al.* (1994) Foot and Ankle problems in rheumatoid arthritis. Foot Ankle Int 15: 608-13
79. Michelson J, Easley M, Wigley FM, *et al.* (1995) Posterior tibial tendon dysfunction in rheumatoid arthritis. Foot Ankle Int 16: 156-61
80. Miehlke W, Gschwend N, Rippstein P, *et al.* (1997) Compression arthrodesis of the rheumatoid ankle and hindfoot. Clin Orthop 340: 75-86
81. Miller HG, Abadesco L, Heaney J (1983) Morton's neuroma symptoms from a rheumatoid nodule. J Am Podiatr Assoc 73: 311-2
82. Minaker K, Little H (1973) Painful feet in rheumatoid arthritis. CMA Journal 109: 724-30
83. Nakano KK (1975) The entrapment neuropathies of rheumatoid arthritis. Orthop Clin North Am 6: 837-60
84. O'Brien TS, Hart TS, Gould JS (1997) Extraosseous manifestations of rheumatoid arthritis in the foot and ankle. Clin Orthop 340: 26-33
85. Ouzounian T (2000) Rheumatoid arthritis of the foot and ankle. In: Myerson MS (ed) Foot and Ankle Disorders. Philadelphia, WB Saunders Company vol 2 1189-204
86. Potter TA, Khus JG (1972) Painful feet. In: Hollander JL (ed) Arthritis and Allied conditions. Philadelphia Lea and Febiger
87. Resnick D (1976) Roentgen features of the rheumatoid mid and hindfoot. J Can Assoc Radiol 27: 99-107
88. Resnick D, Niwayama G, Feingold ML (1977) The sesamoid bones of the hands and feet: participators in arthritis. Radiology 123: 57-62
89. Resnick RN, Jahss MH, Choueka J, *et al.* (1995) Deltoid ligament forces after tibialis posterior tendon ruptures: effect of triple arthrodesis and calcaneal displacement osteotomies. Foot Ankle Int 16: 14-20
90. Resnick D, Niwayama G (1988) Rheumatoid arthritis. In: Diagnosis of bone and joint disorders, 2nd ed., vol 2. Resnick D (ed). Philadelphia, WB Saunders, 259-87
91. Rosenberg ZS, Cheung Y, Jahss MH, *et al.* (1999) Rupture of posterior tibial tendon: CT and MRI imaging with surgical correlation. Radiology, Vol 169, number 1, 229-35
92. Seror P, Claustre J, Kha TD (1983) Les tarsites rhumatoïdes. In: Claustre J, Simon L (eds) Le pied en pratique rhumatologique. Paris, Masson, p 40
93. Serre H, Simon L, Claustre L (1972) Le syndrome douloureux aigu du deuxième espace intermétatarsien. Rev Rhum 39: 495-503
94. Sharp JT, Wilder RR, Hunder RI (1988) The American rheumatism association 1989. Criteria for the classification of rheumatoid arthritis. Arthritis Rheum 31: 315-24
95. Simkin PA, Downey DJ, Richardson ML (1989) Letter: More on the posterior tibial tendon in rheumatoid arthritis. Arthritis Rheum 32: 8
96. Simon L, Claustre J, Allieu Y (1980) Le pied rhumatoïde. Genèse des déformations. Rev Rhum 47: 117-22
97. Smith CA, Arnett FC (1991) Epidemiologic aspects of rheumatoid arthritis, current immunogenetic approach. Clin Orthop: 265: 23-35
98. Spector TD, Scott DL (1988) What happens to patients with rheumatoid arthritis? The long-term outcome of treatment. Clin Rheumatol 3: 315-30

99. Spiegel TM, Spiegel JS (1982) Rheumatoid arthritis in the foot and ankle. Diagnosis, pathology and treatment. Foot Ankle 2: 318-24

100. Stiles RG, Resnick D, Sartoris DJ (1988) Radiologic manifestations of arthritides involving the foot. Clin Podiatr Med Surg 5: 1-16

101. Stiskal M, Szolar DH, Stenzel I, *et al.* (1997) Magnetic resonance imaging of achilles tendon in patients with rheumatoid arthritis. Invest Radiol 32 (10) pp 602-8

102. Stockley I, Betts RP, Rowley Di, *et al.* (1990) The importance of the valgus hindfoot in forefoot surgery in rheumatoid arthritis. J Bone Joint Surg 72B: 705-8

103. Tenoudji-Cohen M, Perez R, Dessauw Ph, Sany J (1983) Apport de l'exploration radiographique du pied dans les rhumatismes inflammatoires. In: Claustre, Simon (eds) Le pied en pratique rhumatologique. Paris, Masson, p 102

104. Thould AK, Simon G (1966) Assessment of radiological changes in hands and feet in rheumatoid arthritis. Ann Rheum Dis 25: 220

105. Tillmann K (1979) The rheumatoid foot. G Thieme, Stuttgart, pp 44-56

106. Tillmann K (1985) Reconstructive foot surgery. Ann Chir Gynaecol 74: 90-5

107. Tillmann K (1987) The mutual interplay between forefoot and hindfoot affections and deformities in RA. Rheumatoid arthritis surgery of the complex foot. Rheumatology 11: 97-9

108. Vahvanen VAJ (1967) Rheumatoid arthritis in the pantalar joint. Acta Orthop Scan Suppl 107: 1-152

109. Vainio K (1956) The rheumatoid foot. A clinical study with pathological and roentgenological comments. In: Kallio, Vara (eds) Ann Chir Gynaecol 45 (suppl 1) 1-107

110. Vannimenus PY, Vannimenus-Hayem C, Thevenon A (1987) Etude radiographique du pied rhumatoïde et comparaison avec l'atteinte de la main. Médecine et Chirurgie du Pied 3: 197-202

111. Viladot A, Viladot R (1983) Biomécanique de l'avant-pied rhumatoïde. In: Claustre J, Simon L (eds) Le pied en pratique rhumatologique, Masson, Paris, p 28

112. Visser H, Le Cessie S, Vos K, *et al.* (2000) How to diagnose rheumatoid arthritis (RA) early: the development of diagnostic criteria. Ann Rheum, 59 (suppl 1), p 35

113. Voutey H, Strauss J, Magnet JL (1980) Résultats dans la chirurgie de l'avant-pied rhumatoïde. Rev Rhum 47: 123-5

114. Wakefields RJ, Gibbon WW, Cnaghan PG *et al.* (2000) The value of sonography in the detection of bone erosions in patients with rheumatoid arthritis. Arthritis Rheum 43: 2762

115. Whitney, Kalan K (1990) Padding and taping therapy. In: Levy LA (ed) Principles and practice of podiatric medicine. Churchill Livingstone, New York, pp 709-46

Additional references

. Bouysset M, Tebib J, Tavernier T and al. (2003) Posterior tibial tendon and subtalar joint complex in rheumatoid arthritis: magnetic resonance imaging study. The journal of rheumatology 30:9

. Chalmers AC, Busby C, Goyert J, Porter B, Schulzer M (2000) Metatarsalgia and rheumatoid arthritis – a randomised, single blind, sequential trial comparing 2 types of foot orthoses and supportive shoes. J Rheumatol. 27(7): 1643-7

. Cracchiolo A 1997 Erd. Rheumatoid arthritis. hindfoot disease. Clin Orthop. jul; (340): 58-68

. Hamilton J, Brydson G, Fraser S, Grant M (2001) Walking ability as a measure of treatment effect in early rheumatoid arthritis. Clin Rehabil. 15(2): 142-7

. Hodge MC, Bach TM, Carter GM (1999) Orthotic management of plantar pressure and pain in rheumatoid arthritis. clinic biomechanics 14(8): 567-75

. Jannick MJ, Van Dijk H, De Vries J, Groothoff JW, Lankhordst GJ (2004) A systematic review of the methodological quality and extent to which evaluation studies measure the usability of orthopaedic shoes. Clin Rehabil. 18(1): 15-26

. Wickman AM, Pinzur MS, Kadanoff R, Juknelis D (2004) Health-related quality of life for patients with rheumatoid arthritis foot involvement. Foot Ankle int. 25(1): 19-26

. Locke M, Perry J, Campbell J, Thomas L (1984) – Ankle and subtalar motion during gait in arthritis patients. Phys. Ther. 64(4): 504-9

. O'Brien T, Hart TS, Gould J (1997) Extra- osseous manifestations of rheumatoid arthritis in the foot and ankle. Clin. Orthop. 340, 26-33

. Thomas JL, Moeini R, Soileau R (2000) The effects on subtalar contact and pressure following talonavicular and midtarsal joint arthrodesis. J. Foot Ankle Surg. 39(2): 78-88

Some reflections on pathomechanics of the rheumatoid foot and ankle

X. Crevoisier

Introduction

Inflammatory synovitis leads to the weakening of the stabilizing structures of the foot, resulting in pain and deformity and in turn leads to biomechanical abnormalities (121). However, these functional abnormalities also enhance deformity, thus a vicious circle is created (fig. 1).

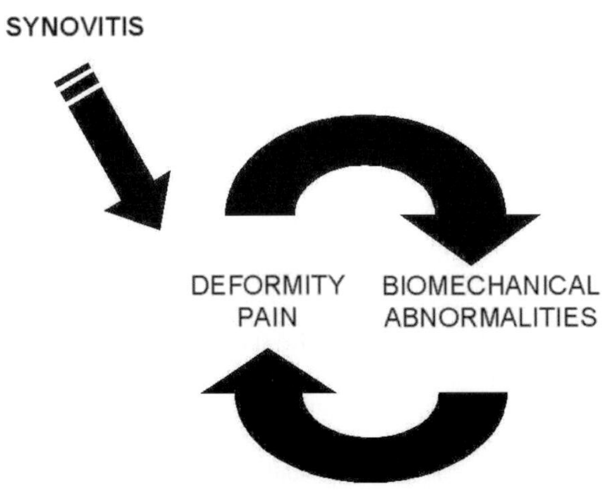

Fig. 1 - Inflammatory synovitis leads to pain and deformities resulting in biomechanical abnormalities of the rheumatoid foot. Inversely, these functional abnormalities enhance the deformities. Thus, a vicious circle is created.

The aims of the present chapter are:
- to describe the properties and the importance of the main stabilizing structures of the foot;
- to address the most frequent deformities of the rheumatoid foot (31), including valgus deformity of the hindfoot, flattening of the arch, hallux valgus, and typical metatarso-phalangeal joints and toe deformities;
- to emphasize the importance of gait analysis because it not only allows to express the functional abnormalities associated with the rheumatoid foot but also allows to show the compensatory mechanisms developed by the patients.

The stabilizing structures

The forefoot is most frequently affected in patients with rheumatoid arthritis (13, 44, 119, 121). The joints that are first involved are commonly the metatarso-phalangeal (MTP) (119, 121, 133, 134). The forefoot is stabilized by a capsulo-ligamentous complex, which includes the articular capsules and their connections with the plantar plate, the collateral ligaments, the intermetatarsal ligaments and the plantar fascia or plantar aponeurosis (122). The intrinsic muscles are the main musculo-tendinous stabilizers of the MTP joints, but the stability of these joints also indirectly depends on the balance between the extrinsic flexors and extensors.

Usually, midfoot involvement is not predominant in the rheumatoid arthritic patient (7, 121).

The hindfoot is also a major target of rheumatoid arthritis (62, 66, 91, 121). The talo-navicular joint is altered in 40% of cases of hindfoot involvement, the subtalar joint in 30-40% of cases, and the calcaneo-cuboidal joint in 25% of cases (31, 59, 91, 113, 129). Main stabilizing ligaments of the hindfoot include the spring ligament, the long and short plantar ligaments, the talo-calcaneal interosseous ligament, the medial talo-calcaneal ligament and the superficial portion of the deltoid ligament. *In vitro* testing has demonstrated that, as the intact foot is loaded, deformation occurs and includes depression of the arch and rotation of the forefoot as a whole in relation to the hindfoot. In the absence of muscular activity, sectioning of the above mentioned ligaments results in severe plano-valgus deformity when an axial load is applied to the foot in a plantigrade posture (69). Thus, compared to the intact situation, metatarsal-to-talar dorsiflexion, abduction and eversion increase by 10° each, calcaneal-to-talar eversion and abduction respectively by 3° and 2°, and navicular-to-talar abduction and dorsiflexion respectively by 13° and 10° (69). There is also increased plantar flexion (8°) observed at the talar-tibial joint. Of course, these angular values are associated with a severely unstable foot condition. Nevertheless, since plano-valgus deformity in the rheumatoid foot is reported as frequently as in 30-60% of the cases (55, 66, 121), and since this deformity is considered rather as a consequence of alteration of the stabilizing structures by inflammatory synovitis than a consequence of musculo-tendinous deficiency (62, 64, 88), these values are listed here to emphasize the importance of the ligamentous stabilizers of the hindfoot. In foot flat position, the musculo-tendinous stabilization of the hindfoot is less important than the ligamentous stabilization (6, 107), even if the tibialis posterior unit is essential in this position (68). On the other hand, as soon as heel rise occurs, the extrinsic muscles including tibialis posterior, flexor hallucis longus (FHL), flexor digitorum longus (FDL), gastro-soleus and also partially peroneus longus (PL) are essential to transform the foot into a rigid lever for push off (99).

The stabilizers of the subtalar joint

The three major ligamentous stabilizers of the subtalar joint include the talo-calcaneal interosseous ligament, the cervical ligament and the calcaneo-fibular ligament (111). Deficiency of the interosseous and cervical ligaments affects subtalar joint stability up to 15% and deficiency of the calcaneo-fibular ligament up to 20% (71, 73). Cervical and calcaneo-fibular ligaments have been clearly established as stabilizers of subtalar joint inversion. Regarding the talo-calcaneal interosseous ligament, there are some doubts on whether its deficiency affects more stability against inversion (74) or against eversion (72).

The spring ligament

The spring ligament is a major stabilizer of the talo-navicular joint. The spring ligament is not a single structure but should rather be considered as a complex unit which includes the strong supero-medial calcaneo-navicular ligament with its cartilaginous triangular facet, the inferior calcaneo-navicular ligament, and the tibioligamentous portion of the superficial deltoid ligament (28, 118). Based on its histological and biomechanical properties this structure is not elastic and should be considered as a sling rather than as a spring (28). Furthermore, there are separate insertional sites of the posterior tibial tendon into the supero-medial calcaneo-navicular ligament. This suggests a true synergism between the dynamic tendon unit and the static ligament in preventing medial and plantar talar head migration (28, 118). A major deficiency of this unit is associated with a 20% decrease of the talo-navicular joint contact surface during loading response and push off phase (90). During foot flat phase of stance, contact characteristics of the talo-navicular joint are not altered. Nevertheless, an in vitro study has demonstrated that arch stiffness decreases by 2% after sectioning of the spring ligament if an axial load is applied to the foot in a neutral position (49).

The long and short plantar ligaments

Based on their expansions from the calcaneus to the cuboid and to the four lesser metatarsals the long and short plantar ligaments contribute significantly to the stability of the longitudinal arch of the foot. Stiffness of the intact foot decreases by 10% after sectioning of the long and short plantar ligaments (49).

The plantar fascia and the capsulo-ligamentous complex of the forefoot

The plantar fascia, or plantar aponeurosis, is subcutaneous and extends from the plantar aspect of the postero-medial calcaneal tuberosity to the deep and subcutaneous tissues of the forefoot and to the base of the proximal phalanges (11, 45, 82, 83, 110). Its stiffness averages 200N/mm and its failure load is as high as 1200N (70). Thus, the plantar aponeurosis is a very solid structure, and, because of its complex anatomical relationships with the capsulo-ligamentous structures of the forefoot (122), it plays a major role in the stabilization of the foot, including stabilization of the hindfoot, of the longitudinal arch and of the MTP joints.

The plantar fascia, the long and short plantar ligaments and the spring ligament have been recognized as important elements that support the longitudinal arch of the foot. In vitro testing indicates that the relative contributions of these three structures to arch stiffness are 56%, 34%, and 10% respectively (49). Stiffness of the intact foot has also been shown to decrease by 25% after sectioning of the plantar fascia (49).

The plantar fascia acts as a dynamic support of the longitudinal arch of the foot (127). Thus, the longitudinal arch of the foot rises as a result of dorsiflexion of the toes which pulls the distal plantar fascia around the metatarsal heads. This windlass mechanism was described by Hicks (46, 47). Excursion around the first metatarsal head approximates 1 cm by maximal dorsiflexion of the big toe (122). Therefore, since the diameter of the lesser metatarsal heads is smaller than that of the first metatarsal head, the windlass effect is mainly produced by dorsiflexion of the big toe. An in vitro study has demonstrated that, in plantigrade posture, 45° of dorsiflexion of the toes result in a nearly 4° increase of the talar-first metatarsal angle in the sagittal plane. This effect on the longitudinal arch is more important than that resulting from the action of any extrinsic muscle of the foot in this posture (127). During ambulation, dorsiflexion of the toes occurs in the second part of stance phase, as the heel rises. Since the plantar fascia originates rather medially under the calcaneus it contributes to inverting the subtalar joint during heel rise, and therefore to locking the hindfoot complex (104).

Due to its connections with the plantar capsulo-ligamentous structures of the MTP joints the plantar fascia also contributes to active and passive stabilization of the forefoot. The plantar plate is located under the metatarsal head and consists of a thickening of the articular capsule which is firmly attached to the base of the proximal phalanx and which is also anchored to its metatarsal head by the collateral ligaments. The plantar plates and the deep transverse metatarsal ligaments form a continuous band of strong ligamentous tissue across the forefoot (110, 122). The deeper layer of the plantar aponeurosis divides distally into five processes. Each process stretches towards its corresponding toe, and then, close to the metatarsal head, divides again into two strong slips, between which the flexor tendons emerge to come to lie on the plantar surface of the plantar plate. These two slips insert into the medial and lateral side of the plantar plate, and into the sesamoids under the first metatarsal head (11, 110, 122). Some fibers from the plantar fascia bifurcate medially and laterally into the deep transverse metatarsal ligaments, thus creating a connection between the longitudinal and transverse capsulo-ligamentous systems (fig. 2). Both systems and their interconnections control the splay of the forefoot, the longitudinal arch of the foot by the windlass mechanism and the stability of the MTP joints by the reverse windlass mechanism (46, 47). The reverse windlass functions as follows: with weight-bearing the longitudinal arch flattens, the foot lengthens, the plantar fascia tightens and produces plantar flexion of the proximal phalanges, thus stabilizing the MTP joints (112). Since electromyographic activity of intrinsic muscles has been reported to be low during foot flat period of stance phase (6, 41, 85), stabilization of the MTP joints by the reverse windlass mechanism is very important.

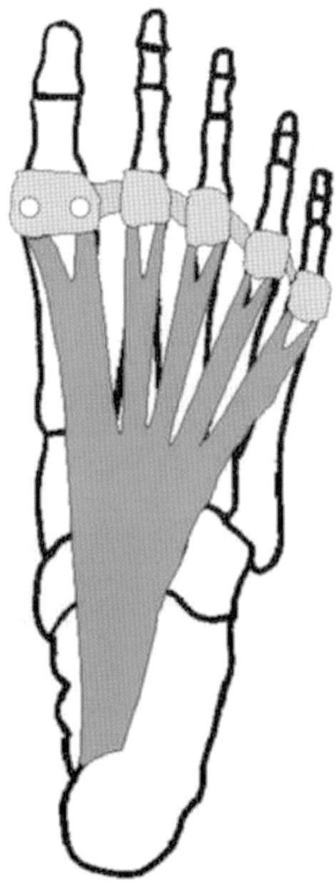

Fig. 2 - The plantar plates and the deep transverse metatarsal ligaments form a strong band of ligamentous tissue across the forefoot. The plantar fascia divides into five processes. Each process stretches towards its corresponding toe. Close to the metatarsal heads, each process divides into two slips. Each slip inserts into the medial and lateral portions of the plantar plate. Fibres from these slips sweep medially and laterally into the transverse metatarsal ligaments. Thus, a connection between the transverse and the longitudinal tie bar systems is established.

The extrinsic muscles

The importance of the extrinsic muscles in stabilizing the arch of the foot is significantly higher from heel rise to push off than during foot flat posture.

Electromyographic studies have shown that extrinsic muscles only play a minor role in stabilization of the arch of the foot in plantigrade posture, and that stability is mainly achieved by passive structures (6, 107). Nevertheless, the effect of the posterior tibial unit must be emphasized in this situation. Thus, if axial load is applied to the foot in neutral position, and if the tibialis posterior muscle is disconnected, ankle dorsiflexion and subtalar joint eversion increase significantly, even if flexor hallucis longus (FHL), flexor digitorum longus (FDL), gastro-soleus, long and short fibular muscles are activated (68).

In the second part of stance phase the foot has to be transformed into a rigid lever for propulsion. To achieve this function the subtalar joint has to be inverted in order to lock the hindfoot complex. As a result of subtalar inversion, the axes of talo-navicular and calcaneo-cuboidal joints converge, transforming the Chopart joint into a rigid segment (84). The inversion capability of the tibialis posterior muscle is twice as high as the inversion capability of the flexor hallucis longus and also twice as high as that of the gastro-soleus (99). Therefore, the tibialis posterior muscle plays a major role in locking the hindfoot. Inversion is balanced by the activity of the peroneal muscles (99). Because of its insertion under the first metatarsal, the peroneus longus also acts as a plantar flexor of the first ray during push off and, therefore, contributes to arch stability.

The intrinsic muscles

Intrinsic muscles, especially interossei and lumbricales, are active stabilizers of the MTP joints. Compared to the extrinsic muscles, intrinsic muscles have the advantage of proximity but they exert less force than the extrinsic muscles because of their lower muscle mass and lever arm (99). Like the extrinsic muscles, intrinsic muscles are more effective during the second part of stance phase. Their electromyographic activity starts at 40% of the gait cycle (65% of stance phase) (85). Because of their insertions at the base of the proximal phalanges, and because their traction axis is located under the transverse rotation axis of the MTP joints, interossei and lumbricales are direct stabilizers of these joints (123). On the other hand, short flexors insert at the middle phalanx and, therefore, are only indirect stabilizers of the MTP joints as long as the balance between flexors ant extensors is maintained.

Deformities

Forefoot deformities

Typical deformities of the rheumatoid forefoot include metatarsus primus varus, hallux valgus, forefoot splaying, dislocation of the MTP joints, lateral deviation of the toes, and clawtoes (16, 23, 40, 60, 91, 114, 120) (fig. 3).

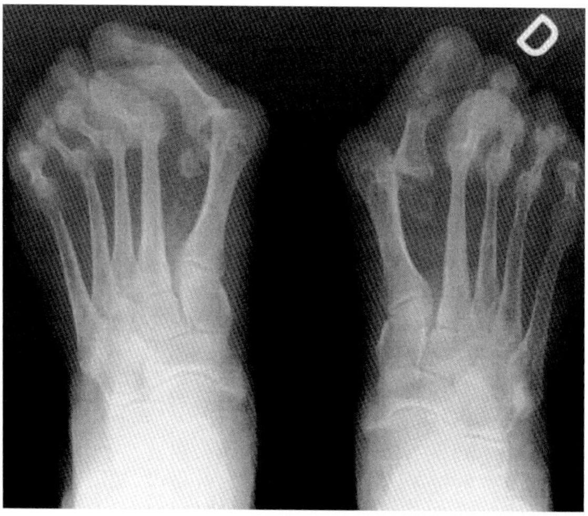

Fig. 3 - Typical deformities of the rheumatoid forefoot: metatarsus primus varus, hallux valgus, splaying of the forefoot, dislocation of the MTP joints, lateral deviation of the lesser toes, clawtoes.

Gender (24), age (121), shoe constraints (4, 33, 115) and heel height of the shoes (25, 89, 101) are well known factors contributing to hallux valgus deformity and these certainly also apply to the development of this deformity in the rheumatoid foot. However, since the medial capsule of the first MTP joint is essential to the stability of this joint (76, 131), inflammatory synovitis probably plays a major role in hallux valgus deformity of the rheumatoid foot (31). Erosion of the metatarsal heads is another factor associated with rheumatoid arthritis. There is a tendency to early erosion of the inferior and lateral surfaces of the metatarsal heads (121, 128). The erosion of the sesamoid crest results from the combined inflammatory and mechanical actions (42, 122). Since increased laxity of the first tarso-metatarsal joint seems to contribute to hallux valgus deformity (34), inflammatory synovitis at this level is likely to be considered as an additional deforming factor.

Functional integrity of the hallux is essential since 40% of bodyweight is supported by the hallux during the final stage of stance phase (124). This load is more than twice the load carried by all lesser toes combined (53). Even a moderate degree of valgus deviation or hallucal pronation causes an eccentric pull of the musculotendinous units acting across the first MTP joint, resulting in decreased functional weight bearing capacity of the hallux (109). With greater deformity, there is a progressive decrease of hallucal loading in favour of increased load bearing on the lateral side of the foot (50, 125). Therefore, the lesser MTP joints undergo higher constraints (86). Furthermore, progression of hallux valgus deformity is associated with a decreased plantarising effect of the plantar aponeurosis on the proximal phalanx. This effect may completely disappear in case of severe hallux valgus (122). In case of hallux valgus deformity, the windlass mechanism of the plantar fascia at the big toe is also markedly impaired. When the hallucal windlass mechanism fails, the control and support of the longitudinal arch of the foot will depend increasingly on the same mechanism of the plantar fascial processes to the lesser toes, particularly the second and the third (122). Even if the plantar plates of the lesser MTP joints are not yet altered by inflammatory synovitis, this additional constraint may accelerate the degenerative process, resulting in instability of these joints.

Functional hallux rigidus of the rheumatoid foot was reported by Clayton and Ries (23). It does not belong stricto sensu to the typical deformities associated with rheumatoid forefeet. However, it has to be mentioned here as a functional deformity. Functional hallux rigidus results from a hyperactivity of the hallucal intrinsic muscles attempting to reduce pressure under the lesser metatarsal heads by the means of excessive plantar flexion of the proximal phalanx of the hallux. Thus, pressure is transmitted to the hallucal interphalangeal joint. This functional deformity can be encountered even in the presence of a well aligned first MTP joint with intact articular surfaces and normal passive range of motion.

Since inflammatory synovitis is considered the most important factor causing foot alterations in rheumatoid arthritis, the close relationship between the articular capsules of the MTP joints and the transverse and longitudinal ligamentous systems explains the high incidence of rheumatoid forefoot deformities, particularly deformities of the MTP joints (86). Synovitis damages the plantar plate, which is particularly weak in its central zone, where it is grooved for the flexor tendons. If this central zone ruptures, both slips of the plantar aponeurosis tend to migrate dorsally around the sides of the metatarsal head (122). Thus, neither the windlass mechanism, nor the reverse windlass mechanism can function because the metatarsal heads no longer play their role as a pulley. Furthermore, since the distal slips of the plantar aponeurosis are now located dorsally from the transverse rotation axis of the MTP joints, it contributes to extension and dorsal dislocation of the proximal phalanx when load is applied to the plantigrade foot. Together with the lesion of the plantar plate the elongation of the deep transverse metatarsal ligaments (27) contribute to forefoot splaying.

The plantar fat pad, which is intimately associated with the soft tissues that insert into the base of the proximal phalanx, migrates distally and the metatarsal head is then exposed to a more direct plantar contact with the ground (86). In an attempt to minimize pain associated with this plantar contact when weight is applied to the forefoot, and also to delay the transfer of bodyweight to the forefoot during stance phase of gait, the extensors exert constant dorsiflectory forces. These forces contribute to progressive subluxation and eventual dislocation of the phalanges on the metatarsals, which also places a plantigrade force on the metatarsals (120).

Dysfunction of the intrinsic musculature is an additional deforming factor. In rheumatoid arthritis, muscular involvement particularly affects interosseous and lumbricales muscles (31, 121, 130). These muscles act as plantar flexors of the proximal phalanges and are, therefore, dynamic stabilizers of the MTP joints. Since they are active in the second part of stance phase (85, 99), their deficiency promotes dorsal dislocation of the proximal phalanx at the end of stance phase (129, 135). Furthermore, even if these muscles are still partially able to contract, their axis of traction can displace dorsally from the transverse rotation axis of the MTP joints because of the deficiency of the capsulo-ligamentous stabilizers. Therefore, from flexors these muscles go on to become extensors. This results not only in the loss of active plantar stabilization of the MTP joints but also in an additional force accentuating dorsal dislocation of the proximal phalanges.

Hindfoot deformities

Cavo-varus deformity of the foot is sometimes associated with rheumatoid arthritis (17, 105) and is reported as a consequence of post-inflammatory soft tissues contracture (17, 27). However, flatfoot deformity is by far the most common hindfoot deformity in rheumatoid arthritis, its incidence being 25 times higher than cavo-varus deformity (44). Etiology of rheumatoid plano-valgus deformity is controversial. Indeed, there have been reports of posterior tibial tendon rupture in rheumatoid arthritis (32, 55, 117), but most authors consider plano-valgus deformity as a consequence of articular laxity resulting from inflammatory lesions that affect the supporting soft tissues (62, 64, 88, 121, 129) without associated impairment of the posterior tibial tendon. In order to clarify the role played by the posterior tibial tendon in plano-valgus deformity, it is important to define the diagnostic criteria that allow to clearly establish a posterior tibial tendon dysfunction. Usual posterior tibial tendon examination includes testing of muscle strength, palpation of the tendon, measurement of arch height, ability to rise the heel off the ground and, thereby, invert the hindfoot, and the too-many-toes sign (37). Michelson *et al.* (92) have demonstrated that, depending upon the diagnostic criteria used, between 13% and 64% of a population satisfying at least four of the seven items proposed in the revised American Rheumatism Association Criteria for rheumatoid arthritis (3) could be considered to have posterior tibial tendon dysfunction. However, using the presence of all three of the most stringent criteria for diagnosis, which include flattening of the longitudinal arch of the foot, inability to perform a heel-rise, and lack of a palpable posterior tibial tendon, only 11% of patients were believed to have posterior tibial tendon dysfunction. There is a complex interaction between hindfoot inflammatory arthropaties and musculo-tendinous dysfunction. Thus, if a significant articular laxity results from inflammatory lesions of the supporting soft tissues, the tendon of the tibialis posterior muscle may become dysfunctional because of the mechanical disturbance of the hindfoot. The influence of hindfoot mechanical dysfunction on the tibialis posterior muscle is well illustrated by the increased electromyographic activity of the tibialis posterior muscle in rheumatoid patients with plano-valgus deformity during stance phase of gait (62) (fig. 4). This increased activity indicates that, during stance phase, the tibialis posterior muscle acts to support the collapsing longitudinal arch and to minimize excessive eversion of the hindfoot (6, 62). Tendons passing behind the medial malleolus include tibialis posterior, flexor digitorum longus (FDL) and flexor hallucis longus (FHL). The posterior tibial tendon is in direct apposition to the tibia. In the intact foot, the gliding resistance of the posterior tibial tendon averages 1.4 N. Thus, the gliding resistance of the posterior tibial tendon is 75% higher than the resistance of FHL and 45% higher than the resistance of FDL. The higher gliding resistance observed in posterior tibial tendon compared with FDL and FHL is consistent with the observations that posterior tibial tendinitis, dysfunction

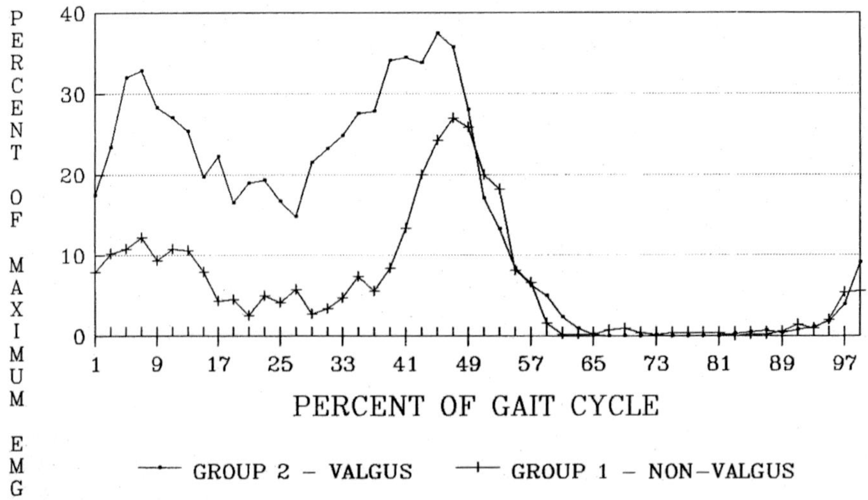

Fig. 4 - Mean quantitated electromyographic data for the tibialis posterior muscle during gait, expressed as a percentage of maximum activity, as determined during a maximum isometric contraction. The activity is increased in Group 2 (rheumatoid patients suffering from valgus deformity of the hindfoot) compared with Group 1 (rheumatoid patients with normal alignment of the foot). This difference indicates that during stance phase (0 to 60 per cent of the gait cycle), the tibialis posterior muscle acts to support the collapsing longitudinal arch in valgus feet. (from Keenan MA, *et al.* (1991) Valgus deformities of the feet and characteristics of gait in patients who have rheumatoid arthritis. J Bone Joint Surg 73A: 237-47, by permission).

and rupture are very common, while tendinopathy of FDL and FHL at the malleolar level is rare. Compared to the intact condition, flatfoot deformity increases gliding resistance by 50% for posterior tibial tendon, but not for FDL and FHL (36), thus potentially favourising posterior tibial tendon degeneration. This mechanical observation, added to the inflammatory tenosynovitis sui generis, is also consistent with the predominance of posterior tibial tendon lesions in the rheumatoid foot compared to FDL and FHL tendinopathy (14).

Articular laxity resulting from inflammatory synovitis and from inflammatory lesions of the soft supporting structures are thought to be the main cause of rheumatoid flatfoot deformity. The most frequently affected joints are the talo-navicular, subtalar and calcaneo-cuboidal joints (31, 59, 91, 113, 129). The ligaments included in these joints, like the talo-calcaneal interosseous ligament and the ligaments intimately associated with these joints are the main stabilizers of the hindfoot. Their respective contributions to stability have been described above. The interactions between the numerous ligamentous and articular lesions accelerate the deforming process (31). A three-dimensional biomechanical model was used to demonstrate that, relative to the neutral foot, five degrees of eversion in the subtalar joint result in a 22% increase in load to the longitudinal arch, in a 47% increase in moment at the talo-navicular joint, and in a 58% increase in moment at the navicular-first cuneiform joint when bodyweight is applied to the foot (2). Furthermore, loading of the unstable foot is associated with abnormal joint contact features. An in vitro study has demonstrated that, with physiologic loading of the unstable foot, the contact area of the talo-navicular joint decreases by 35% compared to normal and that there is a shift in contact distribution towards more dorsal and central regions of the navicular bone (67).

Interactions between forefoot and hindfoot deformities

Severity of hallux valgus correlates with forefoot splaying, particularly with increased M1-M2 and M1-M5 angles (15, 16, 114) and also with the severity of lesser toes deformities (91). It is more difficult to establish a correlation between forefoot deformities and midfoot or hindfoot deformities. Flattening of the longitudinal arch does not seem to depend upon forefoot splaying (114). However, there is a significant correlation between first ray deformities, particularly increased M1-M2 angle, and flatfoot deformity (16). There is also a significant correlation between hindfoot posture and plantar pressures at the metatarsal heads (136). In valgus heel deformity, lateral metatarsal heads are frequently non-weightbearing, producing gross loading patterns with a dominant medial distribution and also a higher prevalence of callosities under the medial metatarsal heads (136). Flattening of the longitudinal arch does not directly influence forefoot splaying (15, 126). Nevertheless, since flattening of the longitudinal arch is associated with forefoot abduction (69), the traction axis of the extensors is displaced laterally, thus contributing to lateral deviation of the toes.

Influence of hindfoot deformities on the ankle joint

In rheumatoid arthritis, the ankle joint is affected later, less frequently, and less severely than the hindfoot and forefoot (12, 40, 65, 129, 132). Degenerative lesions at the tibio-talar joint may result directly from inflammatory synovitis, but they may also be the consequence of valgus deformity of the hindfoot. Thus, a severe plano-valgus deformity results in a lateral shift in global contact surface of the tibio-talar joint (75). This lateral shift may be as high as 5 mm; even a 11 mm lateral shift in peak pressure location has been reported (35). Mean contact area of the tibio-talar joint may decrease by 35% and peak pressure may increase by 13% (35).

Gait analysis

Modern gait analysis requires evaluation of kinematics, kinetics and temporal-distance parameters. Additional or related assessments include electromyography, accelerometry, and podobarometry.

Gait analysis in rheumatoid foot assessment dates back to over twenty years. During this period of time, however, no standardized measurement methods and evaluation criteria have been developed. Therefore, the literature is difficult to interpret. Nevertheless, even if little precise information is available, clear tendencies can be seen in the most rigorous studies.

Gait abnormalities associated with foot and ankle impairment in rheumatoid arthritis include reduced cadence and velocity, shorter stride length, shorter single-limb support period, delayed heel rise, reduced movement of the ankle joint excursion, and excessive hindfoot eversion (31, 54, 62, 81, 87). Even in early stages of rheumatoid involvement, step length, velocity, duration of stance phase, and vertical ground reaction forces are altered (43). Pain is reported to alter variables of gait more than structural deformities of the foot (103). Table 1 and 2 summarize abnormalities of temporal-distance parameters and of kinematics associated with the rheumatoid foot. To some extend, it is possible to differentiate gait abnormalities associated with forefoot dysfunction from those resulting from the whole foot and ankle impairment.

Table I - Temporal-distance parameters: comparison between normal and rheumatoid foot (8, 26, 43, 54, 58, 61, 62, 81, 87, 97, 103, 116).

Temporal-distance parameters	Normal foot	Rheumatoid foot
Cadence (steps/min)	106-124	90-112
Velocity (m/s)	1.2-1.38	0.6-0.98
Double stance (% of gait cycle)	10-15	17-28
Heel rise (% of stance phase)	53-60	70-90
Stance phase (% of gait cycle)	61-63	67-80

Table II - Ankle and hindfoot kinematics: comparison between normal and rheumatoid foot (26, 52, 54, 62, 77, 81, 97, 103, 106).

Kinematics during stance phase of gait	Normal foot	Rheumatoid foot
Ankle sagittal motion (°)	18-20	15-16
Ankle maximal plantar flexion (°)	8-15	1-8
Ankle maximal dorsiflexion (°)	5-11	10-14
Hindfoot coronal motion (°)	11-12	11-14
Hindfoot maximal inversion (°)	2-8	-8-2
Hindfoot maximal eversion (°)	3-9	9-20

Gait abnormalities associated with the rheumatoid forefoot

Gait abnormalities associated with forefoot impairment in rheumatoid arthritis result from the efforts produced by the patient to compensate for forefoot pain by delaying and reducing forefoot loading.

Decreased ankle joint excursion is most noticeable during the period of ankle plantar flexion in late stance phase (54, 81, 97). As a result of diminished ankle plantar flexion, heel rise is delayed and limited in late stance phase. Thus, heel rise is delayed until 70% of stance phase instead of 40-60% of stance phase in normal subjects (61, 94, 97). Hindfoot kinematics are characterized by reduced adduction and internal rotation during push off (54). Maximal hindfoot eversion occurs in the second part of stance phase and can be as much as 10° (62). This is more than twice as high as maximal functional eversion in the normal foot (21, 51, 52, 94). Analysis of ground reaction forces demonstrates less energetical gait pattern. Thus, compared to normal (22), alternation of vertical force peaks is less contrasting (97) in rheumatoid patients (fig. 5). The most noticeable alteration of ground reaction forces associated with a rheumatoid forefoot is a significantly decreased propulsion force, down to 10% of bodyweight during push off (fig. 6) (97), instead of 20-30% of bodyweight in normal (22, 52). Therefore, maximal plantar flexion moments during push off are also markedly reduced. This minimizes the use of the foot as a rigid lever for push off (97). In other terms, the foot becomes more of a pedestal and less of a lever of propulsion (120). Gait velocity may be reduced to 60-70% of normal

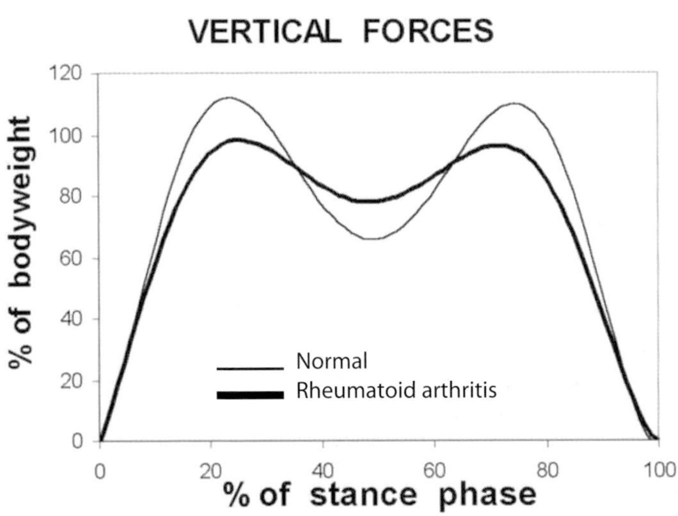

Fig. 5 - Vertical ground reaction forces: alternation of vertical force peaks is less contrasting than in normal subjects. (Thin black curve: normal. Bold curve: rheumatoid arthritis).

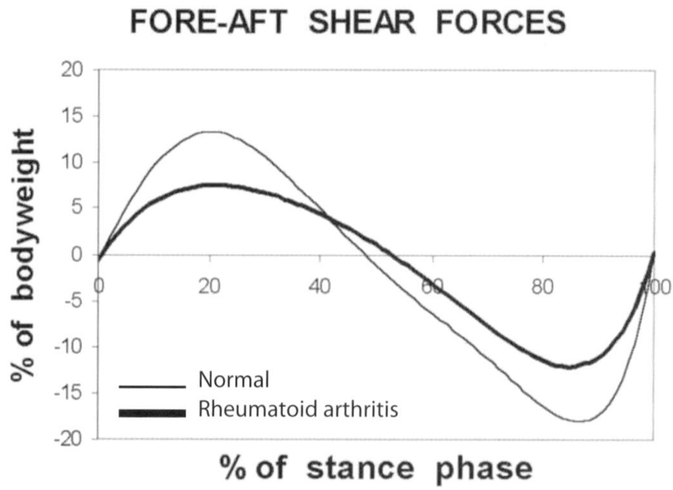

Fig. 6 - Fore-aft ground reaction shear forces: amplitude of braking forces and of propulsion forces is markedly reduced in rheumatoid patients.

and walking cadence decreases by 10% compared to normal (62, 97). Mean duration of single-limb support may decrease to 80% (62); this means also that duration of double-limb support, which is normally 11% of the gait cycle (22, 116), may increase to 16% of the gait cycle (62, 87).

Gait abnormalities associated with the rheumatoid hindfoot

Most of gait abnormalities observed in the case of rheumatoid impairment of the forefoot are also present, and usually more accentuated, in the case of hindfoot involvement, which mainly consists in plano-valgus deformity.

Maximal hindfoot eversion in the second part of stance phase may reach 20° and the hindfoot never assumes inversion throughout stance phase (81) (fig. 7). On the other hand, normally, maximal hindfoot eversion during stance phase usually do not exceed 6°, and a 2-8° of hindfoot inversion is observed in terminal stance (26, 52, 62, 94, 106). In the rheumatoid hindfoot, heel rise may be delayed until double-limb support. Velocity (50% of normal) and cadence (85% of normal) are further reduced compared to the rheumatoid foot without deformity (62). Duration of single-limb support may become as low as 75% of normal (62, 81, 87).

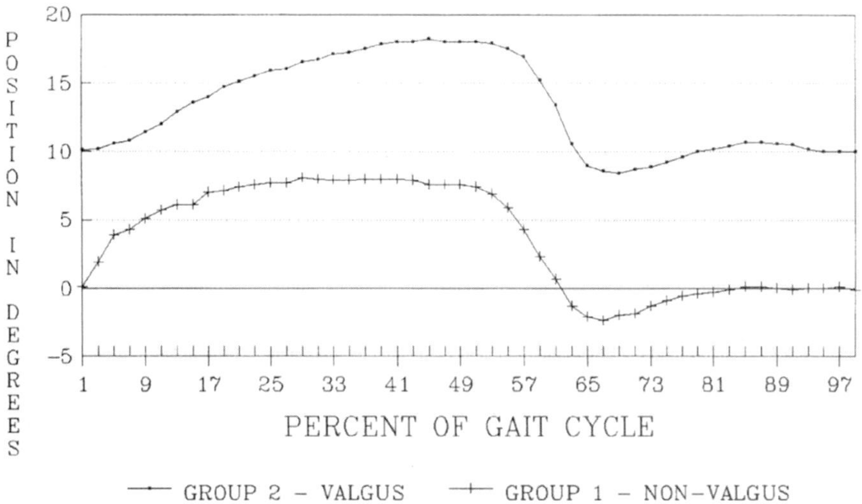

Fig. 7 - Mean electrogoniometric measurements of subtalar motion during gait. In the patients who have valgus deformity of the hindfoot (Group 2), the foot is maintained in an extreme valgus position throughout stance phase (0 to 60 per cent of the gait cycle) and never assumes a varus position. In the patients who have normal alignment (Group 1), valgus positioning of the hindfoot is also increased compared with normal, but there is some varus positioning at the beginning of swing phase (61 to 100 per cent of the gait cycle). (from Keenan MA, *et al.* (1991) Valgus deformities of the feet and characteristics of gait in patients who have rheumatoid arthritis. J Bone Joint Surg 73A: 237-47, by permission).

Muscular activities during gait in rheumatoid plano-valgus deformity

In case of rheumatoid plano-valgus deformity, activity of the extrinsic musculature is markedly altered, compared to its activity in the non-deformed rheumatoid foot. Modified muscular activity compensates for hindfoot valgus and flattening of the arch during stance phase. There is an increased electromyographic (EMG) activity of the invertor muscles (posterior tibial, FHL, FDL) and a decreased EMG activity of the evertors, particularly of peroneus brevis.

- Tibialis posterior: during loading response, EMG activity averages more than 30% of the maximal electrical activity (62) (fig. 4); this is three times higher than normal activity during this period of stance phase (6, 41). This activity remains three times higher than normal during the initial 60% of stance phase. At push off, EMG activity averages 40% of maximal electrical activity, which is 25% more than normal.
- Flexor hallucis longus (FHL): FHL tendon passes behind and under the medial malleolus, and FHL contributes also to hindfoot inversion, even if its mechanical efficiency is less than that of the tibialis posterior muscle (99). In plano-valgus deformity, its EMG activity is 100% higher than normal at heel rise, and 60% higher than normal at push off (62).

- Flexor digitorum longus (FDL): like tibialis posterior and FHL, FDL also contributes to hindfoot inversion. Its EMG activity increases by 100% during loading response and by 30-50% at heel rise.
- Tibialis anterior: EMG activity is slightly increased at heel strike and during initial loading response. During the rest of stance phase, there is no alteration compared to the non-deformed rheumatoid foot.
- Peroneus longus: there is no significant difference between EMG activity in the deformed and in the non-deformed foot.
- Peroneus brevis: EMG activity decreases by 50% throughout stance phase in the deformed foot compared to the rheumatoid foot without deformity.

Podobarometry

Hindfoot deformities are three-dimensional (69). Therefore, they cannot be assessed using plantar pressure measurements which give information in only one or two dimensions. Thus, it is not surprising to find almost no podobarometric evaluation of plano-valgus deformity in the literature. Nevertheless, it is possible to establish a correlation between hindfoot malalignment and forefoot plantar pressures during stance phase of gait. In normal subjects and in rheumatoid patients with normal hindfoot alignment, the highest peak plantar pressures are located at the central metatarsal heads, while in rheumatoid patients with valgus hindfoot deformity, peak pressures follow a medial to lateral distribution in order of magnitude (136), which also occurs in the non-rheumatoid flatfoot (79).

Evaluation of rheumatoid forefeet using plantar pressure measurements is also associated with some difficulties, particularly because of the various types of forefoot morphology. It is difficult therefore, to establish normal values for plantar pressures at the forefoot level, either in standing or during stance phase of gait. Furthermore, in the rheumatoid foot, plantar pressures at the metatarsal heads may be inhomogeneously altered as the result of changes in gait in order to attenuate pain (136). Nevertheless, the difference between plantar pressures at the forefoot before and after treatment of metatarsalgia has been reported as a measure of treatment efficacy (5, 9, 30, 39, 48, 80, 102). Based on MTP joints dysfunction in rheumatoid arthritis, toes do not contribute adequately to support bodyweight during the late stance phase of gait. The load is then almost exclusively transferred to the metatarsal heads. Therefore, excessive plantar pressure at the metatarsal heads contributes to metatarsalgia in rheumatoid arthritis (9, 18, 39, 93). This theory was confirmed by Hodge *et al.* (48), who analyzed the efficacy of orthotic management of plantar pressure and pain in rheumatoid arthritis. Indeed, a significant correlation was established between the 2-3 N/cm2 reduction of the plantar pressures beneath the first and second metatarsal heads by orthoses, and the 30-60% of pain alleviation at the metatarsal heads (Visual Analogue Scales based on the Foot Function Index (19). These authors recommend using average plantar pressure rather than peak plantar pressure as a dependent variable for orthoses efficacy because of the significant correlation between average plantar pressure and walking pain. Another recent study, focussing on surgical treatment of the rheumatoid forefoot, has established a significant correlation between changes in plantar pressures and pain alleviation in 80% of patients (30).

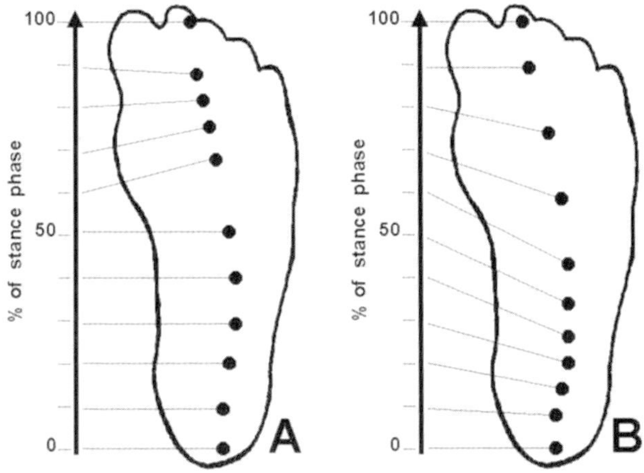

Fig. 8 - Progression of the centre of pressure during stance phase of gait. In the normal foot (A) the center of pressure progresses smoothly and reaches 0.5 foot length at 50% of stance phase, and is then followed by a rapid transfer of the bodyweight to the forefoot. In the rheumatoid foot (B) more time is required for the centre of pressure to reach 0.5 foot length (60% of stance phase). There is a delayed and shortened forefoot loading.

Anterior progression of the center of pressure is delayed in the rheumatoid foot (fig. 8). A recent study has demonstrated that the centre of pressure reaches 0.5 foot length anterior to the ankle at approximately 50% of stance phase in normal subjects, while significantly more time (65%) is required for the centre of pressure to reach the same position under the rheumatoid foot (97). This means that rheumatoid patients compensate for forefoot pain by delaying transfer of bodyweight to the forefoot and by shortening weight bearing duration under the forefoot (116). In flatfoot deformity there is also a medial shift in anterior progression of the centre of pressure (79). These podobarometric observations are consistent with the above mentioned alterations of kinematics and kinetics associated with rheumatoid foot, particularly delayed heel rise, decreased maximal ankle plantar flexion and decreased propulsion forces.

Shock absorption

At the beginning of stance phase, heel strike and loading response are respectively attenuated and controlled by the heel fat pad (1, 29, 95) and by the complex mechanism including hindfoot eversion and flattening of the longitudinal arch (10, 38, 95, 100). Both elements are potentially altered in the rheumatoid foot.

The heel fat pad

The fatty acid composition of the heel fat pad in rheumatoid arthritis reflects an increased fat viscosity, which decreases the ability of the heel to absorb and dissipate energy generated during ambulation (20, 108). This factor may cause degeneration of the heel septal system resulting in fat pad atrophy. In healthy subjects, shock absorbency of the heel in response to an isolated impact averages 45-77% (1, 63). This property declines significantly with heel fat pad atrophy (56, 57, 63).

The hindfoot complex

Since plano-valgus feet typically have an everted calcaneus, these feet may contact with the ground near the end range of motion of the subtalar joint. Therefore, the ability of these feet to attenuate shock may be altered. At least three methods that have been designed to evaluate shock absorbency or loading response of the foot have been reported. They include measurement of impact forces at the lower back (98), angular acceleration of the shank (96), and acceleration of the calcaneus (78). A high-arch foot is reported to be a better shock absorber with regard to the lower back than the low-arch foot (98). However, there is little information regarding true plano-valgus deformity. Calcaneal acceleration at heel strike was demonstrated to be 10% higher in plano-valgus feet than in neutrally aligned feet (78). This difference, however, was not significant.

Conclusion

The foot is the first manifestation of rheumatoid arthritis in 15,7% of cases (44). This high incidence justifies early evaluation and treatment of the foot in rheumatoid arthritis. Understanding pathomechanics of the rheumatoid foot contributes to optimize prevention and treatment of deformities. Indeed, it allows the understanding of the functional relevance of deformities, their interactions, and sometimes their prognosis.

Concerning the biomechanical approaches for the rheumatoid foot and ankle, gait analysis plays an important role because it provides objective and detailed information allowing detection and quantification of functional abnormalities as well as evaluation during treatment. Therefore, gait analysis may be considered as a link between pathomechanics and clinical practice.

Acknowledgments

The author gratefully acknowledges the help of Dr. A. Gray and Dr. O. Borens in editing this chapter.

References

1. Aerts P, Ker RF, De Clercq D, (1995) The mechanical properties of the human heel pad: a paradox resolved. J Biomech 28: 1299-308
2. Arangio GA, Phillippy DC, Xiao D, (2000) Subtalar pronation--relationship to the medial longitudinal arch loading in the normal foot. Foot Ankle Int 21: 216-20

3. Arnett FC, Edworthy SM, Bloch DA, *et al.* (1988) The American Rheumatism Association 1987 revised criteria for the classification of rheumatoid arthritis. Arthritis Rheum 31: 315-24
4. Barnicot NA, Hardy RH (1955) The position of the hallux in West Africans. J Anat 89: 335-61
5. Barrett JP (1976) Plantar pressure measurements. Rational shoe-wear in patients with rheumatoid arthritis. JAMA 235: 1138-9
6. Basmajian JV, Stecko G (1963) The role of muscles in arch support of the foot. An electromyographic study. J Bone Joint Surg 45A: 1184-90
7. Belt EA, Kaarela K, Kauppi MJ (1997) A 20-year follow-up study of subtalar changes in rheumatoid arthritis. Scand J Rheumatol 26: 266-8
8. Benedetti MG, Catani F, Leardini A, *et al.* (1998) Data management in gait analysis for clinical applications. Clin Biomech (Bristol, Avon) 13: 204-15
9. Bitzan P, Giurea A, Wanivenhaus A (1997) Plantar pressure distribution after resection of the metatarsal heads in rheumatoid arthritis. Foot Ankle Int 18: 391-7
10. Blake RL, Ferguson H (1991) Foot orthosis for the severe flatfoot in sports. J Am Podiatr Med Assoc 81: 549-55
11. Bojsen-Moller F, Flagstad KE (1976) Plantar aponeurosis and internal architecture of the ball of the foot. J Anat 121: 599-611
12. Bouysset M, Bonvoisin B, Lejeune E, Bouvier M (1987) Flattening of the rheumatoid foot in tarsal arthritis on X-ray. Scand J Rheumatol 16: 127-133
13. Bouysset M, Bouvier M (1997) Inflammatory foot disease. Rev Prat 47: 43-9
14. Bouysset M, Tavernier T, Tebib J, *et al.* (1995) CT and MRI evaluation of tenosynovitis of the rheumatoid hindfoot. Clin Rheumatol 14: 303-7
15. Bouysset M, Tebib J, Noel E, *et al.* (1991) Rheumatoid metatarsus. The original evolution of the first metatarsal. Clin Rheumatol 10: 408-12
16. Bouysset M, Tebib J, Noel E, *et al.* (2002) Rheumatoid flat foot and deformity of the first ray. J Rheumatol 29: 903-5
17. Braun S (1975) Le pied dans les grands rhumatismes inflammatoires chroniques. Rhumatologie 27: 47-56
18. Brown M, Rudicel S, Esquenazi A (1996) Measurement of dynamic pressures at the shoe-foot interface during normal walking with various foot orthoses using the FSCAN system. Foot Ankle Int 17: 152-6
19. Budiman-Mak E, Conrad KJ, Roach KE (1991) The Foot Function Index: a measure of foot pain and disability. J Clin Epidemiol 44: 561-70
20. Buschmann WR, Hudgins LC, Kummer F, *et al.* (1993) Fatty acid composition of normal and atrophied heel fat pad. Foot Ankle 14: 389-94
21. Carson MC, Harrington ME, Thompson N, *et al.* (2001) Kinematic analysis of a multi-segment foot model for research and clinical applications: a repeatability analysis. J Biomech 34: 1299-307
22. Chao EY, Laughman RK, Schneider E, *et al.* (1983) Normative data of knee joint motion and ground reaction forces in adult level walking. J Biomech 16: 219-33
23. Clayton ML, Ries MD (1991) Functional hallux rigidus in the rheumatoid foot. Clin Orthop 271: 233-8
24. Coughlin MJ, Thompson FM (1995) The high price of high-fashion footwear. Instr Course Lect 44: 371-77
25. Craigmile DA (1953) Incidence, origin, and prevention of certain foot defects. Br Med J 2: 749-52

26. Crevoisier X, Kitaoka HB, Hansen D, Morrow D, Kaufman KR, An KN (2001). Gait abnormalities associated with ankle osteoarthritis. In 48th Annual Meeting of the Orthopaedic Research Society: Dallas, Texas
27. D'Amico JC (1976) The pathomechanics of adult rheumatoid arthritis affecting the foot. J Am Podiatry Assoc 66: 227-36
28. Davis WH, Sobel M, DiCarlo EF, *et al.* (1996) Gross, histological, and microvascular anatomy and biomechanical testing of the spring ligament complex. Foot Ankle Int 17: 95-102
29. De Clercq D, Aerts P, Kunnen M (1994) The mechanical characteristics of the human heel pad during foot strike in running: an in vivo cineradiographic study. J Biomech 27: 1213-22
30. Dereymaeker G, Mulier T, Stuer P, Peeraer L, Fabry G (1997) Pedodynographic measurements after forefoot reconstruction in rheumatoid arthritis patients. Foot Ankle Int 18: 270-6
31. Dimonte P, Light H (1982) Pathomechanics, gait deviations, and treatment of the rheumatoid foot: a clinical report. Phys Ther 62: 1148-56
32. Downey DJ, Simkin PA, Mack LA, *et al.* (1988) Tibialis posterior tendon rupture: a cause of rheumatoid flat foot. Arthritis Rheum 31: 441-6
33. Engle ET, Morton DJ (1931) Notes on the foot disorders among natives of Belgian Congo. J Bone Joint Surg 13: 311-8
34. Faber FW, Kleinrensink GJ, Verhoog MW, (1999) Mobility of the first tarsometatarsal joint in relation to hallux valgus deformity: anatomical and biomechanical aspects. Foot Ankle Int 20: 651-6
35. Friedman MA, Draganich LF, Toolan B, *et al.* (2001) The effects of adult acquired flatfoot deformity on tibiotalar joint contact characteristics. Foot Ankle Int 22: 241-6
36. Fujii T, Kitaoka HB, Uchiyama E, *et al.* (2001). Comparison of gliding resistance of tendons about the ankle. In 47th Annual Meeting of the Orthopaedic Research Society: San Francisco, California
37. Funk DA, Cass JR, Johnson KA (1986) Acquired adult flat foot secondary to posterior tibial-tendon pathology. J Bone Joint Surg 68A: 95-102
38. Genova JM, Gross MT (2000) Effect of foot orthotics on calcaneal eversion during standing and treadmill walking for subjects with abnormal pronation. J Orthop Sports Phys Ther 30: 664-75
39. Gould JS (1982) Conservative management of the hypersensitive foot in rheumatoid arthritis. Foot Ankle 2: 224-9
40. Grace DL (1996) The surgical management of the rheumatoid foot. Br J Hosp Med 56: 473-80
41. Gray EG, Basmajian JV (1968) Electromyography and cinematography of leg and foot ("normal" and flat) during walking. Anat Rec 161: 1-15
42. Haines RW, McDougall A (1954) The anatomy of hallux valgus. J Bone Joint Surg 36B: 272-93
43. Hamilton J, Brydson G, Fraser S, Grant M (2001) Walking ability as a measure of treatment effect in early rheumatoid arthritis. Clin Rehabil 15: 142-7
44. Harris R (2001) Le pied rhumatoïde aux Etats-Unis. Med Chir Pied 17: 199-200
45. Henkel A (1913) Die Aponeurosis plantaris. Arch fuer Anat und Physio Anat 113 (suppl): 113-23
46. Hicks JH (1954) The mechanics of the foot. II. The plantar aponeurosis and the arch. J Anat 88: 25-30
47. Hicks JH (1955) The foot as a support. Acta Anat 25: 34-45

48. Hodge MC, Bach TM, Carter GM (1999) novel Award First Prize Paper. Orthotic management of plantar pressure and pain in rheumatoid arthritis. Clin Biomech (Bristol, Avon) 14: 567-75
49. Huang CK, Kitaoka HB, An KN, *et al.* (1993) Biomechanical evaluation of longitudinal arch stability. Foot Ankle 14: 353-7
50. Hughes J, Clark P, Klenerman L (1990) The importance of the toes in walking. J Bone Joint Surg 72B: 245-51
51. Hunt AE, Smith RM, Torode M (2001) Extrinsic muscle activity, foot motion and ankle joint moments during the stance phase of walking. Foot Ankle Int 22: 31-41
52. Hunt AE, Smith RM, Torode M, (2001) Inter-segment foot motion and ground reaction forces over the stance phase of walking. Clin Biomech (Bristol, Avon) 16: 592-600
53. Hutton WC, Dhanendran M (1981) The mechanics of normal and hallux valgus feet--a quantitative study. Clin Orthop 157: 7-13
54. Isacson J, Brostrom LA (1988) Gait in rheumatoid arthritis: an electrogoniometric investigation. J Biomech 21: 451-7
55. Jernberg ET, Simkin P, Kravette M, (1999) The posterior tibial tendon and the tarsal sinus in rheumatoid flat foot: magnetic resonance imaging of 40 feet. J Rheumatol 26: 289-93
56. Jorgensen U, Bojsen-Moller F (1989) Shock absorbency of factors in the shoe/heel interaction--with special focus on role of the heel pad. Foot Ankle 9: 294-9
57. Jorgensen U, Larsen E, Varmarken JE (1989) The HPC-device: a method to quantify the heel pad shock absorbency. Foot Ankle 10: 93-8
58. Kadaba MP, Ramakrishnan HK, Wootten ME (1990) Measurement of lower extremity kinematics during level walking. J Orthop Res 8: 383-92
59. Kainberger F, Bitzan P, Erlacher L, *et al.* (1999) Rheumatic diseases of the ankle joint and tarsus. Radiologe 39: 60-7
60. Karbowski A, Schwitalle M, Eckhardt A (1998) Arthroplasty of the forefoot in rheumatoid arthritis: long-term results after Clayton procedure. Acta Orthop Belg 64: 401-5
61. Katoh Y, Chao EY, Laughman RK, *et al.* (1983) Biomechanical analysis of foot function during gait and clinical applications. Clin Orthop 177: 23-33
62. Keenan MA, Peabody TD, Gronley JK, (1991) Valgus deformities of the feet and characteristics of gait in patients who have rheumatoid arthritis. J Bone Joint Surg 73A: 237-47
63. Kinoshita H, Francis PR, Murase T, (1996) The mechanical properties of the heel pad in elderly adults. Eur J Appl Physiol Occup Physiol 73: 404-9
64. Kirkham BW, Gibson T (1989) Comment on the article by Downey *et al.* Arthritis Rheum 32: 359
65. Kirkup Jr (1974) Ankle and tarsal joints in rheumatoid arthritis. Scand J Rheumatol 3: 50-52
66. Kitaoka HB (1989) Rheumatoid hindfoot. Orthop Clin North Am 20: 593-604
67. Kitaoka HB, Luo ZP, An KN (1996) Contact features of the talonavicular joint of the foot. Clin Orthop 325: 290-295
68. Kitaoka HB, Luo ZP, An KN (1997) Effect of the posterior tibial tendon on the arch of the foot during simulated weightbearing: biomechanical analysis. Foot Ankle Int 18: 43-46
69. Kitaoka HB, Luo ZP, An KN (1998) Three-dimensional analysis of flatfoot deformity: cadaver study. Foot Ankle Int 19: 447-451
70. Kitaoka HB, Luo ZP, Growney ES, Berglund LJ, An KN (1994) Material properties of the plantar aponeurosis. Foot Ankle Int 15: 557-560

71. Kjaersgaard-Andersen P, Wethelund JO, Helmig P, *et al.* (1987) Effect of the calcaneofibular ligament on hindfoot rotation in amputation specimens. Acta Orthop Scand 58: 135-138
72. Kjaersgaard-Andersen P, Wethelund JO, Helmig P, *et al.* (1988) The stabilizing effect of the ligamentous structures in the sinus and canalis tarsi on movements in the hindfoot. An experimental study. Am J Sports Med 16: 512-6
73. Kjaersgaard-Andersen P, Wethelund JO, Nielsen S (1987) Lateral talocalcaneal instability following section of the calcaneofibular ligament: a kinesiologic study. Foot Ankle 7: 355-61
74. Knudson GA, Kitaoka HB, Lu CL, *et al.* (1997) Subtalar joint stability. Talocalcaneal interosseous ligament function studied in cadaver specimens. Acta Orthop Scand 68: 442-6
75. Kura H, Kitaoka HB, Luo ZP, *et al.* (1998) Measurement of surface contact area of the ankle joint. Clin Biomech (Bristol, Avon) 13: 365-70
76. Kura H, Luo ZP, Kitaoka HB, (1998) Role of medical capsule and transverse metatarsal ligament in hallux valgus deformity. Clin Orthop 354: 235-40
77. Kuster M, Sakurai S, Wood GA (1995) Kinematic and kinetic comparison of downhill and level walking. Clin Biomech (Bristol, Avon) 10: 79-84
78. Ledoux WR, Hillstrom HJ (2001) Acceleration of the calcaneus at heel strike in neutrally aligned and pes planus feet. Clin Biomech (Bristol, Avon) 16: 608-13
79. Ledoux WR, Hillstrom HJ (2002) The distributed plantar vertical force of neutrally aligned and pes planus feet. Gait Posture 15: 1-9
80. Li CY, Imaishi K, Shiba N, *et al.* (2000) Biomechanical evaluation of foot pressure and loading force during gait in rheumatoid arthritic patients with and without foot orthosis. Kurume Med J 47: 211-7
81. Locke M, Perry J, Campbell J, Thomas L (1984) Ankle and subtalar motion during gait in arthritic patients. Phys Ther 64: 504-9
82. Loth E (1907) Die Plantaraponeurose beim Menschen und den uebrigen Primaten. Korr Bl Deutsch Anthrop Ges
83. Loth E (1913) Étude anthropologique sur l'aponévrose plantaire. Bull Mem Soc Anthro Paris 4: 601
84. Mann RA (1999). Biomechanics of the foot and ankle. In Surgery of the foot and ankle (Mann, R.A. & Coughlin, M.J., eds.), 7 ed. pp. 2-35, Mosby: St Louis
85. Mann RA, Inman VT (1964) Phasic activity of intrinsic muscles of the foot. J Bone Joint Surg 46A: 469-81
86. Mann RA, Thompson FM (1997) Arthrodesis of the first metatarsophalangeal joint for hallux valgus in rheumatoid arthritis. 1984. Foot Ankle Int 18: 65-7
87. Marshall RN, Myers DB, Palmer DG (1980) Disturbance of gait due to rheumatoid disease. J Rheumatol 7: 617-23
88. Masterson E, Mulcahy D, McElwain J, McInerney D (1995) The planovalgus rheumatoid foot--is tibialis posterior tendon rupture a factor? Br J Rheumatol 34: 645-6
89. McBride ID, Wyss UP, Cooke TD, Murphy L, Phillips J, Olney SJ (1991) First metatarsophalangeal joint reaction forces during high-heel gait. Foot Ankle 11: 282-8
90. McCormack AP, Niki H, Kiser P, *et al.* (1998) Two reconstructive techniques for flatfoot deformity comparing contact characteristics of the hindfoot joints. Foot Ankle Int 19: 452-61
91. Michelson J, Easley M, Wigley FM, *et al.* (1994) Foot and ankle problems in rheumatoid arthritis. Foot Ankle Int 15: 608-13

92. Michelson J, Easley M, Wigley FM, *et al.* (1995) Posterior tibial tendon dysfunction in rheumatoid arthritis. Foot Ankle Int 16: 156-61
93. Minns RJ, Craxford AD (1984) Pressure under the forefoot in rheumatoid arthritis. A comparison of static and dynamic methods of assessment. Clin Orthop 187: 235-42
94. Moseley L, Smith R, Hunt A, *et al.* (1996) Three-dimensional kinematics of the rearfoot during the stance phase of walking in normal young adult males. Clin Biomech (Bristol, Avon) 11: 39-45
95. Nack JD, Phillips RD (1990) Shock absorption. Clin Podiatr Med Surg 7: 391-7
96. Nester CJ, Hutchins S, Bowker P (2000) Shank rotation: A measure of rearfoot motion during normal walking. Foot Ankle Int 21: 578-83
97. O'Connell PG, Lohmann Siegel K, Kepple TM, *et al.* (1998) Forefoot deformity, pain, and mobility in rheumatoid and nonarthritic subjects. J Rheumatol 25: 1681-6
98. Ogon M, Aleksiev AR, Pope MH, *et al.* (1999) Does arch height affect impact loading at the lower back level in running? Foot Ankle Int 20: 263-6
99. Perry J (1992). Gait analysis: Normal and Pathological Function. Slack: Thorofare, NJ
100. Perry SD, Lafortune MA (1995) Influences of inversion/eversion of the foot upon impact loading during locomotion. Clin Biomech (Bristol, Avon) 10: 253-7
101. Phillips RD, Reczek DM, Fountain D, *et al.* (1991) Modification of high-heeled shoes to decrease pronation during gait. J Am Podiatr Med Assoc 81: 215-9
102. Phillipson A, Dhar S, Linge K, *et al.* (1994) Forefoot arthroplasty and changes in plantar foot pressures. Foot Ankle Int 15: 595-8
103. Platto MJ, O'Connell PG, Hicks JE, *et al.* (1991) The relationship of pain and deformity of the rheumatoid foot to gait and an index of functional ambulation. J Rheumatol 18: 38-43
104. Pontious J, Flanigan KP, Hillstrom HJ (1996) Role of the plantar fascia in digital stabilization. A case report. J Am Podiatr Med Assoc 86: 43-7
105. Potter TA, Khus JG (1972). Painful feet. In Arthritis and Allied conditions (Hollander, J.L., ed.), Lea and Febiger: Philadelphia
106. Rattanaprasert U, Smith R, Sullivan M, *et al.* (1999) Three-dimensional kinematics of the forefoot, rearfoot, and leg without the function of tibialis posterior in comparison with normals during stance phase of walking. Clin Biomech (Bristol, Avon) 14: 14-23
107. Reeser LA, Susman RL, Stern JT, Jr. (1983) Electromyographic studies of the human foot: experimental approaches to hominid evolution. Foot Ankle 3: 391-407
108. Resnick RB, Hudgins LC, Buschmann WR, *et al.* (1999) Analysis of the heel pad fat in rheumatoid arthritis. Foot Ankle Int 20: 481-484
109. Saltzman CL, Aper RL, Brown TD (1997) Anatomic determinants of first metatarsophalangeal flexion moments in hallux valgus. Clin Orthop 339: 261-9
110. Sarrafian SK (1983). Anatomy of the foot and Ankle: Descriptive, Topographic, Functional. J.B. Lippincott: Philadelphia
111. Sarrafian SK (1993) Biomechanics of the subtalar joint complex. Clin Orthop 290: 17-26
112. Scheck M (1977) Etiology of acquired hammertoe deformity. Clin Orthop 123: 63-9
113. Seltzer SE, Weissman BN, Braunstein EM, *et al.* (1985) Computed tomography of the hindfoot with rheumatoid arthritis. Arthritis Rheum 28: 1234-42
114. Shi K, Tomita T, Hayashida K, *et al.* (2000) Foot deformities in rheumatoid arthritis and relevance of disease severity. J Rheumatol 27: 84-9
115. Sim-Fook L, Hodgson AR (1958) A comparison of forms among the non-shoe and the shoe wearing Chinese population. J Bone Joint Surg 40A: 1058-62

116. Simkin A (1981) The dynamic vertical force distribution during level walking under normal and rheumatic feet. Rheumatol Rehabil 20: 88-7
117. Simkin PA, Downey DJ, Richardson ML (1989) More on the posterior tibial tendon in rheumatoid arthritis. Arthritis Rheum 32: 1050
118. Smith EB (1896) The astragalo-calcaneo-navicular joint. J Anat Physiol 30: 238
119. Smyth CJ, Janson RW (1997) Rheumatologic view of the rheumatoid foot. Clin Orthop 340: 7-17
120. Solomon MG, Fillinger EB (1999) Reconstruction of the rheumatoid forefoot. Clin Podiatr Med Surg 16: 285-301
121. Spiegel TM, Spiegel JS (1982) Rheumatoid arthritis in the foot and ankle--diagnosis, pathology, and treatment. The relationship between foot and ankle deformity and disease duration in 50 patients. Foot Ankle 2: 318-24
122. Stainsby GD (1997) Pathological anatomy and dynamic effect of the displaced plantar plate and the importance of the integrity of the plantar plate-deep transverse metatarsal ligament tie-bar. Ann R Coll Surg Engl 79: 58-68
123. Staubesand J (1985). Untere Gliedmassen. In Benninghoff: Makroskopische und mikroskopische Anatomie des Menschen (Staubesand, J., ed.), vol. 1, 14 ed. pp. 328-417, Urban & Schwarzenberg: München-Wien-Baltimore
124. Stokes IA, Hutton WC, Stott Jr (1979) Forces acting on the metatarsals during normal walking. J Anat 129: 579-90
125. Stokes IA, Hutton WC, Stott JR, Lowe LW (1979) Forces under the hallux valgus foot before and after surgery. Clin Orthop 142: 64-72
126. Swoboda B, Martus P, Kladny B, *et al.* (1994) The significance of inflammatory changes in the tarsometatarsal joints for development of rheumatic splayed foot: a radiologic follow-up. Z Rheumatol 53: 299-306
127. Thordarson DB, Schmotzer H, Chon J, *et al.* (1995) Dynamic support of the human longitudinal arch. A biomechanical evaluation. Clin Orthop 316: 165-72
128. Thould AK, Simon G (1966) Assessment of radiological changes in the hands and feet in rheumatoid arthritis. Their correlation with prognosis. Ann Rheum Dis 25: 220-8
129. Tillman K (1979). The pathomechanics of rheumatic foot deformities. The rheumatoid foot. Diagnosis, pathomechanics and treatment. Georg Thieme Publishers: Stuttgart
130. Toolan BC, Hansen ST, Jr. (1998) Surgery of the rheumatoid foot and ankle. Curr Opin Rheumatol 10: 116-9
131. Uchiyama E, Kitaoka HB, Luo Z, *et al.* (2001). Biomechanics and immunohistochemical study of MCL of big toe. In 47th Annual Meeting, Orthopaedic Research Society. pp. 8-32: San Francisco, CA
132. Vahvanen VA (1967) Rheumatoid arthritis in the pantalar joints. A follow-up study of triple arthrodesis on 292 adult feet. Acta Orthop Scand 107 (Suppl): 3
133. Vainio K (1956) The rheumatoid foot: A clinical study with pathologic and roentgenological comments. Ann Chir Gynaecol 45 (Suppl): 1-107
134. Vainio K (1991) The rheumatoid foot. A clinical study with pathological and roentgenological comments. Clin Orthop 265: 4-8
135. Viladot A, Viladot R (1983). Biomécanique de l'avant-pied rhumatoïde. In Le pied en pratique rhumatologique (Claustre, J. & Simon, L., eds.). Paris Masson: pp. 28
136. Woodburn J, Helliwell PS (1996) Relation between heel position and the distribution of forefoot plantar pressures and skin callosities in rheumatoid arthritis. Ann Rheum Dis 55: 806-10

CT and MRI in rheumatoid arthritis (midfoot, hindfoot and ankle)

Th. Tavernier

Except the indication of these procedures due to the common pathology, the sectional imaging in RA is chiefly interesting on the mid-hind-foot and the ankle in RA.
On the forefoot, CT may help to study metatarsal bone involvement (plantar erosions for instance). MRI may particularly help to observe inter-capito-metatarsal bursae if necessary.

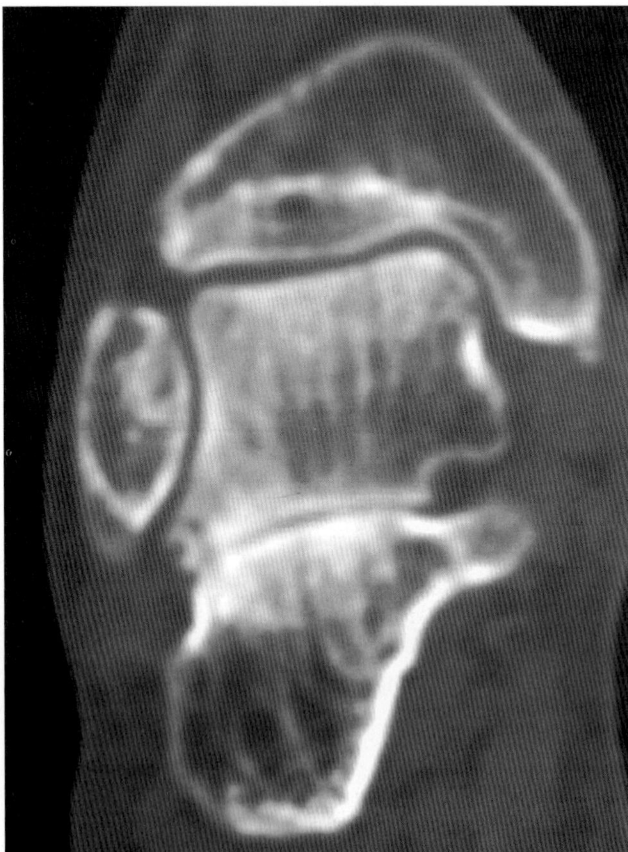

Fig. 1 - CT: coronal slice. Bone window. Subtalar arthritis (joint narrowing).

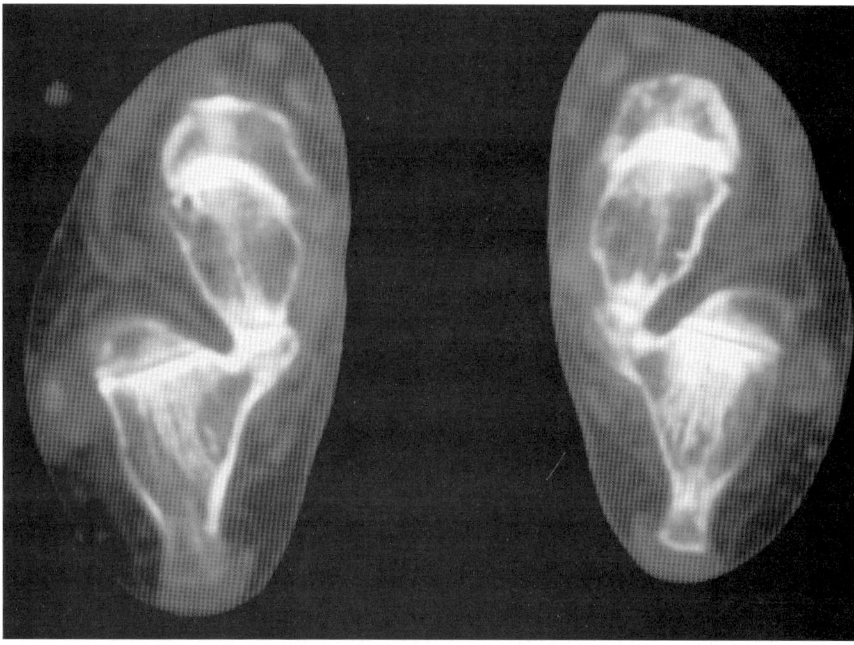

Fig. 2 - CT: axial slice. Bone window. Bilateral talo-navicular arthritis.

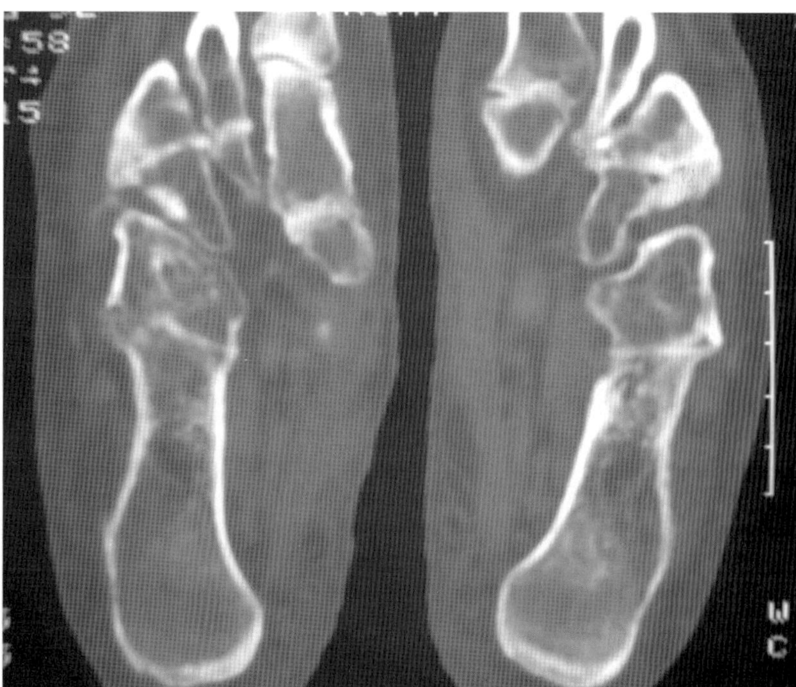

Fig. 3 - CT: bilateral tarso-metatarsal arthritis.

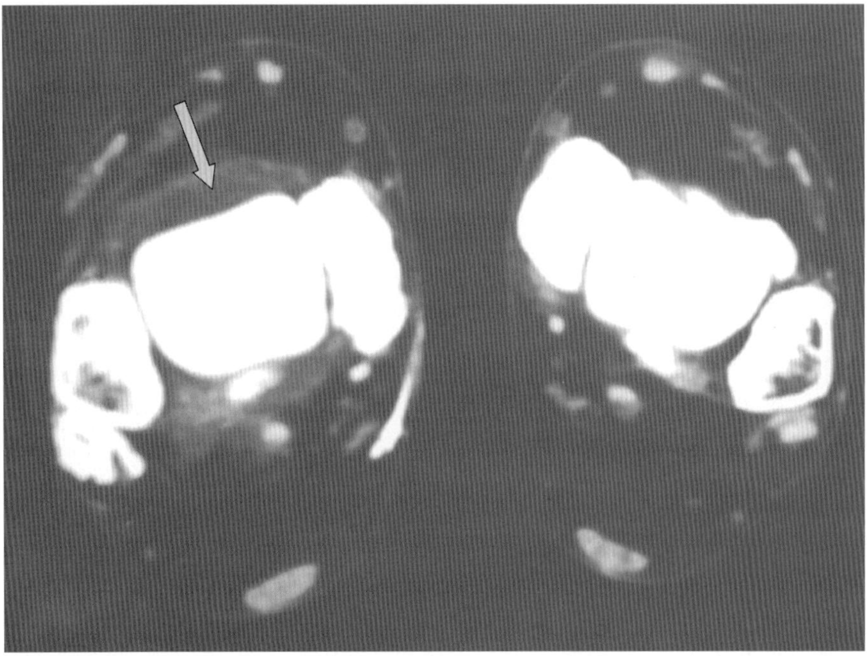

Fig. 4 - CT: soft tissue window. Right talo-crural rheumatoid pannus (arrow).

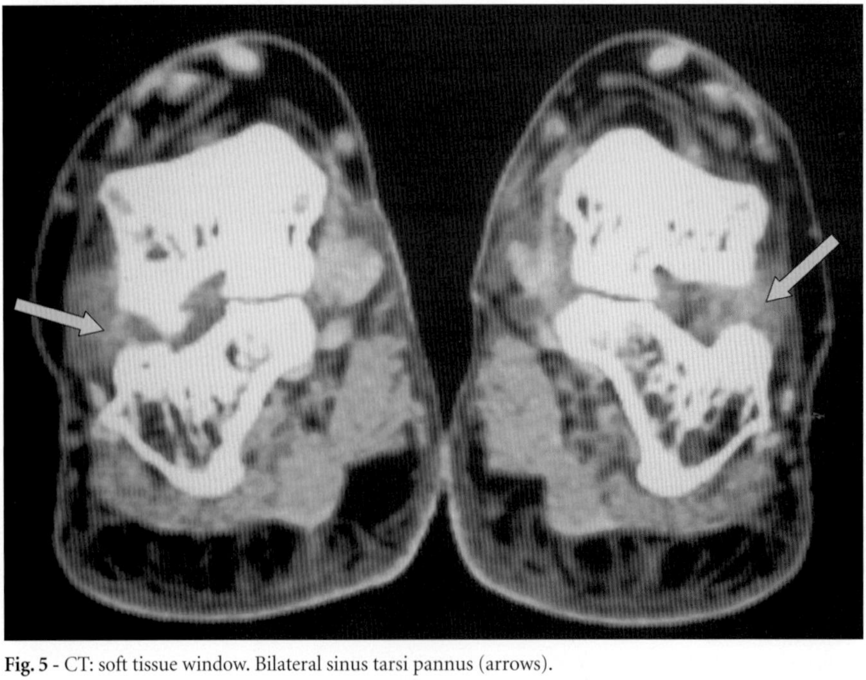

Fig. 5 - CT: soft tissue window. Bilateral sinus tarsi pannus (arrows).

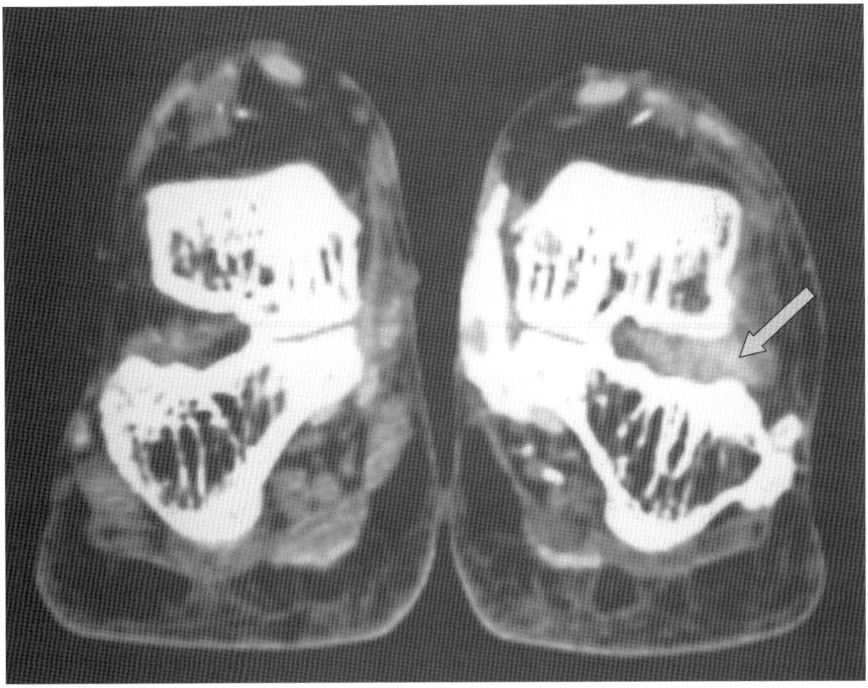

Fig. 6 - CT: soft tissue window. Sinus tarsi pannus on the left side (arrow).

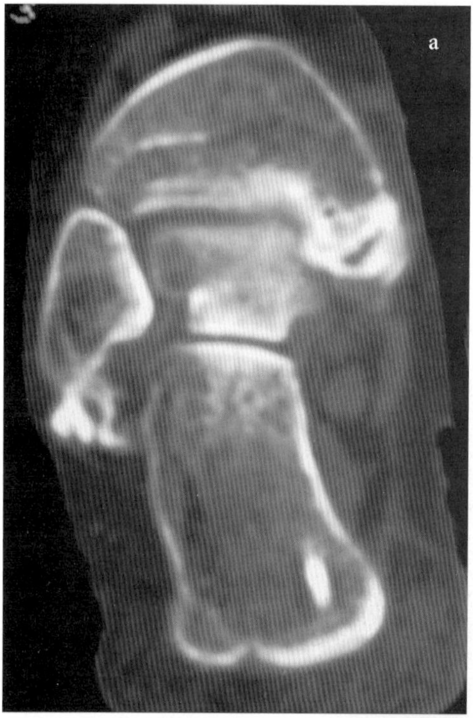

Fig. 7 - CT tenography. a) Tenosynovitis of fibularis tendons and posterior tibial tendon (ptt). b) Stage 2 tendinopathy of posterior tibial tendon.

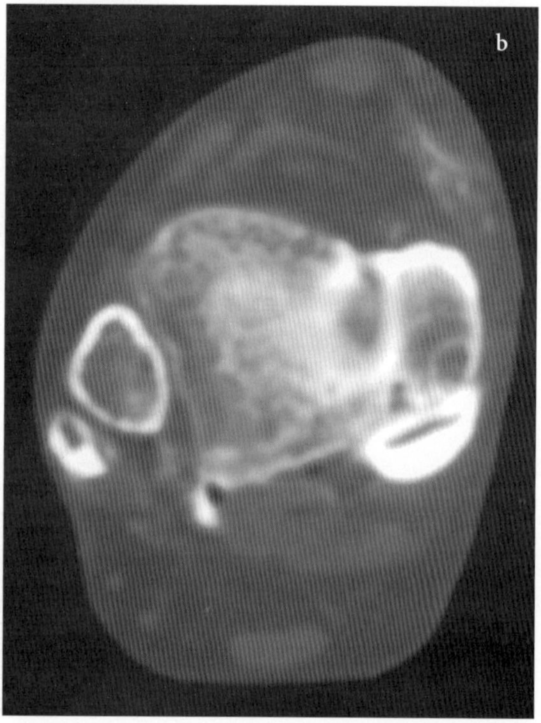

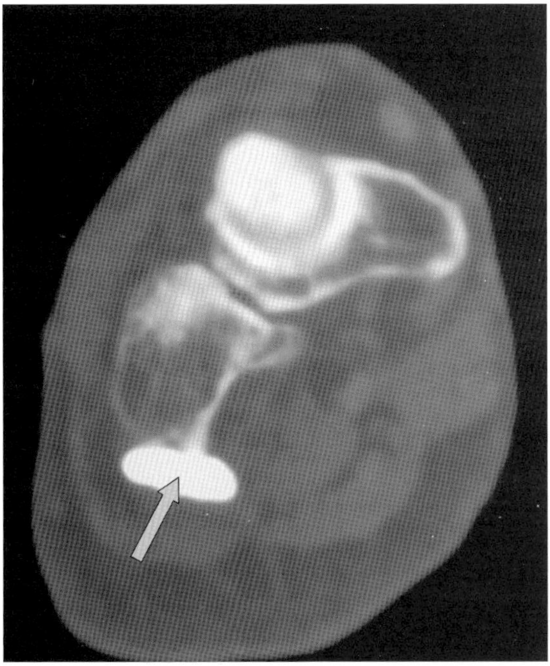

Fig. 8 - CT tenography. Long fibularis tendon ruptured (empty sheath). (Arrow).

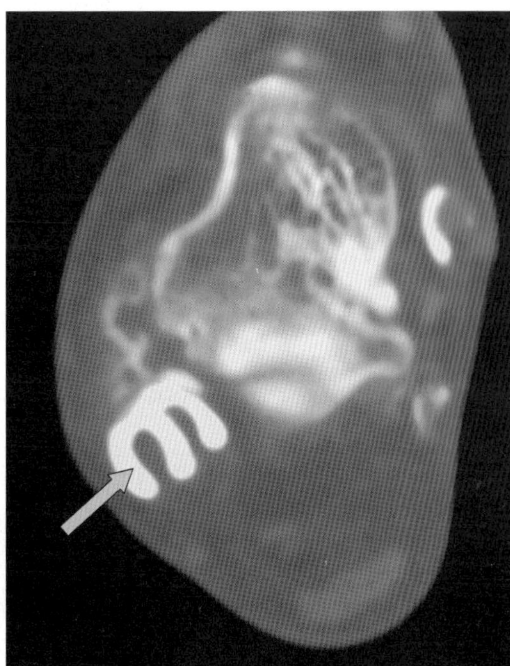

Fig. 9 - CT tenography. Tenosynovitis and tendinopathy of fibularis tendons: thinned aspect of tendons (arrow).

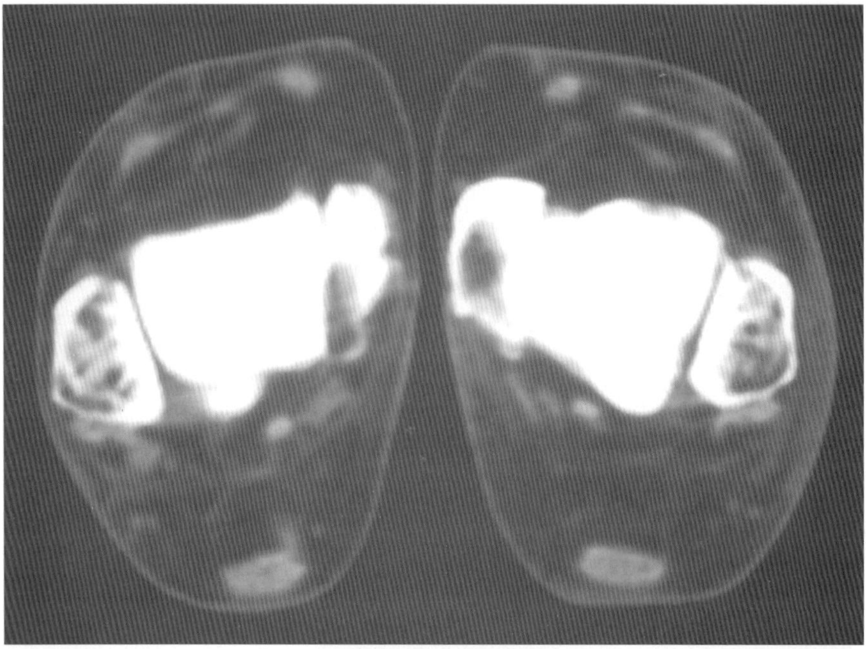

Fig. 10 - CT soft tissue window. Bilateral rupture of posterior tibial tendon. *The ptt is not visible in its sheath.*

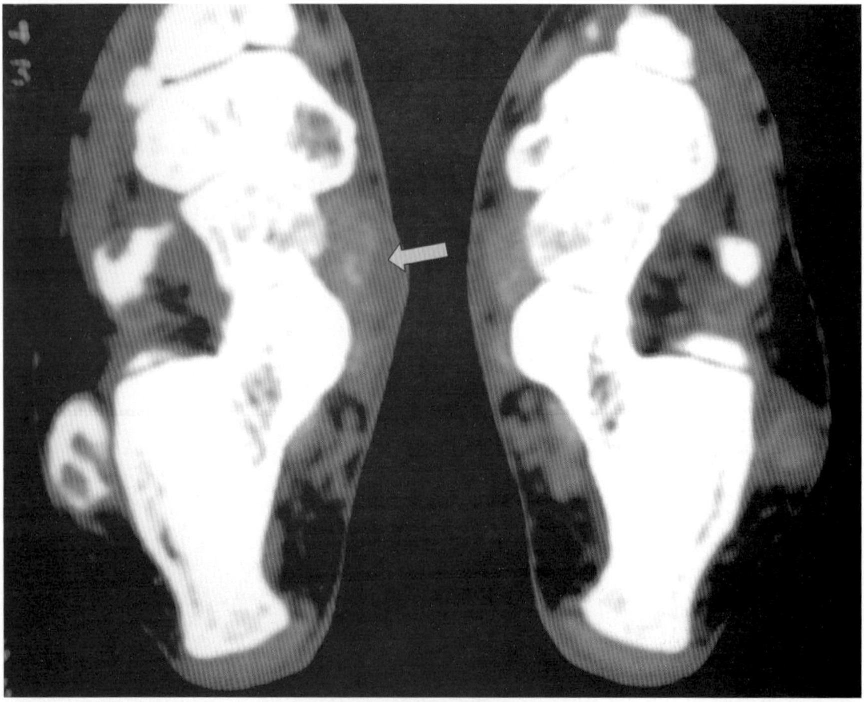

Fig. 11 - CT soft tissue window. Right posterior tibial tendon. Tenosynovitis and stage 1 tendinopathy (arrow).

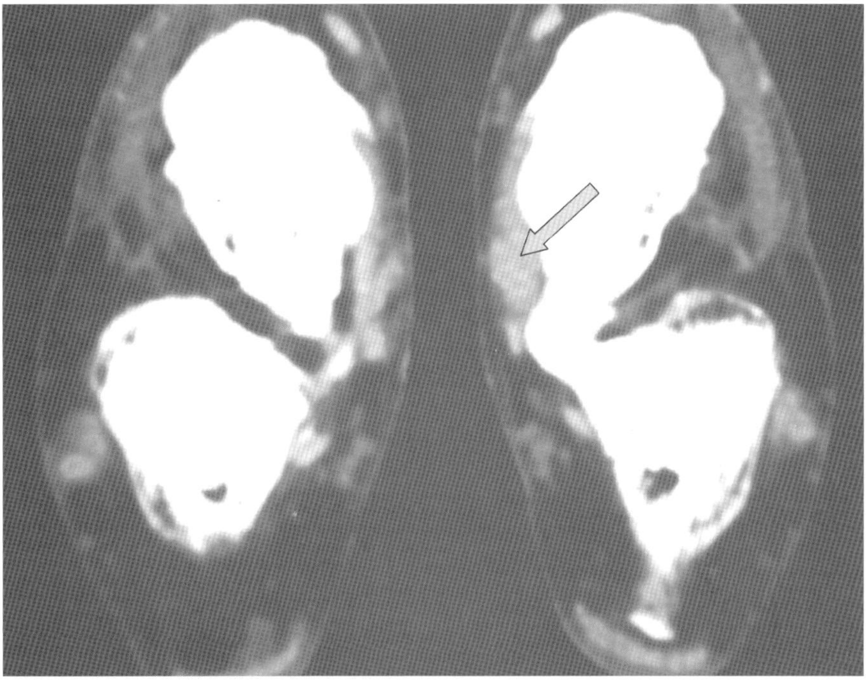

Fig. 12 - CT soft tissue window. Left ptt: stage 1 tendinopathy (arrow).

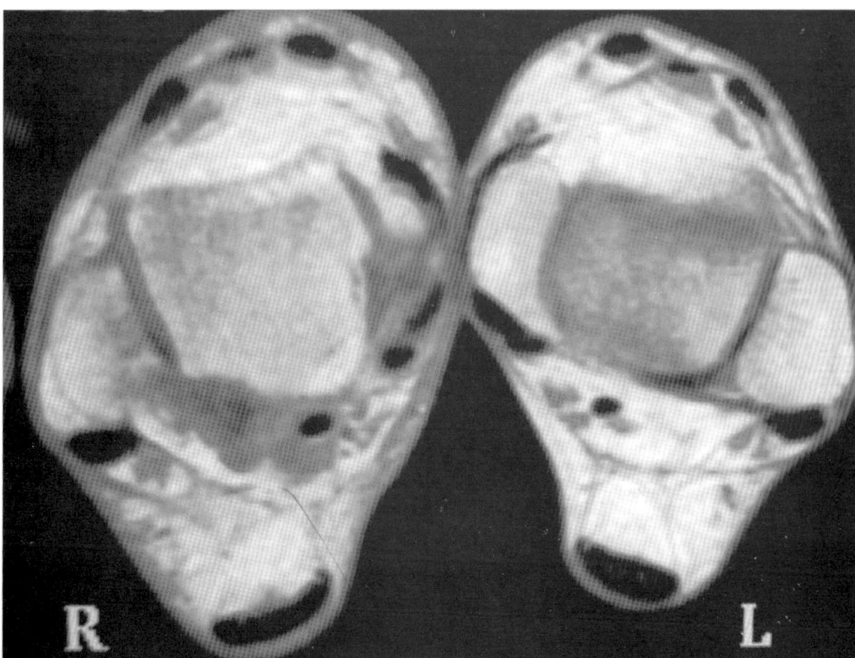

Fig. 13 - Same patient, MRI: T1 gadolinium (1995). Right ptt: tenosynovitis and stage 2 tendinopathy. Left ptt: stage 1 tendinopathy.

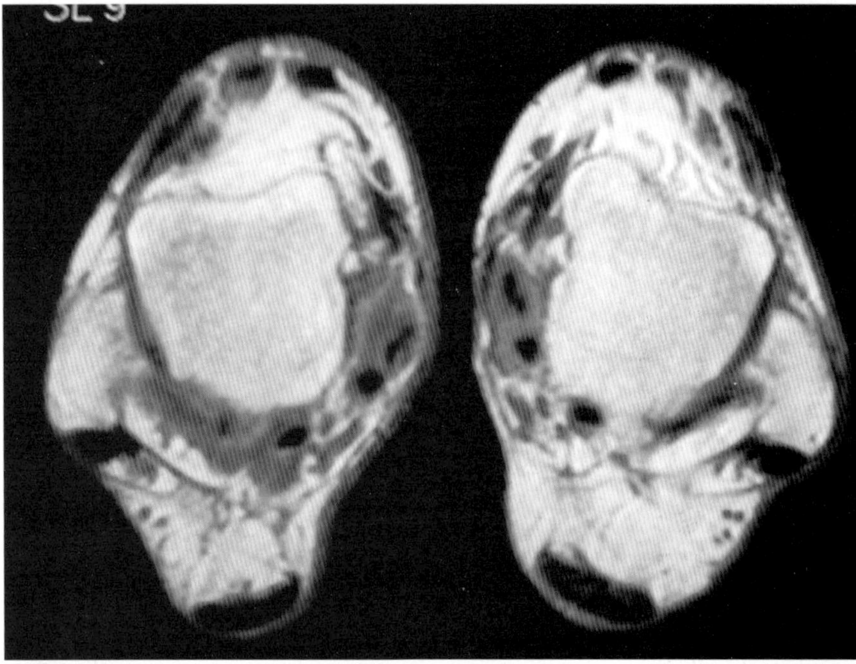

Fig. 14 - Same patient MRI, T1 (1999). Ptt bilateral stage 2 tendinopathy.

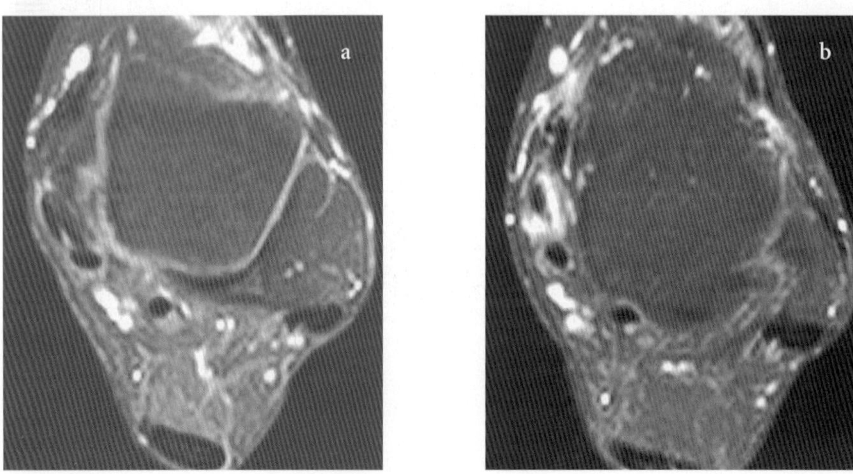

Fig. 15 - Same patient. MRI. T1 fat-sat gadolinium (2002). The tendinopathy of the left ptt has worsened: there is a longitudinal retromalleolar fissure (fig. a) and a stage 2 tendinopathy under medial malleoli (fig. b).

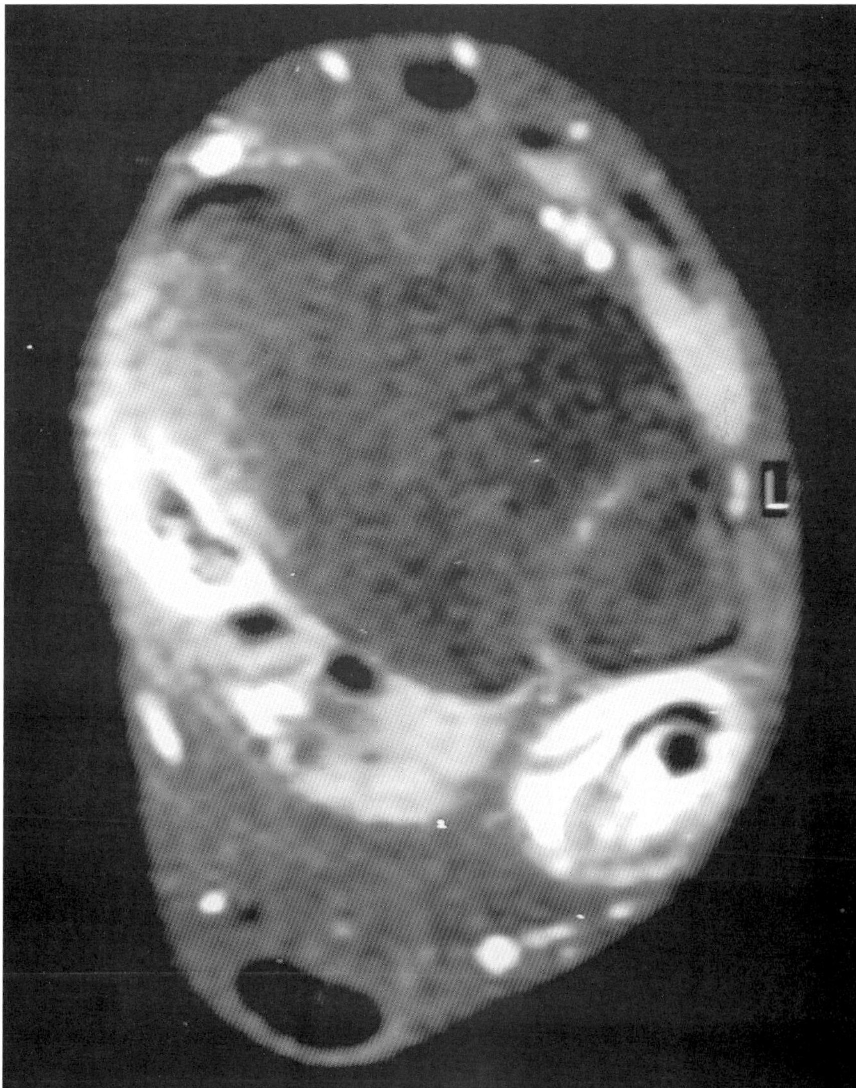

Fig. 16 - MRI. T1 fat-sat gadolinium. Tenosynovitis and stage 2 tendinopathy of the ptt, and stage 2 longitudinal fissure of fibularis brevis tendon *(SOBEL classification)*.

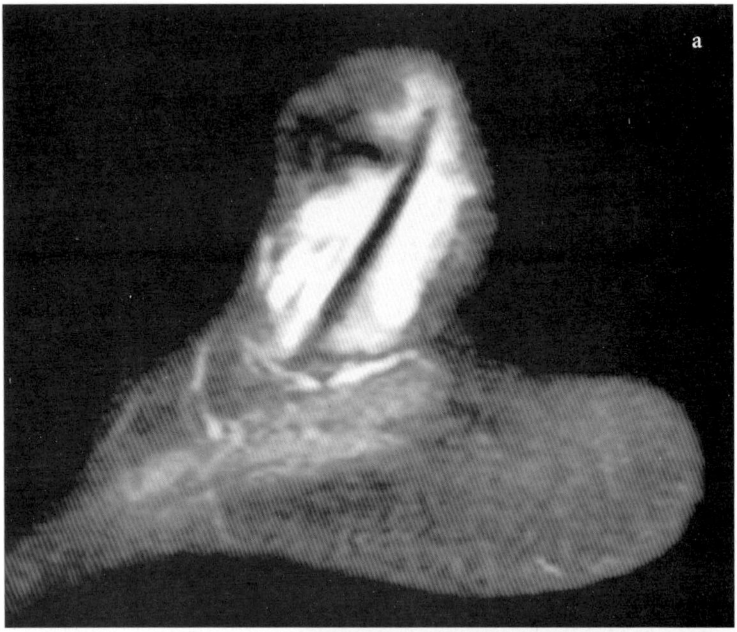

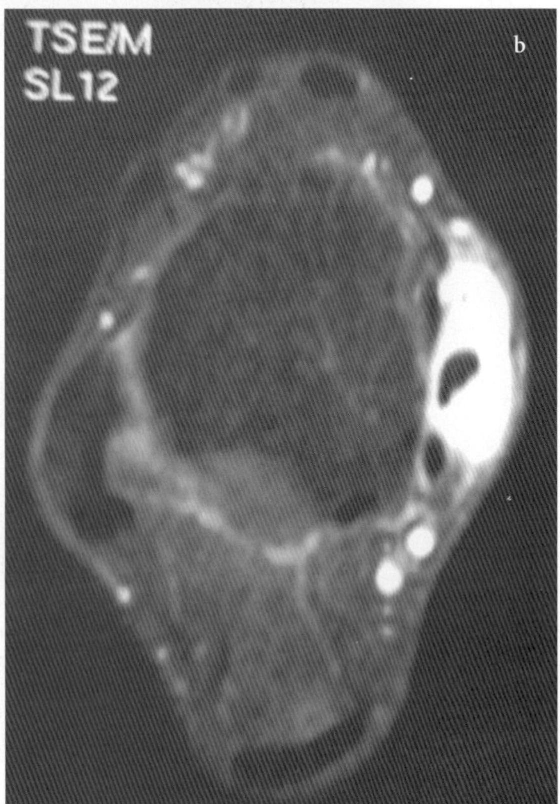

Fig. 17 - MRI: T1 fat sat gadolinium. Pannus of the sheath of the ptt. No pathology of the tendon itself (fig. a and fig. b).

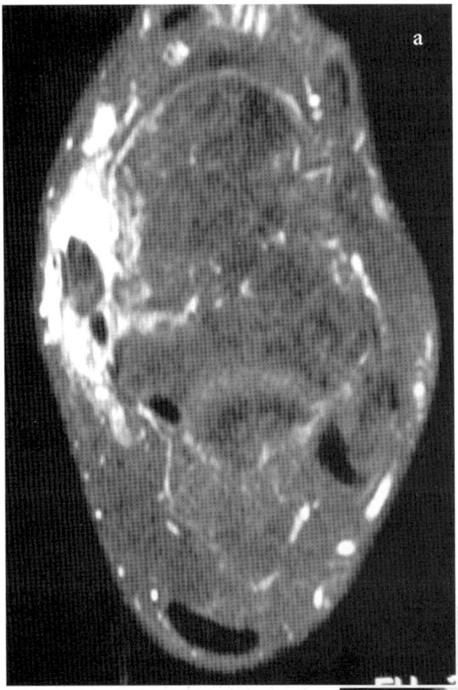

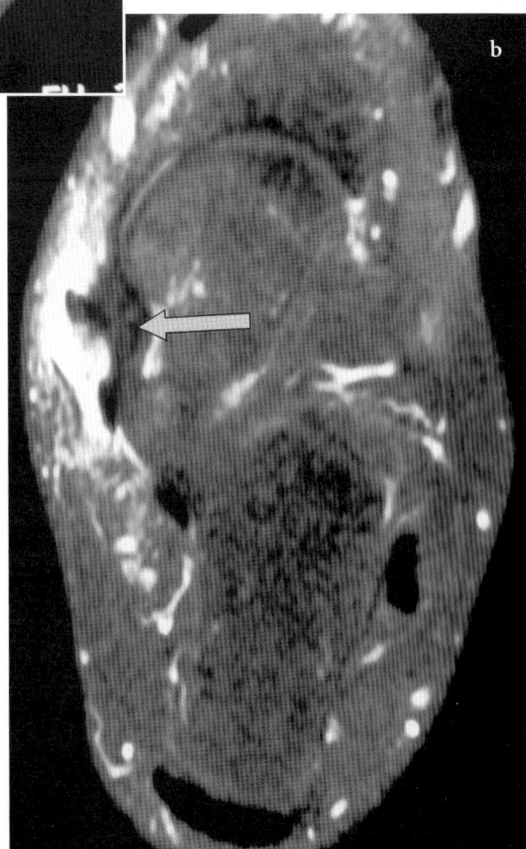

Fig. 18 - MRI: T1 fat sat gadolinium. Ptt: pannus of the sheath of the tendon and stage 2 tendinopathy (fig. a). Normal spring ligament (arrow) (fig. b).

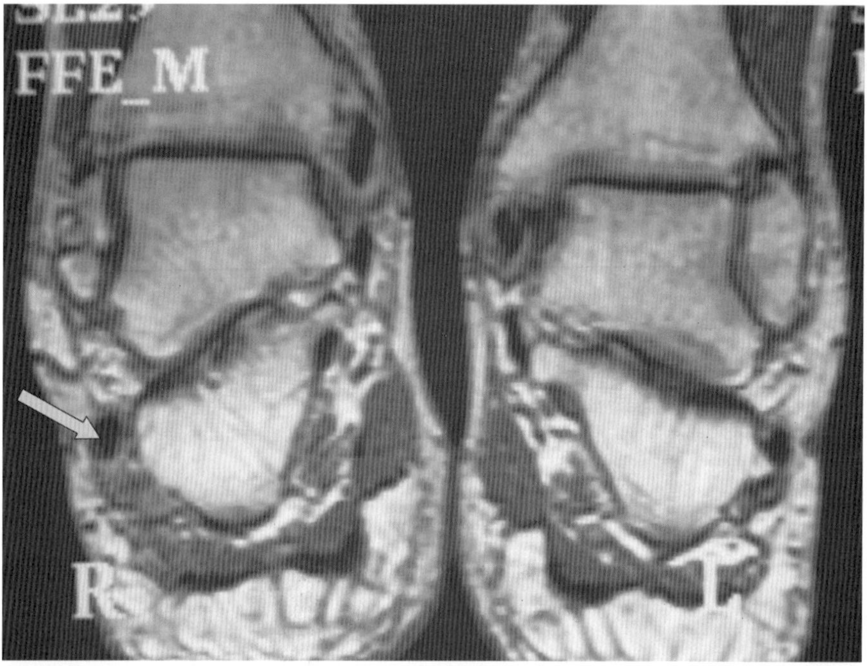

Fig. 19 - MRI: T1 gadolinium. Fibularis longus tendon ruptured. We can only see the fibularis brevis tendon (arrow).

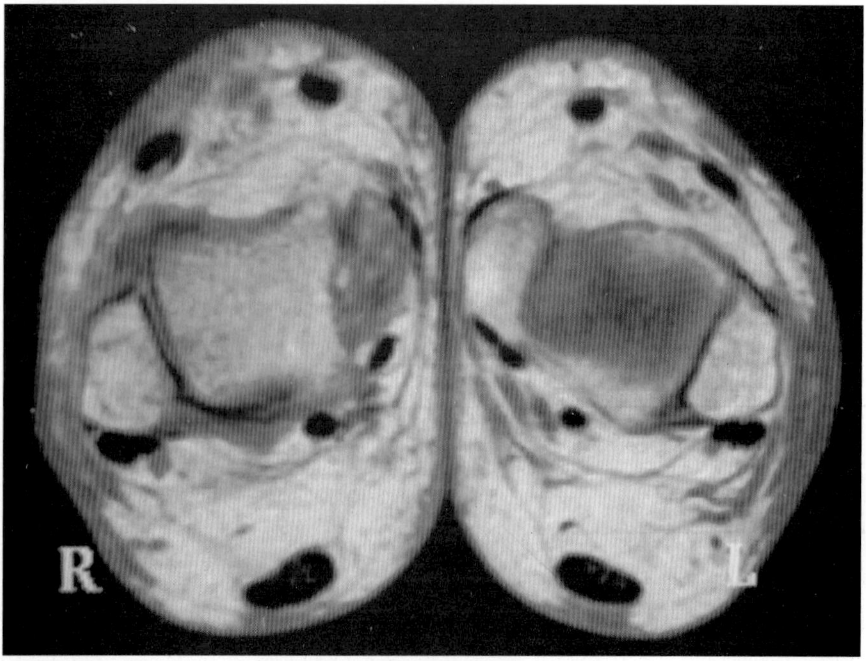

Fig. 20 - MRI: T1 weighted image. Rupture of the right ptt and stage 2 tendinopathy of the left ptt.

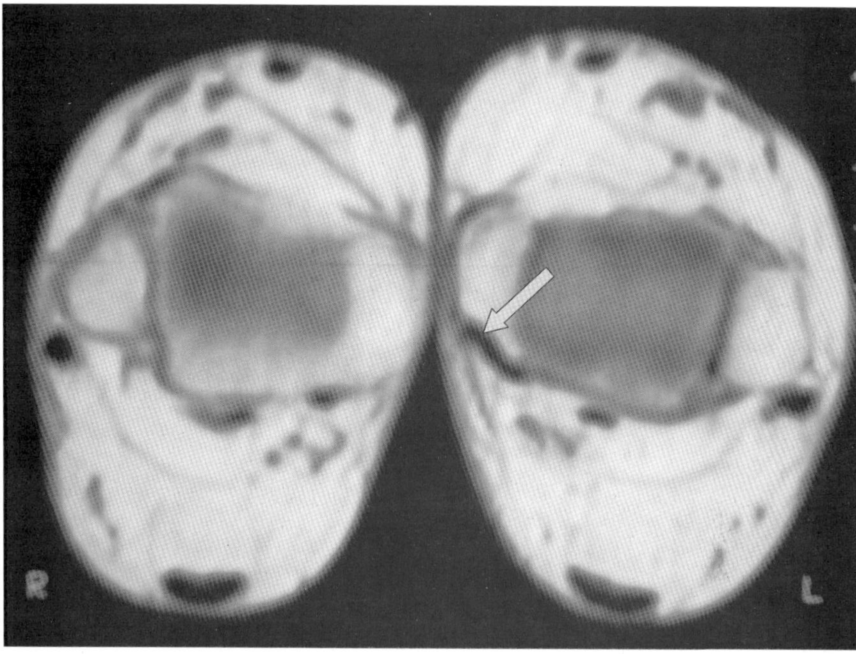

Fig. 21 - MRI: T1. Rupture of the right ptt (not visible). The left ptt is normal (arrow).

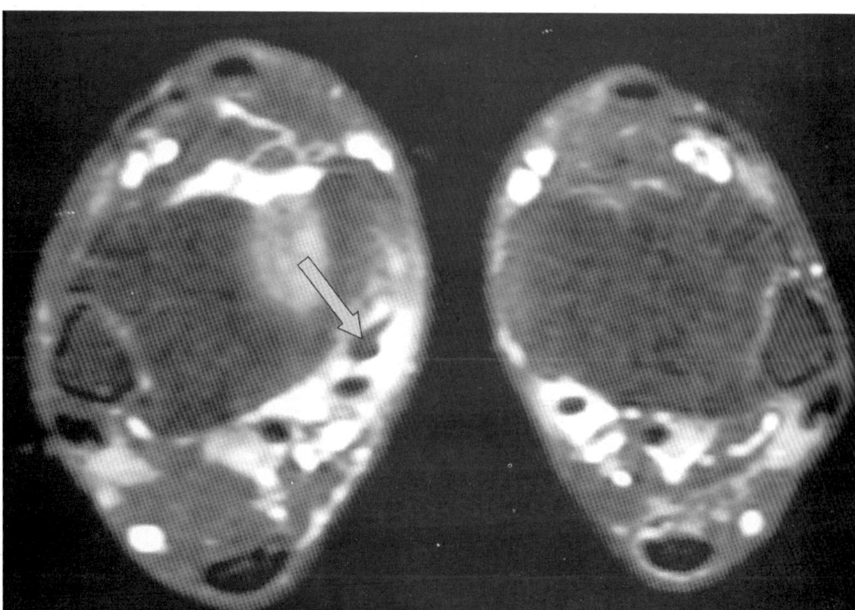

Fig. 22 - MRI. T1 fat-sat gadolinium. Left ptt ruptured (not visible) et stage 2 tendinopathy of the right ptt (arrow). Bilateral tenosynovitis of the flexor tendons.

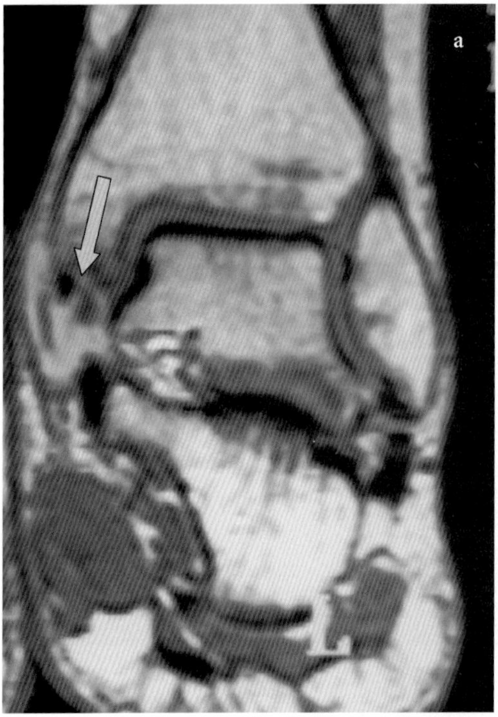

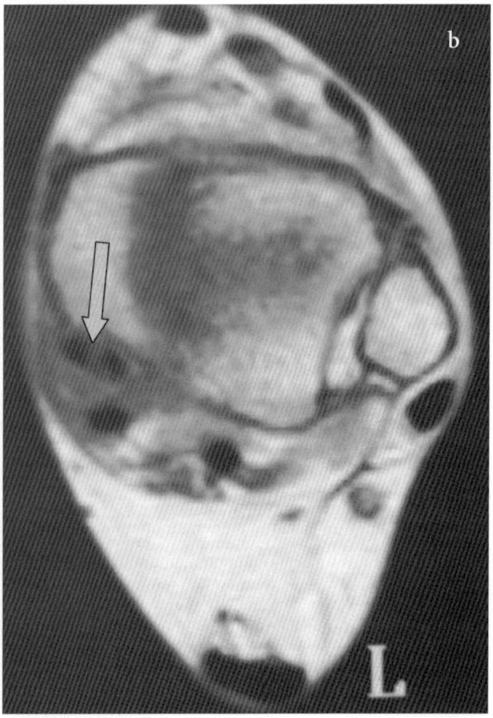

Fig. 23 - MRI: T1 gadolinium. Ptt splitting tendinopathy (arrow) and tenosynovitis (fig. a and fig. b).

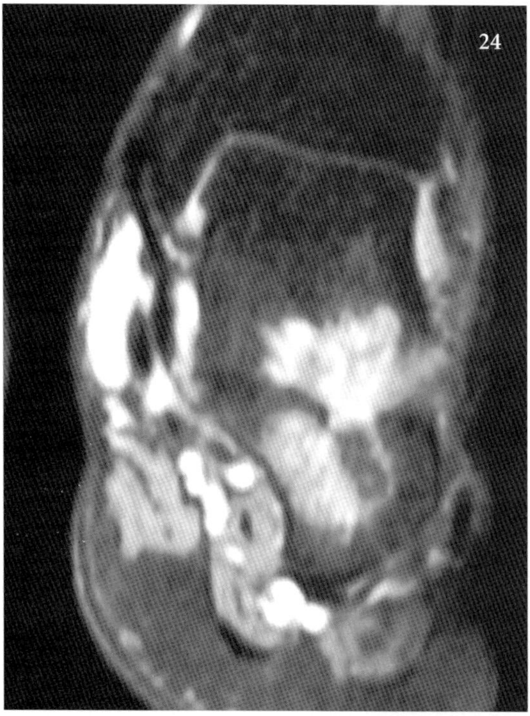

Fig. 24 - MRI: T1 fat-sat gadolinium. Sinus tarsi pannus. Ruptured interosseous talo-calcaneal ligament (itcl).

Fig. 25 - MRI: T1 gadolinium. Right sinus tarsi pannus and ruptured itcl (asterik). On the left side the itcl is normal (arrow).

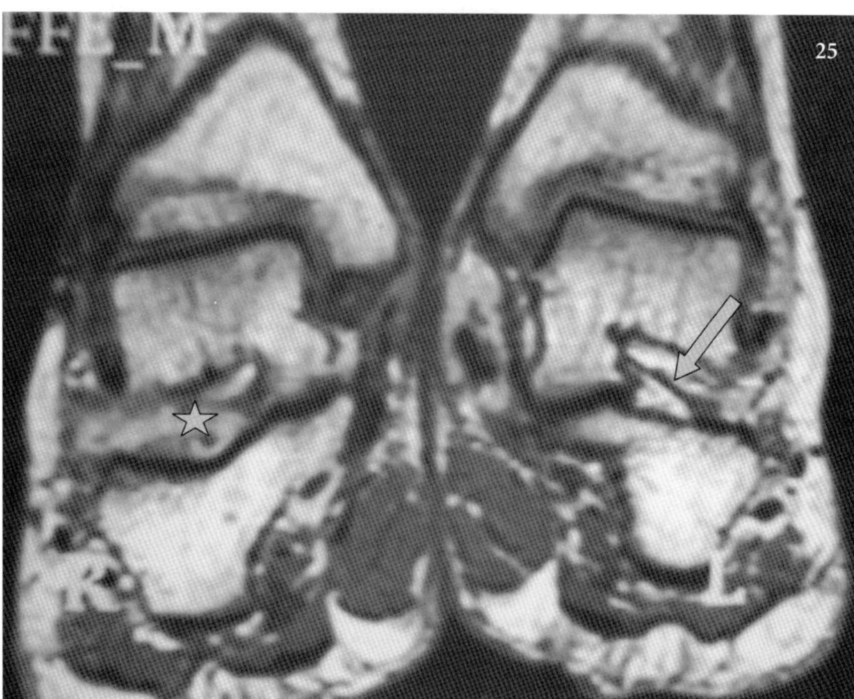

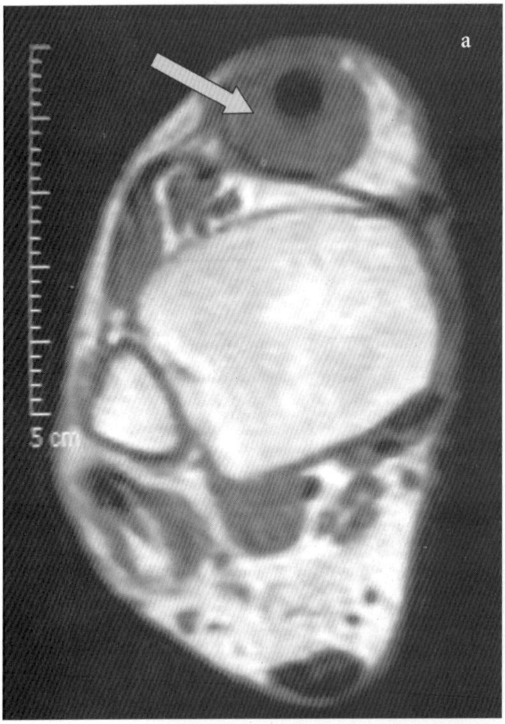

Fig. 26 - MRI: T1 (fig. a): tenosynovitis of the tibialis anterior tendon (arrow). T1 fat-sat gadolinium (fig. b): retro-calcaneal bursitis (white arrow) and plantar bursitis (grey arrow).

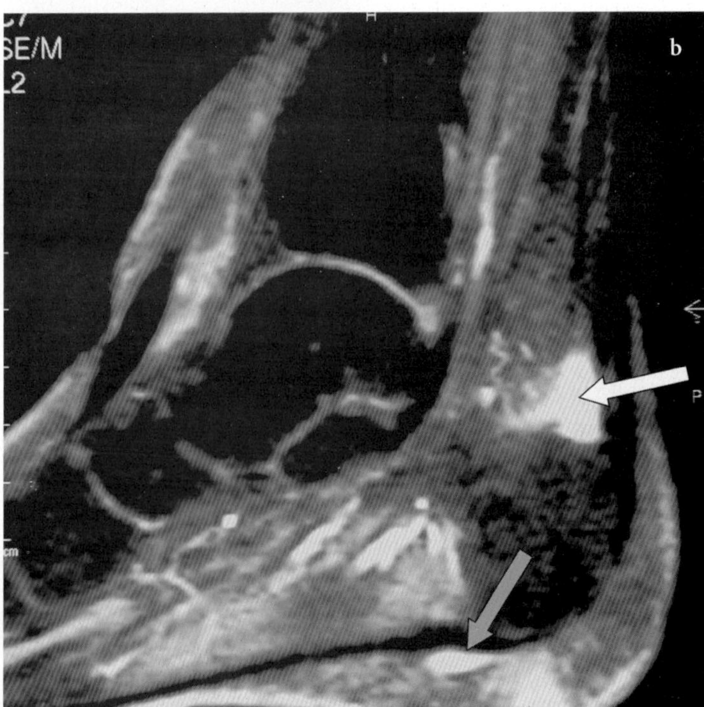

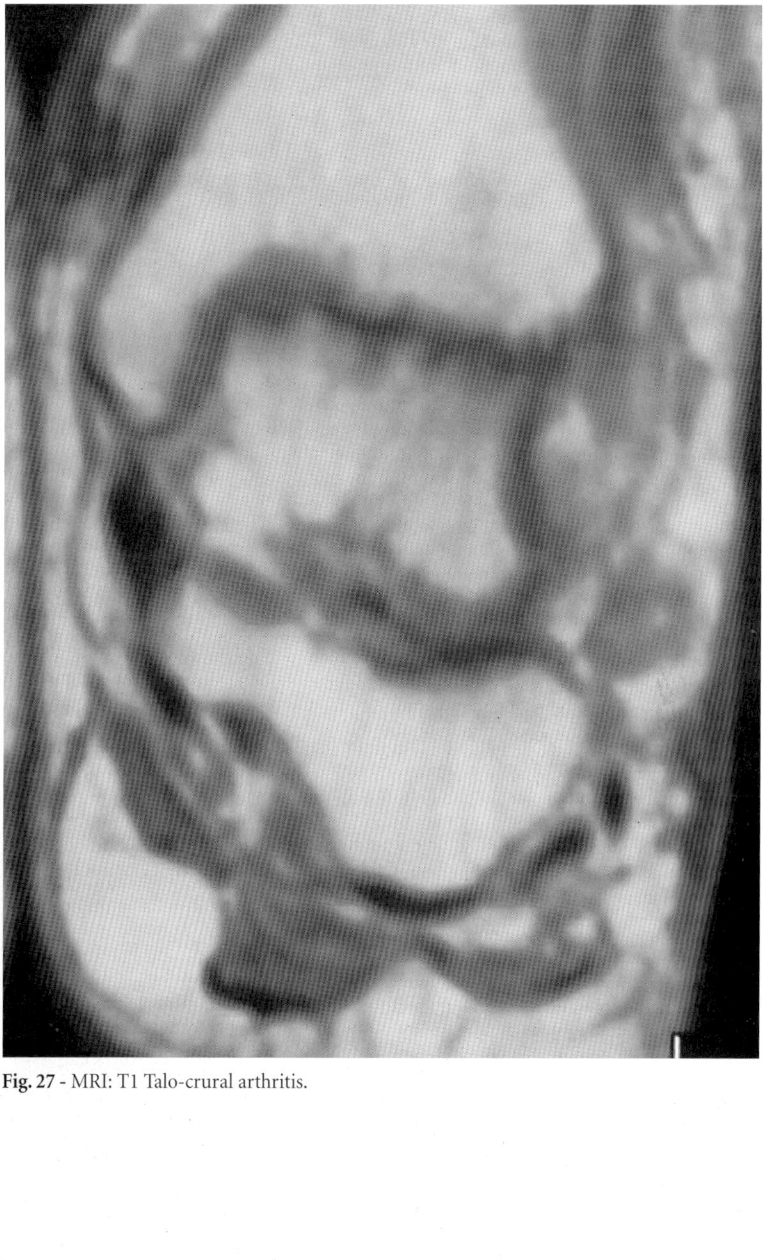

Fig. 27 - MRI: T1 Talo-crural arthritis.

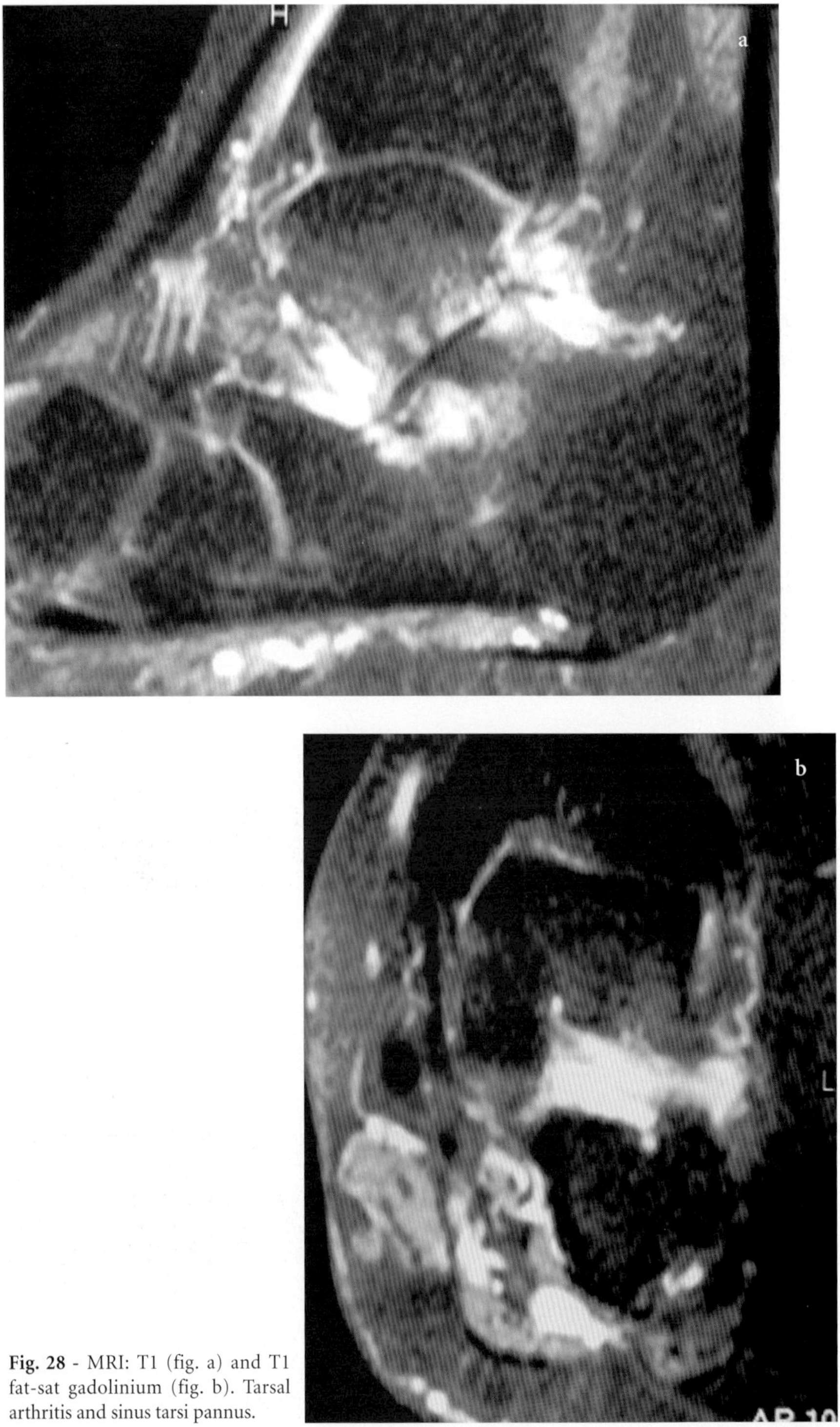

Fig. 28 - MRI: T1 (fig. a) and T1 fat-sat gadolinium (fig. b). Tarsal arthritis and sinus tarsi pannus.

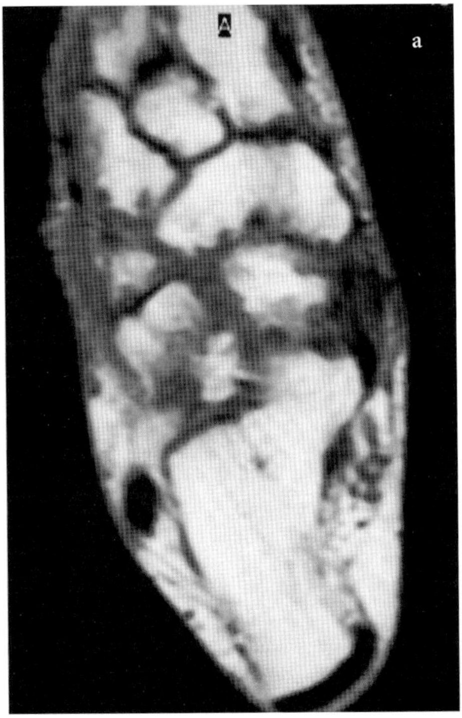

Fig. 29 - MRI: T1 (fig. a, left side). T1 fat-sat gadolinium (fig. b, right side). Talo-navicular arthritis, and strong enhancement after gadolinium injection.

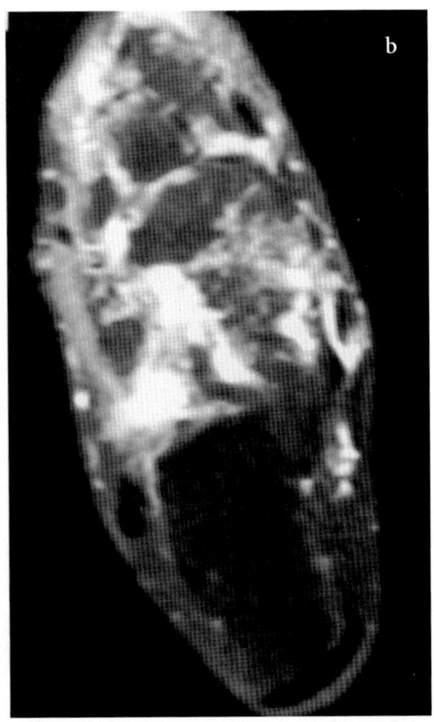

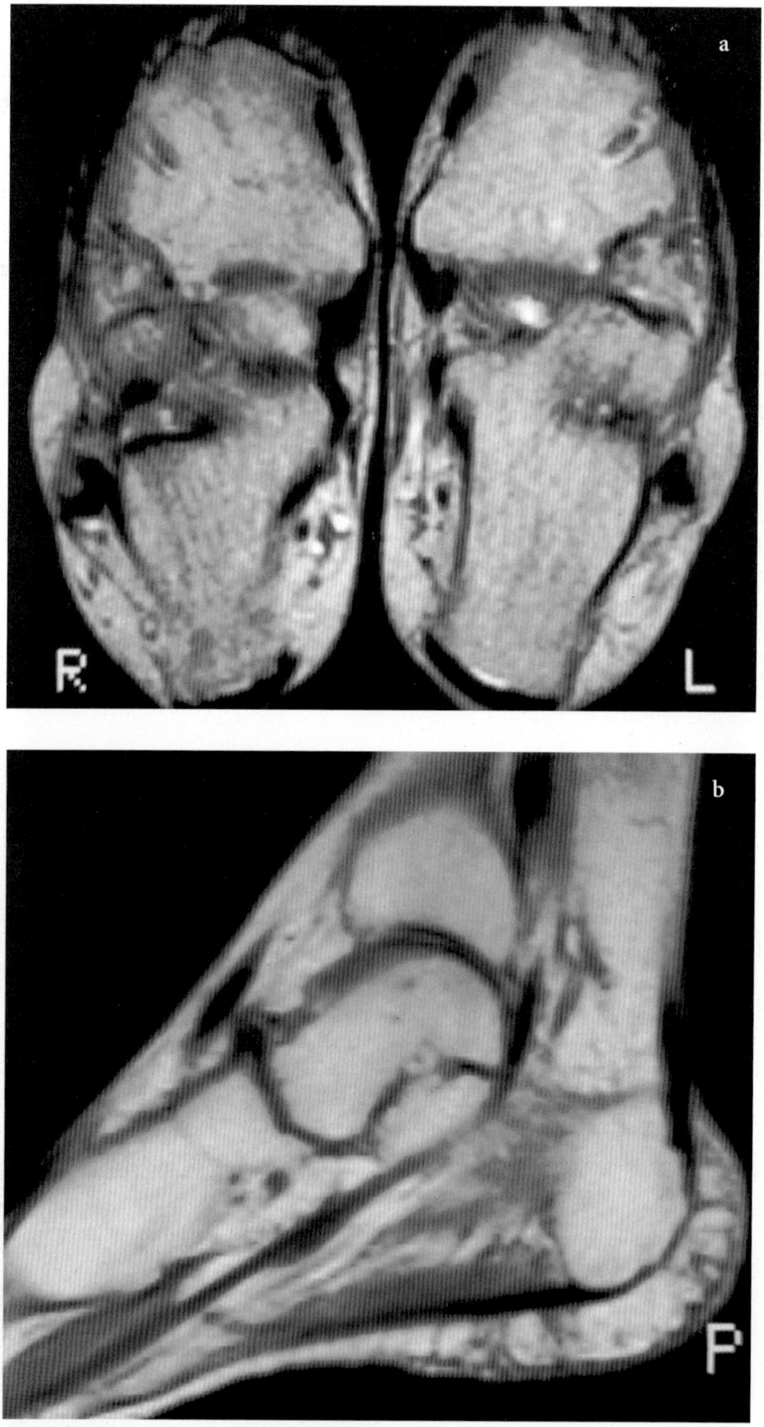

Fig. 30 - MRI: T2 (fig. a) and T1 (fig. b). Tarsal ankylosis. No tendon pathology.

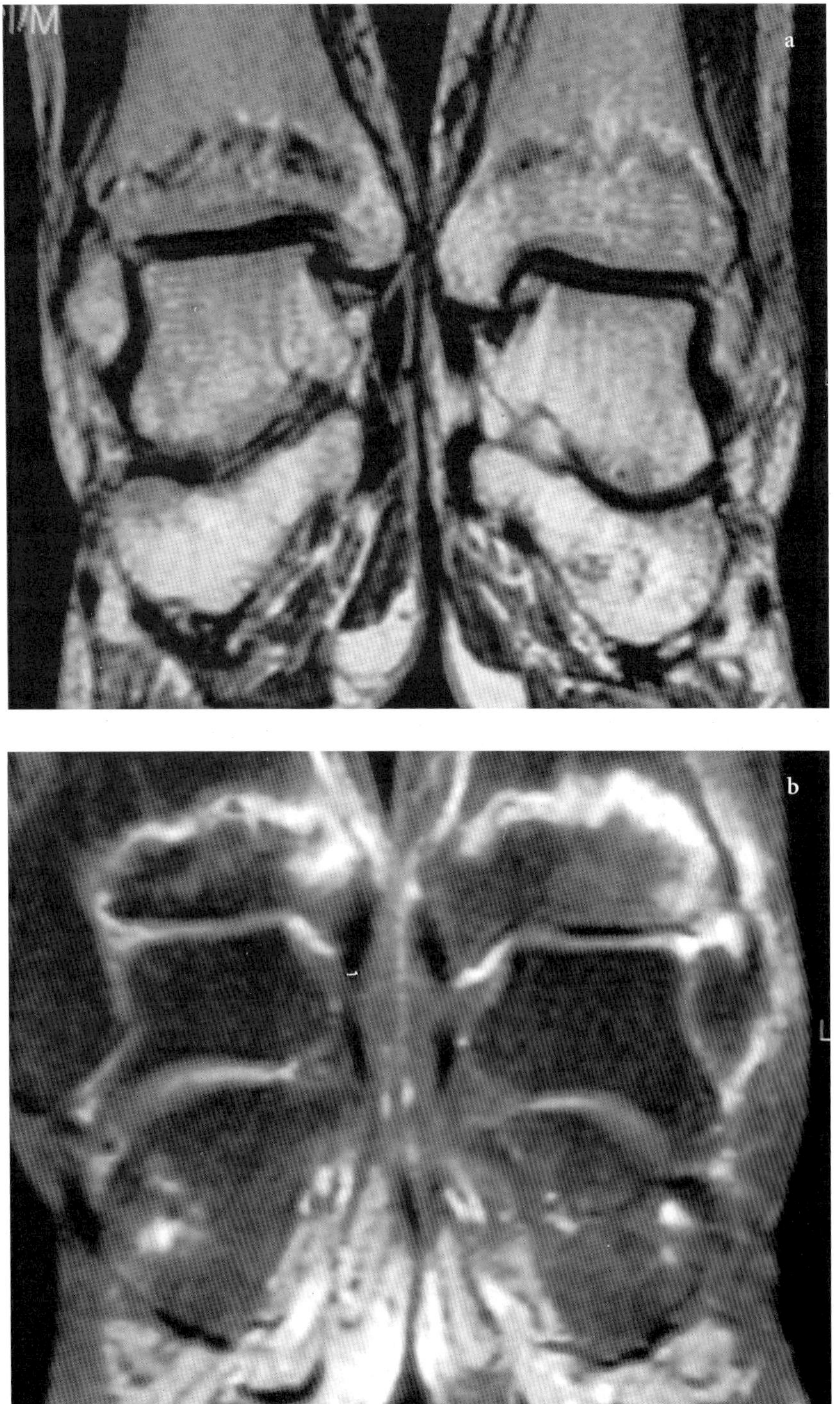

Fig. 31 - MRI: T1 (fig. a) and T1 fat-sat gadolinium (fig. b). Bilateral stress fracture of the lower parts of the tibias.

Management of the patient with rheumatoid arthritis

J.-G. Tebib and P. Miossec

Changing perceptions

Until the early eighties, the treatment of rheumatoid arthritis (RA) was based on the principle of responding to the damage caused by disease progression at the time when the damage actually occurred. In this strategy, known as the "pyramid approach", the physician responded to the patient's worsening condition by initiating a possibly more effective therapeutic option, always at a late stage in disease progression. As the efficacy and toxicity of the medications available were poorly known, such a strategy generally led to inevitable deterioration of the patient's autonomy because the decision to treat necessarily lagged behind the progress of the disease in spite of the contributions made by prosthetic surgery (1). In the eighties, three lines of research led to a complete change in planning the management of RA. Methotrexate was rediscovered as a long-acting drug and meticulous comparative studies were carried out on the efficacy and toxicity of all disease-modifying anti-rheumatic drugs (DMARD). They finally concluded on the supremacy of methotrexate both for controlling flares and for the prevention of joint destruction (2). A second line of research confirmed the importance of early diagnosis by demonstrating the rapidity of joint damage at the very onset of the disease (3) and as a corollary the need for effective, appropriate treatment started as soon as possible (4). The relative inefficacy of the basic DMARDS in arresting structural joint destruction finally led to the search for other modes of treatment. The most immediate option consisted in applying the principles of synergistic action of different treatments to fight the same entity; an approach which had yielded encouraging results against cancer or infectious diseases (5). The second mode of treatment was based on advances in our knowledge of the RA process, in particular relating to the central role of the pro-inflammatory cytokines, IL-1 and

TNF-α, where specific antagonists demonstrated spectacular effectiveness in arresting not only the inflammatory phenomenon, but also structural joint damage (6).

Today, thanks to such advances, we have a well-grounded vision of the management of an RA patient which takes into account many sociological, clinical, biological and also economic parameters. Integration of these parameters is a complex process but it is at this cost that we can hope to see the natural outcome of RA gradually improve in the coming years.

Patient assessment

Thanks to advances in the knowledge of the disease, we can now plan a specific treatment strategy for a given patient at a given time in his or her disease. This treatment program is worked out on the basis of a certain number of prognostic factors.

RA status

The treatment program varies according to whether the patient is in the early stages of RA or has established or advanced disease. While the aim is always to relieve pain and to ensure the best possible quality of life for the patient, the methods used to reach these objectives differ depending on the RA status. With a patient who is at the onset of disease, the accent is placed on strict control of disease progression. With a patient who already has severe joint damage, our ambition must be maintenance of optimal functional ability. The following stages can be distinguished:

- the patient with early RA: this is considered as chronic inflammatory rheumatism with a duration of more than 6 weeks but less than 3 months. The clinical, biological or radiological profile may not allow us to classify this rheumatism as being of rheumatoid origin and the current tendency is to disregard its origin and to base treatment simply on potential gravity (see prognostic factors below);
- classic RA: here the rheumatoid origin is established and is based on the ACR criteria (table I) (7) or on later attempts to improve these criteria (8). This diagnostic method concerns patients whose disease has progressed for more than three months and up to two years. In such circumstances, signs of joint damage are frequently observed and must be taken into account when considering the use of DMARDs. These first two groups require treatments which are sufficiently aggressive to arrest disease progression;
- end-stage RA: by calling upon focused treatments, whether infiltrations or orthopaedic surgery, management of these patients must take account of the inflammatory component and in particular of the joint damage which worsens functional status.

Evaluation of patient status at the time he or she is first seen requires specialized tools for optimal classification and to ensure the most appropriate treatment. These tools aim at measuring the inflammatory process or disease activity, as well as joint damage or disease progression. The findings of prospective studies have provided us with a certain number of prognostic factors.

Table I - The ACR criteria (7) compared with the criteria proposed by Visser *et al.* (8).

ACR criteria Duration of signs on first examination at least 6 weeks		Criteria of Visser *et al.* Duration of signs on first examination at least 6 weeks and not more than 6 months	
1	Morning stiffness lasting more than one hour	1	Morning stiffness lasting more than one hour
2	Arthritis of at least 3 joints	2	Arthritis of at least 3 joints
3	Arthritis affecting the hand	3	Bilateral pain on MTS pressure
4	Symmetrical arthritis	4	Compatible radiological appearance
5	Compatible radiological appearance	5	Rheumatoid factors
6	Rheumatoid nodules	6	Presence of antifilagrin antibody
7	Rheumatoid factors		

The 1987 ACR criteria (7) are compared with Visser's criteria, proposed recently but not yet validated (8). The latter repeat nearly all the clinical arguments, simplifying the analysis of the joint manifestations while regarding joint pain and not only arthritis as a criterion. A duration of more than 6 weeks which was a requirement for the first 4 criteria of the ACR becomes a criterion in its own right. Finally, Visser at al. take into account the good discriminating value of antifilagrin antibodies.

Disease activity

Clinical and paraclinical measurements make it possible to assess the inflammatory state at a given time and also the response to the treatment.

Clinical scales (9)

These take into account the subjective experience of the patient and the clinical investigations.

Measurement of subjective experience

Several measurements have been proposed and their sensitivity and specificity have been analysed. Duration of morning stiffness is often poorly quantified by the patient but can easily be assessed in clinical practice. Stiffness lasting longer than 45 minutes must be regarded as abnormal. Pain is adequately measured by patient self-rating on a 100-mm visual analogue scale; the same method can be used to quantify disability at a given time. Measurements greater than 45 mm must be regarded as abnormal. More accurate but more difficult to carry out in clinical practice, questionnaires such as the Health Assessment Questionnaire (HAQ) are the cornerstone of assessment of subjective experience in all therapeutic trials. Simplified forms can be used in clinical practice (table II).

Table II - Follow-up questionnaire for patients with rheumatoid arthritis.

The questions which you are asked will enable us to better know your disease and the effect it has on your daily activity. Please try to answer as accurately as possible, even if some of the questions do not seem to you to correspond exactly to your condition. If you have a problem understanding the questions, the nurse in attendance will be able to help you. Thank you for your collaboration.	Affix patient label here Date : / / Consulting doctor: ....

• **What drugs are you taking at the moment? Refer to your prescription and ask the nurse or receptionist for help if necessary.**

Name of drug	Dose	Adverse effects
1.		
2.		
3.		
4.		
5.		
6.		
7.		

• **Tick the box which corresponds best to your present condition.**

Today, are you able...	**without any difficulty**	**with some difficulty**	**with great difficulty**	**incapable of doing it**
To dress without help, including tying shoelaces and fastening buttons?	❐	❐	❐	❐
To raise a full cup or glass to your mouth?	❐	❐	❐	❐
To walk outside on even ground?	❐	❐	❐	❐
To wash yourself all over and dry yourself?	❐	❐	❐	❐
To bend and pick up an object on the ground?	❐	❐	❐	❐
To use an ordinary water tap?	❐	❐	❐	❐
To get in and out of a car?	❐	❐	❐	❐

- **How severe do you consider your joint pain has been this week? Indicate severity by putting a cross on the line below, between no pain at all (to the left) and intense pain (to the right).**

No pain ———————————————— Unbearable pain

- When you got up this morning, were your joints stiff?

  Yes ❑ No ❑

  If you answered yes, how long did it take for your joints to warm up?

  . . . . .minutes or . . . . hours.

- How severe do you consider your rheumatism has been this week? Indicate severity by putting a cross on the line below, between no rheumatism at all (to the left) and severe rheumatism (to the right).

No rheumatism ———————————————— Unbearable

THIS PART TO BE COMPLETED BY THE MEDICAL TEAM ONLY

JOINT PAIN AND SWELLING COUNT

	RIGHT			LEFT	
	Pain	**Swelling**		**Pain**	**Swelling**
temporo-mandibular			■■		
sterno-clavicular			■■		
acromio-clavicular			■■		
shoulder			■■		
elbow			■■		
wrist			■■		
MCP 1/2/3/4/5	/ / / /	/ / / /	■■	/ / / /	/ / / /
IP(P) 1/2/3/4/5	/ / / /	/ / / /	■■	/ / / /	/ / / /
IPD 2/3/4/5	/ / /	/ / /	■■	/ / /	/ / /
■■■■■■■■■■■■■	■■■■■■	■■■■■■	■■	■■■■■■	■■■■■■
Hip		■■■■■■	■■		■■■■■■
Knee			■■		
Ankle			■■		
Tarsus			■■		
MTP	/ / / /	/ / / /	■■	/ / / /	/ / / /
IP(P) & IPD	/ / / /	/ / / /	■■	/ / / /	/ / / /
Total					

TOTAL PAIN : SWELLING :

DAS :

This questionnaire is given to the patient during the consultation. The first part is completed by the patient who reports his or her status by answering a certain number of items: the simplified Health Assessment Questionnaire (HAQ) measures the general status of the patient in daily life. Replies are scored from zero to 3 points depending on the answer selected. A visual analogue scale is proposed to measure pain intensity and also the severity of rheumatism. The second part of the questionnaire is completed by the physician who counts the number of painful and swollen joints. From these results, several indices can be calculated, including the DAS if the ESR is available.

Objective measurement

Examination of the joints remains the keystone of clinical analysis. The number of painful and swollen joints is the usual index. Several methods are used in clinical practice. The simplest method should be used (assessment of 28 joints), but more complete counts exist. In a first clinical approximation, counts higher than 12 for pain and 8 for swelling indicate significant joint activity.

The search for extra-articular manifestations, in particular rheumatoid nodules or Sjögren syndrome, completes this examination which, of course, forms part of a full clinical check-up, during which particular attention must be paid to weight loss.

The contribution of laboratory tests

These serve to confirm the analysis of the activity rather than to provide any decisive information, since in RA the clinical signs are strongly correlated with the inflammatory syndrome. Sometimes, dissociation between biological signs of inflammation and relative clinical latency may suggest that a concomitant disorder should be sought. Measurement of the active phase reactants and in particular of C-reactive protein is very informative. The erythrocyte sedimentation test remains the most useful investigation, even if it is only moderately sensitive and above all non-specific. Other laboratory tests are not directly useful for measurement of disease activity. Thus, immunological tests such as the presence (and a fortiori the quantification) of rheumatoid factors (RF) have no place here.

The contribution of imaging

Simple radiography is not informative concerning disease activity. More recent techniques such as ultrasonography (10) or magnetic resonance imaging (11) may enable very early diagnosis of arthritis or tenosynovitis. These investigations are not yet current practice.

Disease progression

Assessment of disease progression attempts to measure structural joint damage over time, which depends mainly on the severity of disease flares. Nowadays, it is carried out by quantitative analysis of informative radiographs, primarily of the hands and the feet. Several increasingly sensitive quantification techniques have been proposed as knowledge of joint damage and analytical tools has advanced. Currently, the Sharp van der Heijde count is the most used (12). While it is very sensitive (0 to 348) and reproducible, it is impossible to use in clinical practice because of the time-consuming measurement which separately analyses narrowing and erosion of sensitive sites of the hands and feet.

These measurements of activity and progression help to define RA status at any given time and so to decide on an appropriate treatment option.

Here, the DAS (disease activity score) can prove to be of practical use since it yields an overall score representative of disease activity (13). It is obtained by regression studies which retain the most important confounding factors. This yields a complex formula: $DAS^{28} = 0.56 \times \sqrt{}$ (number of painful joints/28) + $0.28 \times \sqrt{}$

(number of swollen joints/28) + 0.7 x log (VS) + 0.014 x patient assessment of his or her RA state. The higher the score, the greater the disease activity. Briefly, a DAS $\leq$ 3.2 is considered to indicate low activity, between 3.2 and 5.1 intermediate activity and > 5.1 high activity. However, this index is not very meaningful and its calculation requires an abacus or a programmed calculator. It can also be sufficient to classify disease activity according to the same parameters. Depending on the number of affected joints, RA is defined as moderate (less than 3 affected joints, with arthralgia but without joint damage), active (4 to 12 inflammatory joints, moderate joint damage) or severe (more than 12 inflammatory joints, possibility of extra-articular signs and proven joint damage).

Prognostic factors

Prognostic factors are taken into account in order to develop a therapeutic strategy according to the probable course of the disease. Such an approach requires that the physician should anticipate the course the disease will take in a specific case. During recent decades many studies have addressed this question. Certain results still lack adequate confirmation and the findings of some authors are contradictory. In particular, we are as yet unable to correctly weigh each prognostic factor against the others for a given individual. In spite of these drawbacks, a certain number of decisive factors have to be taken into account.

Socio-epidemiological data

Late onset of the disease or onset in men aged less than 50 years appear to indicate a poor prognosis and RA in the young women is likely to be severe (14, 15).

Low socio-economic status and, in particular, low formal education is a very significant unfavourable factor (15).

Characteristics of the disease

Persistent or extensive RA of more than 6 months duration, tenosynovial involvement of the hands or the early appearance of rheumatoid nodules are factors of poor prognosis, as is a marked inflammatory syndrome persisting for more than 6 months (14).

Early radiological lesions appearing before 8 months are a sign of severe RA.

Biological markers

HLA-DR1 and DR4 antigens indicate a poor prognosis (14). Although the importance of these factors is still debated, homozygosity (DR1/DR1 or DR4/DR4) or heterozygosity (DR1/DR4) appear more prejudicial than a single allele of the type DR1/x or DR4/x (15).

The presence of rheumatoid factors marks the most severe RA and its association with HLA groups further worsens the unfavourable prognosis of this characteristic (16).

Treatments of RA

In the current approach to RA, therapy must be selected according to the state of the disease and in particular according to its prognosis. Some significant points must be stressed:
- All proven cases of RA must benefit from basic treatment appropriate to the disease prognosis, the principal objective being to control flares of activity;
- Global management of the patient is crucial. The cornerstones of management are patient education and surgery as well as the use of sophisticated treatments. These treatments must also take into account the peculiar nature of this disease. It may present spontaneous remissions lasting several years or, on the contrary, can evolve very unfavourably, and treatment will have to be adjusted depending on disease reponse to the strategies undertaken.

Patient education

This addresses significant issues with the sole objective of familiarising the patient with his or her disease and thus achieving better compliance with treatment. The physician must make clear to the patient the rationale for the therapeutic strategy chosen this should be based on a simple explanation of the origin of the disease and available treatments, explaining not only their mode of action but also, in particular, their adverse effects. Such contact can best take place in the course of patient education day courses where the patient will be able to meet various actors in treatment (doctors, nurses, physiotherapists, ergotherapists, etc.).

Symptomatic treatment

This classically includes anti-inflammatory drugs and analgesics. They are regarded today as adjuvant treatments, alleviating symptoms while awaiting the cure broughtby DMARDs. Beside stage II analgesics, morphine and its more convenient derivatives appear today to take a greater place. Anti-cyclooxygenase-2 (anti-COX-2), better tolerated than traditional anti-inflammatory drugs, is a logical option. However, it has the same renal toxicity and recenthly some contra-indications, must be known.

Algorithm for current use of DMARDs (fig. 1)

This is the centre of the entire treatment strategy. Briefly, the early management of the patient, RA with a favourable prognosis and RA with poorer prognosis must all be considered. Early management may be in accordance with the diagnosis of chronic inflammatory rheumatism which does not yet have RA status. In the latter case, hydroxychloroquine or salazopyrine have their place; the first allowing for the possibility of arthritis in the setting of a lupus disease, and the second for that of peripheral arthritis belonging to the seronegative spondylarthropathies.

In a patient with inflammatory rheumatism affecting the small joints and presenting signs of severity, synthetic purine or pyrimidine inhibitors should be started, methotrexate being currently used more than leflunomide for historical reasons and because it is equally effective at a more moderate cost. The accepted dose of methotrexate is 7.5 to 20 mg weekly, while 10 to 20 mg daily is the dose suggested for leflunomide. Treatment is adjusted after 4 to 6 weeks according to the effect on the signs of activity, within limits which depend on the duration of disease, the age of the patient and the tolerance, while always attempting to reduce activity as closely as possible to a state of remission. In case of failure it will be necessary to resort to combination therapy, still centred on the nucleotide synthesis inhibitors and methotrexate in particular. At the present time at least four possible combination regimens have been validated:

- methotrexate and cyclosporine (17) have been shown to be more effective through the synergistic action of the two drugs. The suggested dose of cyclosporine is 2.5 mg/kg/day;

Fig. 1 - Algorithm for current use of DMARDS in rheumatoid arthritis.

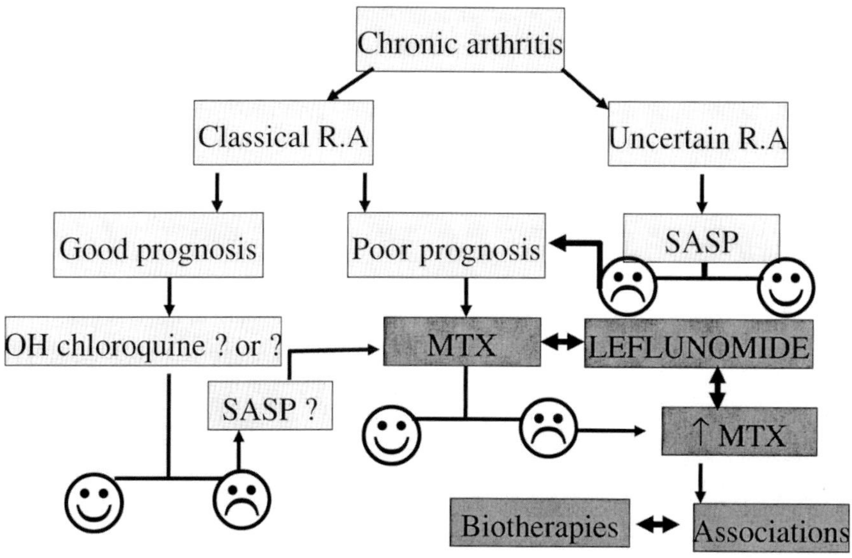

In the case of chronic proven inflammatory rheumatism, after vasculitis has been ruled out, two situations are possible.

If the clinical profile is that of proven RA (7, 8), then introduction of a DMARD is imperative. The choice of DMARD will be made after assessing the prognosis (15) and methotrexate is still the drug of choice if the disease is potentially severe. If the patient does not respond to this treatment or if this strategy is not effective even with increased doses, its replacement by leflunomide and combination therapies must be considered, which may be conventional or which may include biological treatments (see text). These recommendations are likely to be modified in the future, depending on the findings of current studies on the immediate use of biological treatments in the hope of arresting the RA process at its onset.

If RA is uncertain, the debate will mainly concern the diagnosis of peripheral forms of spondylarthropathies and while waiting for an established diagnosis, salazopyrine can be proposed as it is effective in both diseases.

- methotrexate, salazopyrine, hydroxychloroquine and cortisone (18). This quadruple combination is more effective in terms of control of disease activity and progression than methotrexate alone. Moreover, there is no significant increase in side effects;
- the combination of methotrexate and meflunomide (19) appears to be of interest in inadequate control of RA which is refractory of methotrexate;
- combination therapy with methotrexate and infliximab (20) seems one of the most effective alternatives today. However, the physician must take into consideration the cost of the treatment (approximately 10 000 euros per year). This combination is the only one which after two years demonstrated arrest of structural degradation.

Steroids are less used today than in previous decades because of improved knowledge of the efficacy of DMARDs. However, steroids given in low doses effectively reduce the progression of joint damage (21), without involving significant bone damage if given at less than 10 mg/day. With the exception of some limited indications, steroids are now generally used in association (see above).

Biological treatments, which are recent developments, are the therapeutic application of current knowledge on the imbalance between the production of pro-inflammatory cytokines such as IL-1 or TNF-α and their physiological inhibitors. These drugs appear very effective in controlling disease activity and reducing progression, but they have the disadvantage of being costly. Considerable efforts are being made to decrease cost through less complex production techniques. Moreover, etanercept (Enbrel) which has recently been authorised in the USA for the treatment of early RA, offers the possibility of using these drugs before joint damage has occurred. However, these new molecules have not yet proven their total safety in the treatment of young patients.

Surgery

The role of surgery has decreased to some extent while patient management has progressed. Prosthetic surgery is still irreplaceable. However, the aim of the current advances in surgery is to prevent the joint destruction which is inevitable once the process has begun.

Adjuvant treatments

Like surgery, the indications of local treatment have significantly decreased. Today, infiltrations and synoviortheses still have a place in the local treatment of a particular joint and form an integral part of overall management of the disease. Physiotherapy or ergotherapy also belong to the arsenal available to improve the status of already degraded patients. Along the same lines, protective devices such as plantar splints aim at reducing the mechanical factor of damage induced by weakening of the tendon or articular structures secondary to the RA process. As with surgery, prospective studies of the process of destruction have led to significant progress in damage prevention, for example by use of suitable plantar ortheses (22).

Follow-up of RA

Follow-up includes regular monitoring of the patient at least twice a year, with more rapid intervention if a flare-up occurs. This implies flexible organisation of the department or clinic and staff who are familiar with these practice methods. Clinical examination is an essential part of patient surveillance, comparing current and previous results to measure activity intensity and response to the therapeutic regimen. Overall, it can be considered that every patient who presents signs which classify his or her disease as active RA requires reassessment of therapeutic strategy with the aim of arresting joint destruction, which is an overwhelming event (4). With this goal in mind, the DAS we have presented above can be of value. Thus, an improvement of the score from 0.6 to 1.2 indicates moderate response and improvement > 1.2 a good response, whereas a decrease to < 0.6 shows that treatment is ineffective.

Conclusion

Significant advances have been made in recent decades. They are the consequence of better analysis of the RA process rather than of progress due to discovery of new treatments, even though today we can reasonably have real hope in biological treatments (23).

References

1. Amor B, Herson D, Cherot A, Delbarre F. Analyse du suivi de patients affectés de polyarthrite rhumatoïde sur une période supérieure à 10 ans (1966-1978): analyse de la progression et des traitements sur 10 cas. Ann Med Interne (Paris) 1981; 132 (3): 168-73
2. Felson DT, Anderson JJ, Meenan RF. The comparative efficacy and toxicity of second-line drugs in rheumatoid arthritis. Results of two metaanalyses. Arthritis Rheum 1990; 33 (10): 1449-61
3. Fuchs HA, Kaye JJ, Callahan LF, Nance EP, Pincus T. Evidence of significant radiographic damage in rheumatoid arthritis within the first 2 years of disease. J Rheumatol 1989; 16 (5): 585-91
4. Guidelines for the management of rheumatoid arthritis. American College of Rheumatology Ad Hoc Committee on Clinical Guidelines. Arthritis Rheum 1996; 39 (5): 713-22
5. O'Dell JR. Combination DMARD therapy for rheumatoid arthritis: a step closer to the goal. Ann Rheum Dis 1996; 55 (11): 781-3
6. Lipsky PE, van der Heijde DM, St Clair EW *et al.* Infliximab and methotrexate in the treatment of rheumatoid arthritis. N Engl J Med 2000; 343 (22): 1594-602

7. Arnett FC, Edworthy SM, Bloch DA, McShane DJ, Fries JF, Cooper NS, Healey LA, Kaplan SR, Liang MH, Luthra HS, *et al.* The American Rheumatism Association 1987 revised criteria for the classification of rheumatoid arthritis. Arthritis Rheum 1988; 31 (3): 315-24
8. Visser H, Le Cessie S, Vos K, Breedveld FC, Hazes JMW. How to diagnose rheumatoid arthritis (RA) early: the development of diagnostic criteria (abstract). Ann Rheum 2000; 59 (suppl 1): 35
9. American College of Rheumatology Ad Hoc Committee on Clinical Guidelines. Guidelines for the management of rheumatoid arthritis. Arthritis Rheum 1996; 39 (5): 713-22
10. Wakefield RJ, Gibbon WW, Conaghan PG, O'Connor P, McGonagle D, Pease C, Green MJ, Veale DJ, Isaacs JD, Emery P. The value of sonography in the detection of bone erosions in patients with rheumatoid arthritis: a comparison with conventional radiography. Arthritis Rheum 2000; 43: 2762-70
11. McGonagle D, Conaghan PG, O'Connor P, Gibbon W, Green M, Wakefield R, Ridgway J, Emery P. The relationship between synovitis and bone changes in early untreated rheumatoid arthritis: a controlled magnetic resonance imaging study. Arthritis Rheum 1999; 42 (8): 1706-11
12. van der Heijde DM, van Leeuwen MA, van Riel PL, van de Putte LB. Radiographic progression on radiographs of hands and feet during the first 3 years of rheumatoid arthritis measured according to Sharp's method (van der Heijde modification). J Rheumatol 1995; 22 (9): 1792-6
13. van der Heijde DM, van't Hof M, van Riel PL, van de Putte LB. Development of a disease activity score based on judgment in clinical practice by rheumatologists. J Rheumatol 1993; 20 (3): 579-81
14. van Zeben D, Hazes JM, Zwinderman AH, Cats A, Schreuder GM, D'Amaro J, Breedveld FC. Association of HLA-DR4 with a more progressive disease course in patients with rheumatoid arthritis. Results of a followup study. Arthritis Rheum 1991; 34 (7): 822-30
15. Combe B, Eliaou JF, Daures JP, Meyer O, Clot J, Sany J. Prognostic factors in rheumatoid arthritis. Comparative study of two subsets of patients according to severity of articular damage. Br J Rheumatol 1995; 34 (6): 529-34
16. Rau R, Herborn G, Zueger S, Fenner H. The effect of HLA-DRB1 genes, rheumatoid factor, and treatment on radiographic disease progression in rheumatoid arthritis over 6 years. J Rheumatol 2000; 27 (11): 2566-75
17. Tugwell P, Pincus T, Yocum D, Stein M, Gluck O, Kraag G, McKendry R, Tesser J, Baker P, Wells G. Combination therapy with cyclosporine and methotrexate in severe rheumatoid arthritis. The Methotrexate-Cyclosporine Combination Study Group. N Engl J Med 1995; 333 (3): 137-41
18. Mottonen T, Hannonen P, Leirisalo-Repo M, Nissila M, Kautiainen H, Korpela M, Laasonen L, Julkunen H, Luukkainen R, Vuori K, Paimela L, Blafield H, Hakala M, Ilva K, Yli-Kerttula U, Puolakka K, Jarvinen P, Hakola M, Piirainen H, Ahonen J, Palvimaki I, Forsberg S, Koota K, Friman C. Comparison of combination therapy with single-drug therapy in early rheumatoid arthritis: a randomised trial. FIN-RACo trial group. Lancet 1999; 353 (9164): 1568-73
19. Weinblatt ME, Kremer JM, Coblyn JS, Maier AL, Helfgott SM, Morrell M, Byrne VM, Kaymakcian MV, Strand V. Pharmacokinetics, safety, and efficacy of combination treatment with methotrexate and leflunomide in patients with active rheumatoid arthritis. Arthritis Rheum 1999; 42 (7): 1322-8

20. Lipsky PE, van der Heijde DM, St Clair EW, Furst DE, Breedveld FC, Kalden JR, Smolen JS, Weisman M, Emery P, Feldmann M, Harriman GR, Maini RN; Infliximab and methotrexate in the treatment of rheumatoid arthritis. Anti-Tumor Necrosis Factor Trial in Rheumatoid Arthritis with Concomitant Therapy Study Group. N Engl J Med 2000; 30; 343 (22): 1640-1

21. Kirwan JR. The effect of glucocorticoids on joint destruction in rheumatoid arthritis. The Arthritis and Rheumatism Council Low-Dose Glucocorticoid Study Group. N Engl J Med 1995; 333 (3): 142-6

22. Bouysset M, Tebib J, Noel E, Eulry F, Bonnin M, Nemoz C, Bouvier M. When should orthopaedic treatment be prescribed to avoid the flattening of the rheumatoid foot? Clin Rheumatol 1992; 11 (4): 580-2

23. Pincus T, O'Dell JR, Kremer JM. Combination therapy with multiple disease-modifying antirheumatic drugs in rheumatoid arthritis: a preventive strategy. Ann Intern Med 1999; 131 (10): 768-74

Footwear for the rheumatoid foot and ankle

M. Bouysset, P. Hugueny, G. Guaydier-Souquières and F. Lapeyre

Rheumatoid arthritis (RA) is a destructive disease leading to deformity. The medical treatment of RA includes, among other options, drugs and adequate footwear. It requires careful monitoring of the foot. The principal deformities of the rheumatoid foot are due to two main factors: inflammatory synovitis which plays a major role, followed by mechanical stresses (and among them static disorders in particular). Now the disease-modifying antirheumatic drugs play an essential role against the inflammatory process, helped if necessary by intra-articular corticosteroid or isotopic injections. Local treatment with appropriate footwear aims to decrease the influence of these harmful factors which cause pain and deformity.

The aim of prescription footwear (1, 16, 19) is to:

- control the mobility of certain joints, particularly the subtalar joint. In most cases it is an attempt to decrease the tendency to hyperpronation during the gait cycle;
- accommodate the foot, above all by embedding of the plantar surface and use of soft materials or external shoe modifications that can compensate for lost joint motion.
- relieve areas of increased pressure, especially under the metatarsal heads, to prevent pain, hyperkeratosis, plantar bursitis and possible ulceration;
- reduce shock and shear, decrease the overall amount of vertical pressure particularly at the beginning of the gait cycle and reduce horizontal movement of the foot in the shoe (20);

We will not deal here with postoperative shoes, but will address the principal concepts relating to the appropriate use of adequate footwear and plantar orthoses depending on observation of foot and ankle involvement.

Principal concepts relating to footwear and plantar orthoses

Shoes

- **Consumer guidelines** have been issued in the USA ("10 points of proper shoe fit") (20, 24):

1. Sizes vary among shoe brands and styles. Do not select shoes by the size marked inside the shoe. Judge the shoe by how it fits on your foot.
2. Choose a shoe that conforms as nearly as possible to the shape of your foot.
3. Have your feet measured regularly. The size of the foot changes as you grow older.
4. Have both your feet measured. For most persons, one foot is larger than the other. Fit to the largest foot.
5. Fit at the end of the day when the feet are largest.
6. Stand during the fitting process and check that there is adequate space for your longest toe at the end of each shoe.
7. Make sure the ball of your foot fits snugly into the widest part of the shoe.
8. Do not purchase shoes that feel too tight, expecting them to "stretch" to fit.
9. Your heel must fit comfortably in the shoe with a minimum amount of slippage.
10. Walk in the shoe to make sure it fits and feels right.

These recommendations are even more important where rheumatoid feet are concerned, but further points require attention.

As RA is a progressive disease, the shoe must be changed more often to fit the deformed foot. The size and shape of the foot vary during the course of the disease particularly with the importance of the inflammatory process. Moreover, in RA the deformity frequently differs between the two feet.

When dealing with the rheumatoid foot some points of the shoe are particularly important.

- The counter is a stiffener around the back part of the shoe. It secures or stabilizes the heel of the foot inside the shoe and helps the shoe retain its shape and an aesthetic appearance of the back of the shoe (10, 27). In RA the hindfoot must be reasonably stable within the shoe. The need for a firm counter seems self-evident since the fragile inflammatory structures which maintain the normal shape of the hindfoot are subject to deformity; minimal stresses and torsion are more harmful in structures already liable to stretching. Some conventional shoes contain firm counters, others have small or soft counters, others have no counters at all. Fashion has far more influence on the use and shape of the counter than medical opinion (27). We should bear in mind that in RA the counter must be firm to support the hindfoot, but also comfortable to avoid rubbing.

- The good quality shoe must have a wide forefoot. The toe-cap should be sufficiently large and supple in the upper part to avoid rubbing of the deformed toes. The inside of the shoe must have no seam or stitching which could cause friction. The sole should be firm and the heel not too high (about 2 cm).

- The shank, of wood or metal, supports the midfoot (instep) between the heel and the forefoot (it continues up to the back of the metatarsal heads). It is particularly important in the rheumatoid foot with its tendency to deformity.

Many forefoot deformities are attributed to shoe pressure, but a shoe which is too flexible does not support the foot and leads more so to flattening (11, 17, 28, 30).

Walking can sometimes be made more comfortable by small improvements in the heel or sole of the shoe (2).

- Several external modifications of shoes for the rheumatoid foot may be prescribed (15, 20, 22).

- Rocker soles (20, 26, 29, 31) which aim to decrease stresses on the foot during the different phases of gait. The sole of the shoe is rounded off at the toe and heel to make walking easier, so that the foot rocks during walking. The sole is rigid, which prevents bending of the shoe and restricts motion of the joints of the foot, particularly extension of the metatarsophalangeal joints (9). These rocker soles with an angle at the heel and the forefoot aim to help propulsion at toe-off. They also decrease the intensity of impact at heel strike and reduce the need for ankle motion. In particular, they compensate for a lack of ankle dorsiflexion.

Several important features of rocker shoes should be taken into consideration: for example, the part of the rocker sole which is in contact with the floor when standing, the angle at the toe, the angle of the heel of the shoe to the ground and the height of the sole of the shoe (9, 20).

Cavanagh insists on plantar pressure measurement in conjunction with gait training. This helps to ensure correct use and optimizes the pressure-reducing effect of the rigid bottom of the rocker shoes (9).

- Stabilization (19): when the counter is not sufficient in the rheumatoid foot, a medial stabilizer helps to maintain the proper shape of the hindfoot and midfoot and to limit deformity. High uppers which cover the entire foot and ankle may be useful, even in certain mass-produced shoes (see below) (20).

- Other shoe modifications may be used, such as extended steel shanks, wedge extensions or internal modifications (20). Orthotic inserts (wedges, Thomas bars, etc.) may also be added to the outsole of a mass-produced shoe and so complete the treatment (34).

Finally, footwear for the rheumatoid foot should be attractive, light, easy to put on and to close. It must also be comfortable, causing no pressure or excessive rubbing (4, 11). These conditions may be difficult to reconcile; mass-produced shoes are sometimes not wide enough to contain a specially designed orthosis and so special shoes, whether custom-made or not, become necessary.

Made-to-measure shoes are sometimes a solution. Depending on their construction and the choice of materials, they can more easily correct a tendency to deformity.

Normally the subtalar joint pronates as the leg rotates internally and supinates as the leg rotates externally. If an abnormal pattern of motion arises, stability must be improved and pain reduced. Control of calcaneal eversion and inversion in the frontal plane is better achieved with bimalleolar contact and medial lateral support of the calcaneus. The orthotist must ensure that the heel is maintained in a neutral position. In the sagittal plane, the forward translational movement of the tibia and the fibula on the talus and of the talus on the calcaneus must be controlled particularly by the high part of the high upper shoes. Motion in the transverse plane must be controlled to prevent rotation of the lower part of the leg, using plantar orthoses and the means we have mentioned above.

An adequate stabilizer in customized shoes gives better support to the mid-hindfoot and the ankle, and decreases rotation of the lower part of the leg. These customized shoes can also be adapted to fixed deformities (11).

A leg-hindfoot orthosis may be used (18). Low temperature plastics may fracture after bending stresses. If high temperature plastics are used, additional modifications and devices are necessary. Foam padding placed inside the orthosis will give better cushioning (18) (the same may be done for mass-produced shoes or shoes made to measure).

In certain cases, the orthotic and customized shoe are moulded and give a very satisfactory result if there is good clinical follow-up (13, 17).

Plantar orthoses

These are important in completing the role of the shoe itself. Their indications and design may vary. The orthosis must provide function which is as close as possible to physiological mechanics and must relieve pain. Unfortunately, few objective studies have supported the quality of their therapeutic effect (8, 23, 33). They aim to relieve pain and any existing trophic disorders, and to prevent increasing deformity (8, 21). These two goals are difficult to achieve. The foot must not be constricted which would cause pain, but it must be supported in a satisfactory position. Clinical data are a major reference for the indication and design of foot orthoses (1).

Foot orthoses are usually classified in several categories:

- corrective orthoses, to correct reversible static disorders;
- accommodation orthoses, which are palliative and relieve fixed deformities by being closely fitted to the foot;
- preventive orthoses, which distribute stress and avoid excessive pressure in some areas.

Each foot is individual and there is no such thing as a standard orthosis (or shoe) for a given deformity.

Materials and composition of the orthosis (12, 17, 22)

Three types of materials are used: leather and leatherwork, glues, materials for orthotic inserts.

When choosing a material for the orthotic inserts, its characteristics are assessed: the weight, the density, the shock-absorbing capacity, the strength and the resilience. Various fabrication techniques are also considered, such as baromolding or thermomolding, thermoforming, thermowelding, cutting and polishing.

To make up the orthosis, the practitioner chooses among the various materials available those which seem most suited to each case, depending on the desired therapeutic effect and the condition of the foot (correction of hyperpronation, loss of fatpad or not, bursitis under metatarsal heads).

Plantar orthoses may be rigid to give support and better stability. Soft orthoses give better shock absorption and the movement of the foot when walking is more natural. Flexible and rigid materials may be combined in a composite orthosis (16).

The orthosis must always lend itself to modification at a later stage (2, 8, 28) and it is adjusted according to the patient's observations or after the control examination.

Wearing shoes and orthoses

Variations in size and volume of the rheumatoid foot during the course of the disease and the bulk of the orthosis sometimes make it difficult to wear conventional shoes. A specially adapted mass-produced shoe therefore proves necessary:
- a mass-produced therapeutic shoe for permanent use;
- or another range of material for temporary uses, some models of which are already available.

A custom-made shoe may later be necessary to attempt to correct deformities or provide appropriate footwear. Custom-made shoes have the advantage of being made specially for the individual. They act on the forefoot and on the hindfoot, with specific orthoses and shoes, thus providing an optimal fit. They are chiefly indicated when all the possibilities previously mentioned have proved to be unsuitable and when surgery is not indicated.

Systematic history taking and assessment of the rheumatoid foot before designing shoes and orthoses (cf clinical chapter)

The patient's gait should be observed. Hindfoot valgus deformity everts the forefoot and increases the load on the first metatarsal, the talonavicular joint and navicular-medial cuneiform joint (3, 6), which places stress on the subtalar joint complex and the joints of the medial side of the foot. Antalgic supination may occur (16, 28). The leg axes and hip rotation should be evaluated, as well as the angle of gait: when the latter is increased there can be excessive pressure and even increased midtarsal flattening. However, when the angle of gait is reduced this can result in problems of inversion.

With the foot in weight-bearing and in neutral position, the possibilities for correcting deformities are noted, as well as the mobility or stiffness of joints: subtalar mobility, ankle dorsiflexion, midtarsal joint and toe mobility. The practitioner should observe the reduction of hindfoot pronation when the patient is standing on tiptoe.

Pressure spots (here the foot-print is important), bursitis, callosities, trophic alterations, bony prominences, toe deviation, pulses and atrophy of the plantar fat pad or intrinsic muscles are assessed. The importance of pain, spontaneous or induced by pressure or by mobilisation, and of local inflammation is assessed.

After this thorough evaluation, suitable shoes and orthoses can be prescribed following the recommendations already given and those which will be mentioned later.

Indications

In early RA when there is no foot and ankle involvement, some basic advice on proper footwear must be given.

- Even if no deformity is observed, the patient should already be advised to wear adequate footwear; shoe shape and size are very important considerations for obtaining a good fit. Shoes that are too firm must be avoided, as well as shoes that are too soft. The worst situation is often observed in elderly persons. If they wear slippers or worn-out old shoes they will become unaccustomed to proper shoes, aggravating the causes of deformity mentioned above (30).
- If static disorders are already present the prescription of preventive plantar orthoses is justified (25), particularly if the hindfoot is pronated (fig. 1).

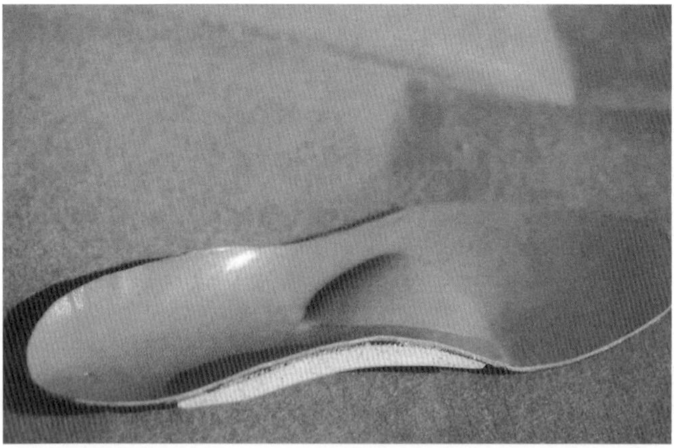

Fig. 1 - Preventive orthose: stabilizing cup, firm arch support and a median support behind the metatarsal heads (courtesy of Philippe Magnin).

Developing metatarsalgia in an inflammatory forefoot without metatarsophalangeal joint erosion.

The patient may spontaneously complain of metatarsalgia or it may only be observed during systematic assessment of the rheumatoid foot (pain on lateral compression of the forefoot, for instance). Suitable shoes and plantar orthoses should be prescribed. The latter should be used early, as soon as there is inflammatory involvement of the foot, for effective correction and relief (14, 21, 28).

The plantar orthosis may have several components. The retrocapital metatarsal bar elevates all the metatarsal heads posteriorly and its shape can modify the statics of the forefoot. When it is flat and uniform it tends to spread the forefoot. A bulge in the median area narrows the metatarsus and relieves the median heads, especially if it is high and abrupt in its front part. Lastly, the metatarsal bar provides frontal stabilization (7).

Orthoses with median cavities beneath the metatarsal heads relieve the forefoot but maintain the forefoot deformity which little by little will become fixed. Such a purely palliative solution, which is better accepted by the patient and therefore easier to implement for the physician, can sometimes have harmful consequences. In this way a stiffened flat forefoot which is not correctable can be created, with its own complications. Cavities are therefore only indicated in cases with severe metatarsophalangeal joint deterioration and fixed deformities, and in cases where surgery is impossible. The aim of these orthoses can only be palliative.

In fixed metatarsophalangeal deformity, inserts under and in front of the metatarsal heads may be added to the inserts described above, on each side of one or several metatarsal heads. The empty space thus created, of varying length, can provide an area of relief. Such inserts are more effective in the last phase of gait. However, they may make the orthosis bulky, which increases the risk of rubbing between the forefoot (particularly the toes) and the shoe.

When there is rheumatoid inflammation of the forefoot, inflammatory involvement of the tarsus must always be looked for (5, 6, 32).

When metatarso-phalangeal joint erosion or clinical midhindfoot involvement is observed.

On an X-ray, metatarsal erosion and midfoot flattening appear at the same stage of disease duration and before narrowing of the tarsal joints can be visualised (5). This emphasizes the value of detecting clinical inflammatory involvement of the tarsus as early as possible. Therefore, as soon as metatarsal erosion is observed it is better to consider that the midhindfoot may begin to flatten and to take steps to prevent deformity.

The patient may sometimes complain of anterior or posterior ankle pain, particularly on uneven ground. In fact this is of midtarsal or subtalar origin. In other cases patients may complain of medial ankle or medial heel pain, and the possibility of a posterior tibial tendon lesion must be considered and looked for. This description of the features which should draw the practitioner's attention to localised inflammatory involvement of the midhindfoot is not exhaustive (cf clinical chapter).

Tarsal collapse and dislocation, often of insidious onset, is particularly disabling at an advanced stage (5, 6). An orthosis must therefore be prescribed very early on when the deformity can still be controlled. Plantar support must be sufficiently firm to be effective (21, 30, 33). However, skin atrophy and wasting of the plantar soft tissues often lead to problems of local tolerance. Thermoformed orthoses can be of help in this case. At the least we can hope to obtain ankylosis of the foot in a functionally acceptable position (6, 21). An orthosis including a stabilizing heel cup with good embedment which firmly holds the calcaneus and decreases subtalar motion aims to avoid pronation. A firm medial arch support prevents midfoot flattening. Finally, support behind the metatarsal heads and increased median support (a bulge) maintains a more physiological shape of the forefoot and relieves pressure on the metatarsal heads. The firm thermomolded polyethylene foam of which the orthosis is made is covered with thinner more supple foam which provides cushioning as needed (figs. 2 and 3). High-upper shoes or leg-hindfoot orthoses may be very useful in this case. Often high-upper shoes with medial and lateral stabilizers are more effective if they are custom-made and therefore give better fit.

If there are talocrural and subtalar lesions, these joints should be supported (11, 17, 21). Leg-hindfoot orthoses or made-to-measure shoes with high uppers are often the chosen solution, when pain and flexible deformities are disabling and when surgery is not indicated (11, 18). Well-made and of suitable materials, they can more easily correct a tendency to deformity.

When the foot deformities are fixed and when surgery is not indicated, the orthosis attempts to give relief by using palliative (and therefore non-corrective) flexible or semi-flexible materials.

Whatever the stage of the lesion, when metatarso-phalangeal pain is important, when dorsiflexion of the ankle is limited, rocker shoes are particularly indicated (fig. 4). However, one must be careful; the pitch on the heel and on the forefoot must not be too important: there is a risk of instability.

Conclusion

Adequate shoes and orthoses are an important tool in the treatment of the rheumatoid foot. They must provide function as close as possible to physiological biomechanics and give relief from pain.

The practitioner must bear in mind the severity not only of the lesions of the foot and ankle, but also of the patient's other joints. Patient care requires optimal planning, particularly regarding surgery at the appropriate time, so management involves a care-team approach.

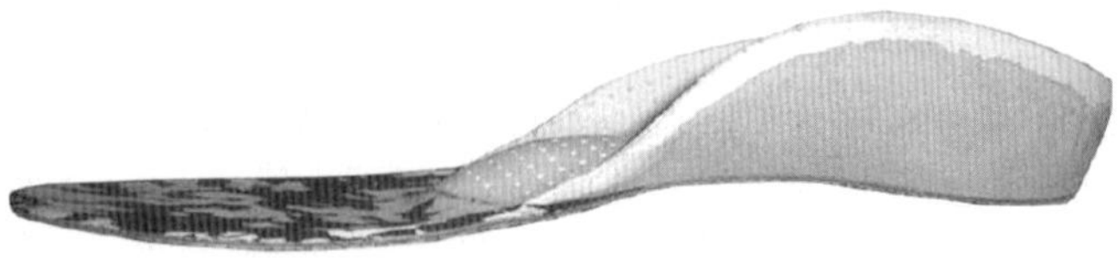

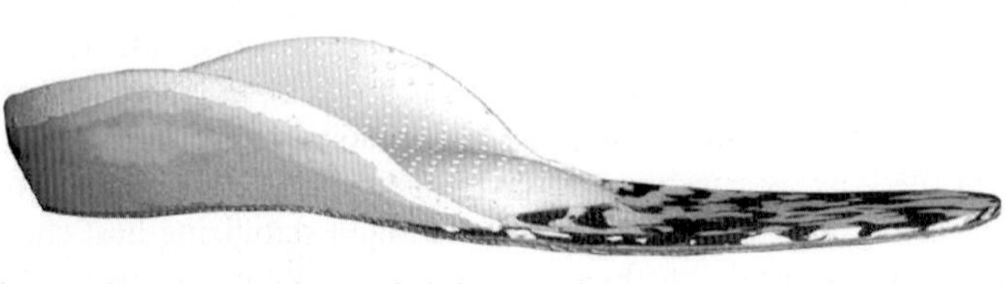

Fig. 2 and 3 - Plantar orthose included in special shoes (custom-made or not): very stabilizing cup, firm medial arch support and median support behind metatarsal heads.

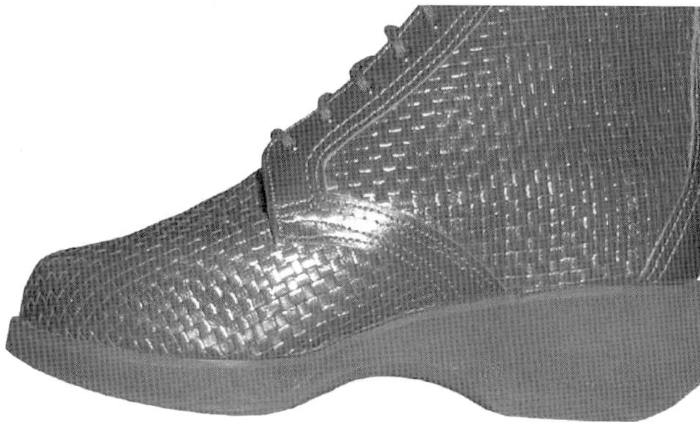

Fig. 4 - High-upper rocker-shoe (courtesy of Jerome Bonnin, DEAGE company).

References

1. Acker D, Bouysset M, Guaydier-Souquières G *et al.* (1998) Foot orthoses. In: Bouysset M (ed) Bone and joint disorders of the foot and ankle. A rheumatological approach. Paris Springer-Verlag France: 329-40
2. Anderson EG (1990) The rheumatoid foot: a sideways look. Ann Rheum Dis 4: 851-857
3. Arangio GA, Phillippy DC, Xiao D, Gu WK, Salathe EP (2000) Subtalar pronation – relationship to the medial longitudinal arch loading in the normal foot. Foot Ankle Int 21 (3): 216-20
4. Blake R, Ferguson H (1992) Limb length discrepancies. J Am Podriatr Med Assoc 82: 33-8
5. Bouysset M, Tebib J, Noel E *et al.* (1992) When should orthopaedic treatment be prescribed to avoid the flattening of the rheumatoid foot? Clin Rheumatol 11 (4): 580-52
6. Bouysset M, Tebib J, Noel E *et al.* (2002) Rheumatoid flat foot and deformity of the first ray. J Rheumatol 29: 903-5
7. Braun S (1995) Orthèses plantaires et métatarsalgies mécaniques. Rhumatologie 47: 95-102
8. Budiman-Mak E, Conrad K, Roach J *et al.* (1993) Can foot orthoses prevent deformity in rheumatoid arthritis? American College of Rheumatology, San Antonio Nov 7-11
9. Cavanagh PR, Ulbrecht JS (1991) Plantar pressure in the diabetic foot. In: Sammarco GJ (ed) The foot in diabetes. Philadelphia, Lea and Febiger, p 947
10. Clancy WG (1980) Runner's injuries. Part one. Am J Sports Med 8: 137-44

11. Claustre J (1979) Le pied rhumatoïde. Problèmes podologiques pratiques. Rev Rhum 46: 673-8
12. Claustre J, Olie L (1982) Orthèses plantaires et matériaux utilisables et techniques. In: Claustre J, Simon L (eds) Troubles congénitaux et statiques du pied. Orthèses plantaires. Monographies de podologie 2. Paris, Masson p. 203
13. Dixon ASJ (1971) The rheumatoid foot. Mod Trends Rheumatol 2: 158-73
14. Gold RH, Basset LW (1982) Radiologic evaluation of the arthritic foot. Foot Ankle 2: 332-341
15. Gould JS (1982) Conservative management of the hypersensitive foot in rheumatoid arthritis. Foot Ankle 2: 224-9
16. Grifka JK (1997) Shoes and insoles for patients with rheumatoid foot disease. Clin Orthop 340: 18-25
17. Henderson WH, Campbell J, Wardossian WH *et al.* (1967) The UC-BL shoe insert: casting and fabrication. Biomechanics Laboratory of the University of California
18. Hunt GC, Fromherz WA, Gerber LH, Hurwitz SR (1987) Hindfoot pain treated by a leg-hindfoot orthosis. Physical Therapy 67 (9): 1384-88
19. Janisse DJ (1998) Prescription footwear for arthritis of the foot and ankle. Clin Orthop 349: 100-7
20. Janisse DJ (2000) Orthoses, shoewear, and shoe modifications. In: Myerson MS (ed) Foot and ankle disorders. Philadelphia, WB Saunders, vol 1: 195-212
21. Kitaoka HB (1989) Rheumatoid hindfoot. Orthop Clin North Am 20: 593-604
22. Lapeyre-Gros F (1996) Le chaussage du pied rhumatoïde. Méd Chir Pied 12: 196-201
23. Mereday C, Dolan C, Lusskin MD (1972) Evaluation of the University of California biomechanics laboratory shoe insert in "flexible" pes planus. Clin Orthop 82: 45-58
24. National Shoe Retailers Association, Prescription Footwear Association, American Orthopaedic Foot and Ankle Society (1995) 10 points of proper shoe fit. Columbia, MD. NSRA/PFA/AOFAS
25. Potter TA, Khus JG (1972) Painful feet. In: Hollander JL (ed) Arthritis and allied conditions. Lea and Febiger, Philadelphia
26. Rosenfield JS, Trepman E (2000) Treatment of sesamoid disorders with a rocker sole shoe modification. Foot Ankle Int 21 (4): 914-5
27. Rossi W (1982) The shoe counter and the foot. J Am Pod Ass 72 (6): 326-7
28. Tillmann K (1979) The rheumatoid foot. G Thieme, Stuttgart, pp 44-56
29. Trepman E, Yeo SJ (1995) Nonoperative treatment of metatarsophalangeal joint synovitis. Foot Ankle Int 16: 771-7
30. Vainio K (1991) The rheumatoid foot. A clinical study with pathological and roentgenological comments. 1956. Clin Orthop 265: 4-8
31. Van Schie C, Ulbrecht JS, Becker MB, Cavanagh PR (2000) Design criteria for rigid rocker shoes. Foot Ankle Int 21 (10): 833-44
32. Vidigal E, Jacoby RK, Dixon J, Ratliff AH, Kirkup J (1975) The foot in chronic rheumatoid arthritis. Ann Rheum Dis 34: 292-5
33. Wenger DR, Mauldin D, Speck G, Morgan D, Lieber RL (1989) Corrective shoes and inserts as treatment for flexible flatfoot in infants and children. J Bone Joint Surg 71A: 800-10
34. Wu KK (1990) Foot orthoses. Williams & Wilkins, Baltimore, pp 71-8 and 328-33

Additional references

. Budiman-Mak E, Conrad KJ, Roach KE (1991) The Foot Function Index: a measure of foot pain and disability. J Clin Epidemiol 44: 561-70

. Dereymaeker G, Mulier T, Stuer P *et al.* (1997) Pedodynographic measurements after forefoot reconstruction in rheumatoid arthritis patients. Foot Ankle Int 18: 270-6

. Jackson L, Binning J, Potter J (2004) Plantar pressures in rheumatoid arthritis using prefabricated metatarsal padding. Journal of the American Podiatric Medical Association (J-Am-Podiatr-Med-Assoc), May-Jun, Vol 94 (3): 239-45

. Kavlak Y Uygur F, Korkmaz C, Bek N (2003) Outcome of orthoses intervention in the rheumatoid foot. Foot and Ankle international (Foot-Ankle-Int), Jun, vol 24 (6): 494-9

. Wickman-Amy M, Pinzur-Michael S, Kadanoff R (2004) Health-related quality of life for patients with rheumatoid arthritis foot involvement. Foot and Ankle international (Foot-Ankle-Int), Jan, 25 (1): 19-26

. Woodbrun J, Helliwell PS, Barker S (J6Rheumatol) 2003 Nov, 30 (11): 2356-64, Changes in 3D joint kinematics support the continuous use of orthoses in the management of painful rearfoot deformity in rheumatoid arthritis.

Corticosteroid injections and synoviortheses of the foot and ankle in rheumatoid arthritis

M. Bouysset, P. Hugueny, B. Gintz, J. Jalby and J. Tebib

There have recently been considerable advances in the medical treatment of rheumatoid arthritis (RA), particularly since the introduction of anti-TNF agents. Nevertheless rheumatoid inflammation may persist in some joints.

Corticosteroid injections give localized concentration of the active drug, resulting in fewer adverse effects than with systemic corticotherapy (27, 33). They were first used in 1951 (15) and, whether intra-articular or periarticular, are a treatment of choice in rheumatology, particularly in the foot and ankle (13). Close compliance with the indications and contraindications and strict asepsis reduce the risk of potentially serious adverse effects.

Synoviorthesis may be useful in some cases if corticosteroid injections are ineffective.

Corticosteroid injections

Indications

The indications are inflammatory rheumatisms when localized acute episodes are not controlled by systemic medication (13). Intra-articular corticosteroids have no effect on the progression of bone erosions, nor on joint destruction due to synovitis (11).

Absolute contraindications (11, 17, 33)

Any infection whether local (joint or skin) or distant, the presence of exogenous material (metal in particular), allergy to an excipient or to the contrast agent which may be used during the procedure, known fracture or osteonecrosis, immune deficiency and coagulation disorders or anticoagulant treatment must be excluded. If the patient is receiving anti-vitamin K medication, extreme care must be taken and the physician who prescribed the treatment must decide if and how it should be interrupted. A free interval must be allowed between discontinuation of anticoagulants and the corticosteroid injection. The prothrombin index must be equal to or greater than 65% before the injection can be given.

Relative contraindications (11)

Diabetes is not an absolute contraindication but there must be no suspicion of any infection (dental, urinary, or mammary). During the procedure of injection the rules of asepsis must be strictly adhered to. The patient must be informed that there is a risk of transient glycaemia increase after injection of corticosteroids. Glycaemia above 2.50 g/l (13.50 mm/l) or unstable diabetes are absolute contraindications.

Corticosteroid injections must be avoided in patients on haemodialysis because of the risk of infection and because their effect is poor.

One month must elapse after healing of an active stomach or duodenal ulcer. The same applies to some current virus infections (particularly hepatitis, herpes, chicken-pox, shingles…) and to psychosis which is not controlled by treatment.

General principles

In the foot, valid antitetanus protection is obligatory. An X-ray of the affected joint must be obtained before injection. Any joint effusion must be drained and analyzed beforehand. If there is no joint effusion, minimal biological tests are prescribed: sedimentation rate and glycaemia, completed by further tests if there is any doubt. Surgery on the involved bone and joint planned within the following six months is a contraindication to intra-articular corticosteroid injection.

Platelet anti-aggregation treatment (salicylic acid, ticlopidine) is not a contraindication for corticosteroid injection particularly in the talocrural joint. The fine needles which are now currently used, with manual compression applied locally for one to two minutes after the injection, make this a feasible procedure. If the patient is receiving clopidogrel, treatment should be discontinued eight days before injection and resumed the evening after injection. Pregnancy is not a contraindication to corticosteroid injection (11, 23).

The minimum effective dose should always be used; this varies depending on the joint.

Injection sites

Intra-articular injections: talocrural, subtalar, midtarsal and metatarsophalangeal joints. The bursae between the phalangeal heads should preferentially be injected as this is less damaging for the joint capsule and the anti-inflammatory effect on the nearby joints is still satisfactory. As the joint capsule of the metatarsophalangeal joints is subject to considerable mechanical stress, it is more likely to be weakened by intra-articular injections (8) and there is a greater risk of deformity.

Peri-articular corticosteroid injections on the foot are done for tenosynovitis (tendon of tibialis anterior and tibialis posterior muscle, tendons of fibularis, flexor and extensor muscles), for retrocalcaneal bursae, the tarsal tunnel and the plantar side of the heel. The specific risks of such injections must be considered before the procedure.

The technical rules for injection must be strictly followed (3, 11, 16, 17, 32). The use of image guidance for intra-articular steroid injection is particularly recommended in patients with hindfoot synovitis (28).

Complete synovial fluid aspiration before corticosteroid injection reduces the risk of relapse (35). The joint should be immobilized for 48 hours afterwards to lessen extra-articular diffusion of the injected drug (9).

Adverse effects

Adverse effects are rare if the above-mentioned recommendations are followed. The main risks are septic arthritis and tendinous lesions (tears caused by the needle in intra-tendinous injection or the side-effects of the corticosteroids themselves).

Local adverse effects

Septic arthritis: its incidence is very low (between 1/14.000 and 1/50.000 injections) but this is a medical and surgical emergency where rapid diagnosis and treatment are essential to limit functional and sometimes fatal damage. It occurs 24 to 48 hours or more after the injection (episodes of inflammatory crystal arthropathy have an earlier onset). Features generally include fever, local manifestations with a red, hot, swollen joint which cannot be mobilized and there may be signs of extension (tenosynovitis, lymphangitis, swollen lymph nodes).

Diagnosis is sometimes difficult because the septic signs are mistaken for a rheumatoid symptom and the clinical features are deceptive (subacute onset, irregular fever), accounting for delayed diagnosis. Laboratory tests show elevated sedimentation rate and C-reactive protein with hyperleucocytosis. If there is a fluid collection or talocrural arthritis, aspiration and analysis of synovial fluid are very helpful for diagnosis and for isolation of bacteria by direct examination or by culture. The possibility of tuberculosis must not be forgotten (11, 12, 33).

Microcrystal arthropathies occur in 1 to 2% of cases, 4 to 12 hours after injection with cortiscosteroid suspensions. Fever and hyperleucocytosis may be observed. Analysis of synovial fluid reveals intracellular crystals which may be observed one month or more after triamcinolone hexacetonide injection. These features decrease spontaneously and resolve in 1 to 3 days.

Apatitic calcifications are sometimes observed after triamcinolone hexacetonide injection. Often they are asymptomatic. *Local allergy* to the excipient is possible. *Destructive arthropathies* have been described but it is uncertain whether they are due to corticosteroids. However, it is prudent not to exceed one injection per month. Localized cutaneous, subcutaneous or muscular *atrophy* are more likely after use of fluorinated corticosteroids. Cutaneous or muscular *necrosis* may occur.

The risk of tendinous lesions or plantar fascia rupture secondary to corticosteroid injection should be borne in mind (18). Intra-tendinous injection is never done because of the possibility of rupture. Peritendinous injection, sometimes very useful, may lead to involvement of tendinous structures, particularly when injections are frequent. Spontaneous tendon rupture after local corticosteroid injection has been noted in several studies (1, 2, 5, 6, 10, 19, 21, 31) and its weakening effect has been documented (19, 25, 34). Kennedy and Willis (19) demonstrated early collagen necrosis and disruption of collagen fibers in rabbit Achilles tendons injected with corticosteroid; they also reported complete biomechanical reconstitution by 6 weeks after injection. For Acevedo (1), there is an average time to rupture after injection of approximately 10 weeks. This would suggest a delayed or inadequate healing response after corticosteroid injection (2, 21, 31). The histopathological changes observed by Kennedy are not very different to those observed in human posterior tibial tendon insufficiency since this pathology displays disruption of collagen bundle structure and orientation (25). These observations suggest degenerative tendinosis and a non-specific repair response to tissue injury which represent significant intrinsic changes in posterior tibial tendon architecture. This may compromise the tendon and predispose it to rupture under physiological loads (24).

These findings indicate that caution is required with corticosteroid injection in tendons subject to high mechanical stresses (particurlaly calcaneal tendon and tendon of the tibialis posterior muscle). Although controversy remains, corticosteroid injections (intra-articular or peritendinous) seem to produce a change in tendons that could ultimately lead to rupture. Should an injection be necessary activity should be reduced or the affected area immobilized for two weeks following injection to decrease the possibility of rupture (18).

Other adverse effects: haematoma even when there is no coagulation disorder. Irritation of a nerve may set off an electrical discharge which ceases when the needle position is changed.

General adverse effects

Anaphylactic shock is very rare but extremely serious (20, 22, 26, 30).

Transient hypotension is less serious and more frequent with malaise, pallor, sometimes nausea and sweating. The patient usually recovers if placed perfectly supine with the legs raised but injection of atropine (1/4 mg) may be necessary, while bearing in mind the contra-indications of this product.

Flushes, headaches and vasomotor disturbances can last several days. A single corticosteroid injection may transiently inhibit or affect the function of the hypothalamo-hypophyseal-adrenal axis. Repeated injections of large amounts of corticosteroids may lead to secondary hypercorticism with cutaneous, vascular, muscular and metabolic features.

Osteonecrosis may be due to hypercorticism. Lymphocytopenia and eosinopenia have also been described.

Synoviortheses (4, 14)

Synoviortheses (medical synovectomy) consist of intra-articular injection of osmic acid or radioactive agents, as a supplement to local corticotherapy. Monitoring with arthrography and an image intensifier is necessary. It is now common practice for synoviortheses to be carried out mainly in the talocrural joint. After failure of one to two injections of triamcinolone hexacetonide, osmic acid or a radioactive agent are injected after xylocaine and followed by a corticosteroid injection. The joint must then be immobilized for 48 hours.

Synoviortheses are more effective in less advanced osteoarticular lesions and is very useful in cases of single joint arthritis when there is no contraindication (allergy to iodine or to local anaesthetics, joint puncture or intra-articular injection less than one week before synoviortheses). The contraindications to corticosteroid injection that we have already mentioned must be respected.

Osmic acid (4) is only indicated in the talocrural joint; there is a risk of retrograde diffusion and this drug is relatively little used. But there is no risk of systemic contamination and osmic acid may be helpful in young patients when use of radioactive agents is contraindicated, in particular in order to avoid exceeding the total radiation dose (4).

Pain and fever may develop during the 24 hours after injection.

Black coloured urine and rare cases of skin pigmentation may be observed. Cutaneous necrosis has been described. The toxic effect of osmic acid on cartilage has been stressed (4).

Radiation synoviortheses (table I): the agent used depends on the joint concerned. Extra-articular irradiation is reduced with use of short-lived radioactive agents but because of the theoretical haematological and cancerigenic risk, the dose injected in each joint and during each injection should be limited.

Rhenium 186 is used for the ankle joint at the dose of 2 mCi.

Erbium 169 is exceptionally used for the metatarsophalangeal joints. In rheumatoid arthritis, this radioisotope seems to be less effective than triamcinolone hexacetonide (7, 29).

Table I - Radioisotopes used in treatment of the rheumatoid foot and ankle.

Isotope	Half-life (days)	Type of radiation	Tissue penetration (mm)	
			Mean	Maximum
Erbium	9.4 j	$\beta\ \gamma$	0.5	0.9
Rhenium	3.7 j	$\beta\ \gamma$	1.2	3.7
Yttrium	2.7 j	β	3.6	11

Conclusion: Corticosteroid injections and synoviortheses are very useful therapeutic procedures in RA. They may precede long-term treatment in single joint arthritis or they may follow it to control one or several inflammatory joints. They make it possible to delay or to avoid a surgical procedure in some cases (particularly synovectomy in rheumatoid arthritis).

References

1. Acevedo JI, Beskin JL (1998) Complications of plantar fascia rupture associated with corticosteroid injection. Foot Ankle 19: 91-7
2. Ahstrom JP (1988) Spontaneous rupture of the plantar fascia. Am J Sports Med 16: 306-7
3. Amor B (1998) Les infiltrations articulaires: technique de préparation et implication médico-légale. La Lettre du Rhumatologue 239: 14-5
4. Ayral X, Menkes CJ (1997) Traitement de la polyarthrite rhumatoïde. Stratégie des gestes locaux. Expansion Scientifique Française, pp. 233-45
5. Balasubramaniam P, Prathap K (1972) The effect of injection of hydrocortisone into rabbit calcaneal tendons. J Bone Joint Surg 54B: 729-34
6. Bedi SS, Ellis W (1970) Spontaneous rupture of the calcaneal tendon in rheumatoid arthritis after local steroid injection. Ann Rheum Dis 29: 494-5
7. Bouvier M, Bouysset M, Bonvoisin B *et al.* (1983) Synoviorthèses à l'erbium 169 et infiltrations d'hexacétonide de triamcinolone dans les arthrites métatarso-phalangiennes des rhumatismes inflammatoires chroniques. Rev Rhum 50 (4): 267-71
8. Chandler GN, Wright V (1958) Deleterious effect of intra-articular hydrocortisone. Lancet II: 661
9. Daragon A (1997) Faut-il imposer une immobilisation après une injection intra-articulaire de glucocorticoïde. La Lettre du Rhumatologue 237: 20-1
10. Ford LT, DeBender J (1979) Tendon rupture after local steroid injection. South Med J 72: 827-30
11. Fritz P (1996) Injection articulaire et périarticulaire de glycocorticoïde et d'anesthésique. In: T Bardin, D Kuntz (ed). Thérapeutique Rhumatologique. Flammarion, pp. 63-89
12. Gaillard F, Rémy G (1997) Les arthrites septiques du pied et de la cheville. In: M Bouysset (ed). Le Pied en Rhumatologie. Springer Verlag France, pp. 103-8
13. Geppert MJ, Sobel M, Bohne WH (1992) The rheumatoid foot: part I. Forefoot. Foot Ankle 13: 550-8
14. Gintz B, Gaudin Ph, Dumolard A, Phelip X (1998) Le traitement médical du pied rhumatoïde. Stratégie thérapeutique. Méd. Chir. Pied14: 49-52
15. Hollander JL, Brown EM, Jessar RA (1951) Hydrocortisone and cortisone injected into arthritic joints. JAMA 147: 1629-35
16. Kahn MF (1990) Les injections intra-articulaires de corticoïdes. Rev Prat (Paris), 40: 531-5
17. Kaplan G (1998) Les accidents infectieux des infiltrations. La Lettre du Rhumatologue. Suppl to n°242, p. 9
18. Karpman RR, McComb JE, Volz RG (1980) Tendon rupture following local steroid injection. Postgrad Med 68: 169-76

19. Kennedy JC, Willis RB (1976) The effects of local steroid injection on tendons: a biomechanical and microscopic correlative study. Am J Sports Med 4: 11-21
20. Larson LG (1989) Anaphylactic shock after intra-articular administration of triamcinolone acetonide in a 35 year old female. Scand J Rheumatol 18: 441-2
21. Leach R, Jones R, Silva T (1978) Rupture of the plantar fascia in athletes. J Bone Joint Surg 60A: 537-9
22. Mace S, Vadas P, Pruzanski W (1997) Anaphylactic shock induced by intra-articular injection of methylprednisolone acetate. J Rheumatol 24: 1191-4
23. Mejjad O, Favre S (1997) Anticoagulants et antiagrégants plaquettaires; l'infiltration est-elle possible, et comment? La Lettre du Rhumatologue - n° 237: 12-3
24. Mosier SM, Lucas DR, Pomeroy G, Manoli A II (1998) Pathology of the posterior tibial tendon in posterior tibial tendon insuffiency. Foot Ankle 19: 520-4
25. Noyes FR, Nussbaum NS, Torvik PJ, Cooper S (1975) Biomechanical and ultrastructural changes in ligaments and tendons after local corticosteroid injections. J Bone Joint Surg 57A: 876-82
26. O'Duffy EK, Clunie GP, Lui D, Edward JC, Ell PJ (1999) Double blind glucocorticoid controlled trial of samarium 153 particulate hydroxyapatite radiation for chronic knee synovitis. Ann Rheum Dis 58: 554-8
27. Rappaport G, Gerster JC (1988) Les injections locales de corticostéroides en pratique rhumatologique. Méd Hygiène 46: 890-6
28. Remedios D, Martin K, Kaplan G, Mitchell R, Woo P, Rooney M (1997) Juvenile chronic arthritis: diagnosis and management of tibio-talar and subtalar disease. Br J Rheumatol 36: 1214-17
29. Ruotsi A, Hypen M, Rekonen A, Oka M (1979) Erbium-169 versus triamcinolone hexacetonide in the treatment of rheumatoid finger joints. Ann Rheum Dis 38: 45-7
30. Saraux A, Garo B, Devauchelle V *et al.* (2000) Choc anaphylactique aux corticoïdes: conduite à tenir. La Lettre du Rhumatologue 264: 20-2
31. Sellman Jr (1994) Plantar fascia rupture associated with corticosteroid injection. Foot Ankle 15: 376-81
32. Seror S, Pluvinager P, Lecoq L *et al.* (1999) Evaluation du risque d'accident après infiltration de dérivés cortisonés en milieu rhumatologique libéral. Enquête portant sur 1160 000 infiltrations. Réflexion Rhumatologique 13: 15-20
33. Vergne P, Bertin Ph, Bonnet Ch, Treves R (1997) Effets secondaires locaux et généraux des infiltrations. La Lettre du Rhumatologue 237: 24-5
34. Vogel HG (1969) Zum Wirkung von hormonen auf physikalische und chemische eigenschaften des binde und stützgewebes. Arzneimittelforschung 19: 96-101
35. Weitoft T, Uddenfeldt P (2000) Importance of synovial fluid aspiration when injecting intra-articular corticosteroids. Ann Rheum Dis 59: 233-5

Additional references

- Csizy M, Hintermann B. (2001) Rupture of the Achilles tendon after local steroid injection ; Case reports and consequences for treatment Swiss-Surg, Vol: 7, P: 184-9
- Gill Sanjitpal S, Gelbke Martin K, Mattson Steve L, Anderson Mark W, Hurwitz Shepard R. (2004) Fluoroscopically guided low volume peritendinous corticosteroid infection for Achilles tendinopathy. A safety study J Bone Joint Surg Am Apr, Vol:86-A (4), P: 802-6

- Kotnis R A, Halstead J C, Hormbrey P J. (1999) Atraumatic bilateral Achilles tendon rupture : an association of systemic steroid treatment J Accid Emerg Med Sep, Vol: 16(5), P: 378-9
- Leppilahti J, Orava S., Total Achilles tendon rupture. A review Sports-Med 1998 Feb, Vol: 25 (2), P: 79-100
- Martin D F, Carlson C S, Berry J, Reboussin B A, Gordon E S, Smith B P., (1999) Effect of injected versus iontophoretic corticosteroid on the rabbit tendon South Med J jun, Vol: 92(6), P: 600-8
- Shrier I, Matheson G O, Kohl H W (1996) 3rd. Achilles tendonitis : are corticosteroid injections useful or harmful ? Clin J Sport Med Oct, Vol: 6 (4), P: 245-50
- Tsai Wen Chung, Tang Fuk Tan, Wong May Kuen, Pang Jong Hwei S. (2003) Inhibition of tendon cell migration by dexamethasone is correlated with reduced alpha-smooth muscle actin gene expression: a potential mechanism of delayed tendon healing J-Orthop-Res Mar, Vol: 21 (2), P: 265-71
- Wong Margaret Wan Nar, Tang Yin Nei, Fu Sai Chuen, Lee Kwong Man, Chan Kai Ming, (2004) Triamcinolone suppresses human tenocyte cellular activity and collagen synthesis Clin-Orthop Apr (421), P: 277-81
- Wong Margaret Wan Nar, Tang Yvonne Yin Nei, Lee Simon Kwong Man, Fu Bruma Sai Chuen, Chan Barbara Pui, Chan Cavor Kai Ming (2003). Effect of dexamethasone on cultured human tenocytes and its reversibility by platelet-derived growth factor J Bone Joint Surg Am Oct, Vol: 85 A (10), P: 1914-20

Forefoot surgery for rheumatoid arthritis

Y. Tourné

Introduction

If the foot is very frequently affected during the evolution of rheumatoid arthritis (between 70 and 90% of the cases according to authors) (1, 10, 11), the forefoot is almost always concerned. It is the way the disease starts in 25% of the cases (12, 54, 58).

Surgical treatment of forefoot lesions and deformities in rheumatoid arthritis is suggested in 30% of the cases (58, 63). Medical treatment whether per os or local prevails but the therapeutic program including surgery must be determined within a multidisciplinary team. Persistence of an aggressive synovial pannus, loss of cartilage, onset or worsening of toe deformities, leading the patient to an increasing functional debilitation are reasons to suggest surgery

Naturally, surgical treatment for the rheumatoid forefoot is included in the global medical therapeutic program (25) but must be discussed, if necessary, for the lower limb (5, 9, 69).

Basic surgical treatment

Physiopathology of deformities (1, 10, 57, 61, 69)

Progressive inflammatory tenosynovitis is responsible for the deformities by weakening the capsulo-ligamentous structures of the foot, by inducing paresis of the intrinsic muscles with disequilibrium between the plantar flexors and the dorsal flexors on one part, and the adductors, abductors on the other part. The extrinsic muscles also participate in the disorganization.

"Physiological" mechanical constraints (body weight, gravity) but also "pathological" (foot morphotype, disorders of the lower limb axes, variations of the hindfoot, inappropriate shoes) act on these destabilized joints and generate deformities then joint destruction.

These long-term deformities usually found in the static foot in this case present a rapid evolution.

Degenerative consequences

Without going back on the anatomo-pathological descriptions of the previous chapter, it seems interesting to present the most common clinical aspects which may help select surgical therapy.

Deformities are essentially fibular orientation of the toes with major hallux valgus, dorsal and lateral dislocation of the metatarso-phalangeal joint (excentered action of the extensor digitorum brevis muscle), clawed toe and triangular forefoot with major metatarsus varus, hallux valgus, quintus varus, and clawed toes with plantar prominence of metatarsal heads.

The bone and joint destructions combine osteolysis and osteoporosis and are located on the metatarsal heads and the proximal part of first phalanges.

Wearing shoes and walking become very difficult because of bursitis and *lateral overloading* which may induce fistulisation (first and fifth metatarsi), but also *plantar overloading* (plantar prominence of metatarsal heads and atrophy of the plantar fat pad) and *dorsal conflicts of* clawed toes with the shoe.

Goals of surgical treatment

Surgery must suppress deformities in a durable way, especially deviation of the great toe and dorsal dislocation of the toes.

It must also suppress lateral, dorsal and plantar conflicts of the foot.

It must improve the state of the plantar fat pad.

It must treat simultaneously bone and joint destructions and inflammatory synovial lesions.

Surgical treatment must restore forefoot function by following Lelievre's "ideal model" for the alignment of metatarsal heads and toes. By improving foot wear and walking, along with surgery of the hind foot, surgical treatment strongly and radically participates in restoring the patient's mobility and is perfectly integrated in the medico- surgical therapeutic strategy.

Various surgical techniques and Their results

History

In 1912, Hoffman (30) suggested using the resection of median metatarsal heads up to the neck, to suppress painful overloading, by a surgical plantar approach.

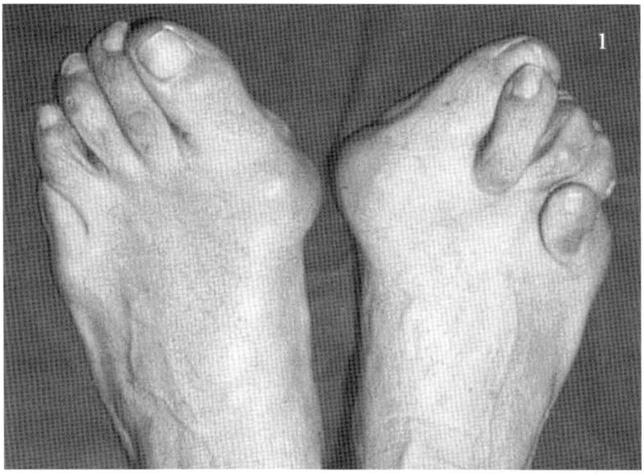

Fig. 1 -

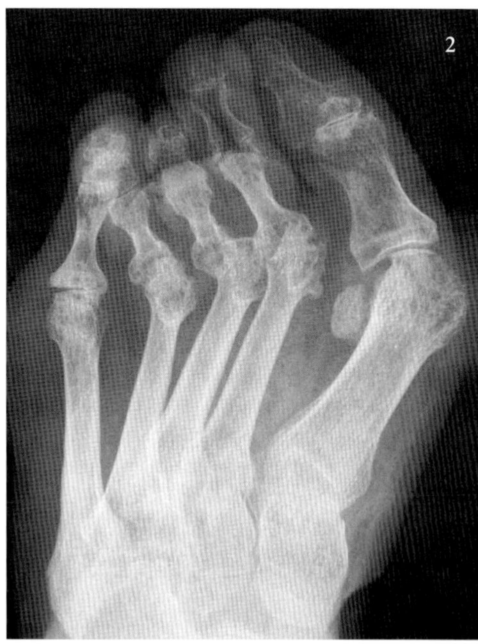

Fig. 2 -

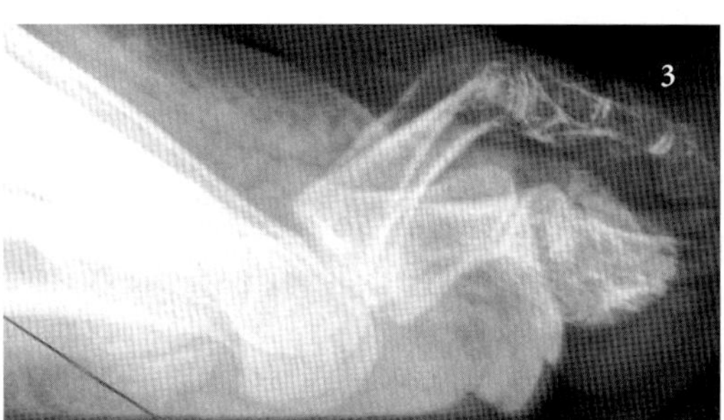

Fig. 3 -

Other authors modified this surgery by varying incision sites or the level of bone resection, whether metatarsal or phalangeal (13, 14, 23, 34, 35).

Lelievre (40) suggested a functional reconstruction by metatarsal realignment.

All authors agreed on the major and motor role of the first ray in the genesis and aggravation of forefoot deformities. Keller's(36, 37) resection arthroplasty was modified by Swanson (60) with a silicone implant arthroplasty of the hallux.

However, secondary disorders generated by this arthroplasty could lead to using arthrodesis of the first metatarso-phalangeal joint (21, 52, 74).

Combining surgery on the first ray and lateral rays has become the choice surgery for deformities of the rheumatoid forefoot.

Surgery of the first ray

Two concepts are still opposed:
- arthrodesis of the first metatarso-phalangeal joint.
- surgery allowing mobility of this joint (simple resection, prosthetic arthroplasty, surgery commonly used for hallux valgus).

Arthroplasty according to Keller

This consists in resecting the base of the hallux proximal phalange combined with a capsulo-ligamentous plasty allowing to reduce the phalangeal valgus.

A metatarso-phalangeal pinning improves the healing of soft parts. Partial or total resection of the metatarsal head improves the joint decompression. Mann (45), Clayton (13), or Johnson (33) have suggested interesting modifications.

However, all authors reported the degradation of results with time. Deformities came back in more than 50% of the cases (33, 51); retraction of the sesamoid belt due to extensive resections of the phalangeal base induced a muscular imbalance and insufficiency of the first ray: the forefoot was unstable and metatarsalgia reappeared. This data was confirmed by baropodometric studies: Stokes (59) compared a series of hallux valgus operated by Keller's resection to a series of healthy controls. Henry and Waugh (29) compared Keller's resection with arthrodesis. Their similar conclusions confirmed the lack of weight bearing under the first metatarsal head and excessive pressure on lateral metatarsal heads.

Silicone implant arthroplasty

This was developed by Swanson (60) to compensate the inconveniency of Keller's resection.

The prosthesis was made of a flexible double stem silicone elastomere implant which replaced the phalangeal base and the metatarsal head. Thus, it replaced the arthritic joint and compensated the deformity both because of its own design and because of the combined plasty of the soft parts.

The good short-term results (37) rapidly degraded in the medium and long term with fractures of implants, macrophage reaction to foreign bodies and loss of "push-off" power of the hallux (19, 26, 27). Some authors have reported frequent septic complications (2, 72).

To increase the life span of these implants, Swanson suggested adding titanium grommets which would decrease the wear of silicone and thus limit the implant fractures and macrophage reaction to foreign bodies with major osteolysis (60). Cracchiolo (17) seemed to be the only one author in favour of these implants reporting 86% of excellent results in the long term.

Clayton (14) did not find any significant difference on a comparative series of resection arthroplasty with or without use of Swanson's prosthesis. Kitaoka (38) suggested dealing with these silicone implant failures by simple excision combined with an extended synovectomy. But he confirms the increase of pressure under the lateral metatarsal heads.

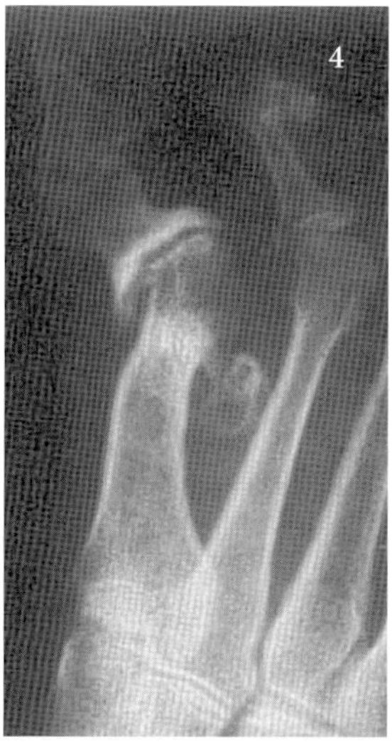

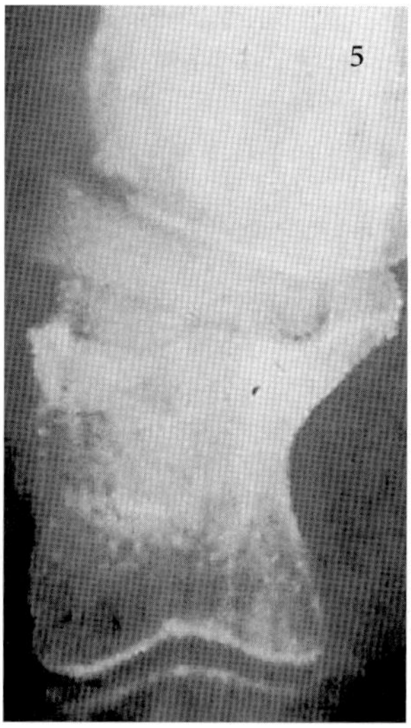

Fig. 4 -

Fig. 5 -

Arthrodesis of the first metatarso-phalangeal joint

Introduced by Watson (74) and DuVries (21), arthrodesis of the first metatarso-phalangeal joint has become the choice surgery in the treatment of deforming and debilitating lesions of the rheumatoid forefoot (44, 64, 65, 68).

The harmonious gait is preserved as long as the tibiotalar joint and inter-phalangeal joint of the hallux remain intact. The integrity of these joints has a strong bearing in the indication of arthrodesis for the great toe (22, 64, 70).

A consensus seems to be established on the position to set, for arthrodesis, between the great toe's proximal phalange and the first metatarsal.

Valgus between 15 and 20° and dorsiflexion between 25 and 35° is a good biomechanical compromise (8, 22, 41, 64). If dorsi-flexion is insufficient, the inter-phalangeal joint is rapidly overloaded. If dorsi-flexion is excessive, the pressure increases under the first metatarsal head.

Arthrodesis is performed by a medial approach. Joint surfaces are resected with a oscillating saw with plane cuts (valgus and dorsiflexion are usually calculated for the metatarsal cut) or by resurfacing using special reamers adapted to the convex metatarsal head and to the concave phalangeal base. Only cartilage is excised. The exact positioning of the 2 bone parts is facilitated by the morpho-adaptation of bony surfaces (15, 49).

Stabilizing the arthrodesis is important both for the quality of post-operative weight bearing and for the percentage of fusion. Various modes of osteosynthesis have been used (15, 46, 65, 69). Pins may migrate and lead to pseudarthrosis. Two crossed medial screws or an axial screw introduced in the medial condyle towards the phalange require good quality bone structures. Memory titanium alloy staples can also be used even when osteoporosis is in a late stage.

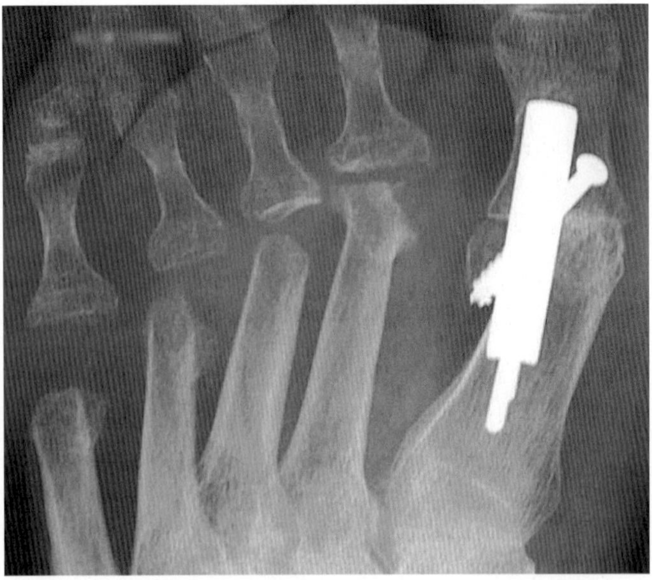

Fig. 6 -

Our team uses a rigid and stable set-up combining a 4.0 mm diameter cancellous bone screw in compression, going from the plantar aspect of the proximal phalange to the lateral side of the first metatarsal with a 4 or 5 hole 1/4 tubular plate. This plate is then positioned on the dorsal aspect of the arthrodesis and secured with 2.7 mm diameter screws. This rigid and stable set-up allows immediate weight bearing and 100% fusion (67).

This arthrodesis gives the destructured and inflammatory rheumatoid forefoot a stable and solid first ray which deals with all the body weight while sparing lateral metatarsal heads. It creates a stable base on which the adjacent toes can be realigned both laterally and vertically.

The level of resection depends on the positioning level of the second metatarso-phalangeal joint. It should spare the great toe's proximal phalange. It is performed and secured after lateral metatarso-phalangeal realignment.

Conventional surgery for hallux valgus

The possible shortening of the first metatarsal using Scarf's osteotomy procedure seems interesting for the correction of phalangeal valgus, combined with surgery on lateral metatarsals (alignment of metatarsal heads or Weil's osteotomies) (71)

But forefoot deformities in rheumatoid diseases have two presentations: static, of course, but also and especially inflammatory. This aspect is completely ignored, thus leading to a relapse of deformities and constitution of the osteo-chondral destruction process.

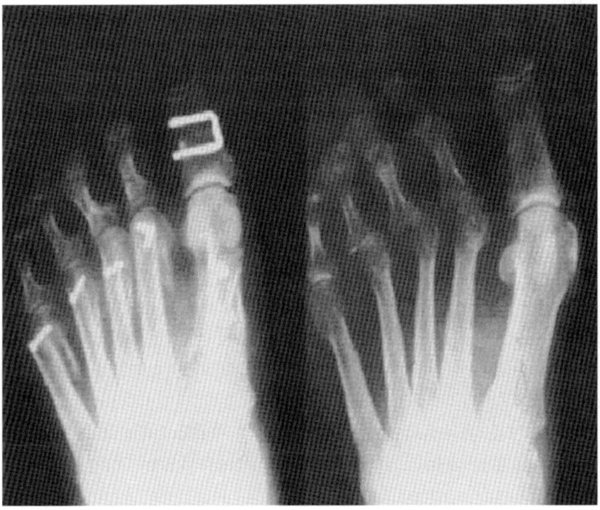

Fig. 7 -

Surgery for lateral rays

Several surgical techniques may be used to treat subluxations or dislocations with osteolysis of lateral rays.

Moderate deformities

Helal (28) suggested using an oblique plane distal shaft osteotomy of the 3 lateral metatarsals. The patient, with immediate weight bearing, was to "adjust" the ideal position of his metatarsal heads and thus attempt to suppress painful hyper weight bearing. But adjustment was not very accurate and pseudarthrosis was often reported.

Lipscomb (41) using 3 dorsal approaches, combined resection of the toes' proximal phalange base, tenotomy of extensors, and excision of metatarsal condyles. Post-operative mobilisation came in early but the partial resection of metatarsal heads exposed to relapse of deformities and metatarsalgia.

Barouk (69) suggested using Weil's osteotomy to loosen subluxated or dislocated lateral metatarso-phalangeal joints but with little osteo-cartilagineous damage. If the short-term result was good, the inflammatory part of deformity was not taken into account and probably one of the main reasons for relapse of deformities. Medium or long- term results are not documented.

Major deformities

They are permanent deformities including capsulo-tendineous retraction and serious osteo-cartilaginous lesions.

Hoffman (30), using a transversal plantar approach in front of the metatarsal heads, resected all metatarsal heads following a smooth arc on a horizontal plane. He sometimes went as far as resecting heads on the neck level. The first metatarsal head was often included in the resection.

Fowler (23) used Hoffman's technique but resections were performed by a transversal elliptical dorsal approach. He also performed a resection of phalangeal bases. Finally, he resected zones of excess plantar skin using a second plantar approach.

Kates *et al.* (34, 35) used the same technique as Fowler but through a single plantar approach and temporarily immobilized the hallux.

Lelievre (40) using these various procedures, determined the "ideal" biomechanical bases for functional reharmonisation of the rheumatoid forefoot. Using 3 longitudinal dorsal approaches, metatarsal resection was performed on the first ray and eventually completed by resection of the proximal phalange of the hallux (presence of hallomegaly). Resection was then continued from the second to the fifth metatarsal.

Special care was taken to avoid any irregular resection that could be in conflict with dorsal or plantar skin. When deformities were very important, Lelievre suggested using a plantar approach.

Thus, Lelievre's realignment allowed suppression of plantar overload and helped correct deformities and loosen soft parts. Arthrolysis and synovectomy were performed at the same operative time. The ideal biomechanical formula, at the end of surgery, was Greek on the digital level, with a great toe shorter than the second toe. The metatarsal formula was of the index-plus or index-plus-minus kind, with a strong first metatarsal able to produce the required efforts for a normal gait.

Gauthier (24) suggested using silicone implants similar to Swanson's for lateral rays. Resection of metatarsal heads was combined with resection of phalangeal bases and a flexible double stem prosthesis linked the 2 bone parts, thus maintaining passive and active mobility, and preventing relapse of metatarso-phalangeal error, sometimes reported with Lelievre's alignment procedure. The prosthesis thus acts as a spacer. Our experience confirmed the adequacy of this alternative to Lelievre's alignment procedure (65, 67). As in Gauthier's study, we did not note on lateral rays any of the silicone's adverse effects reported for the first ray.

All these techniques yielded between 75 and 100% of satisfactory results, despite modifications (4, 6, 25, 31, 32, 50, 70).

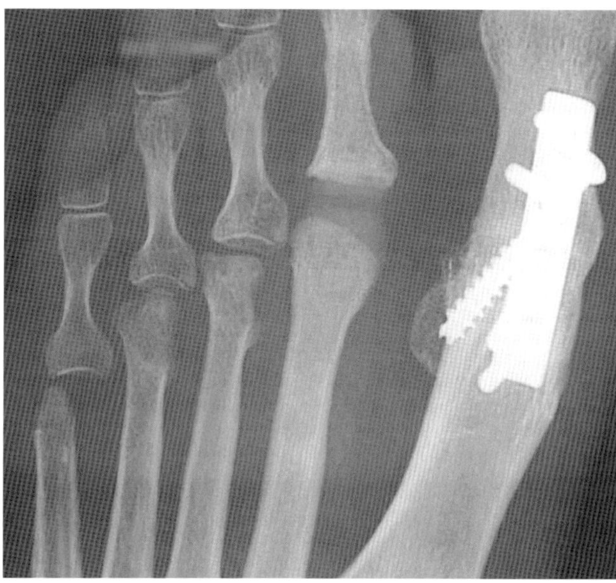

Fig. 8 -

Additional technical data

Surgical approach

Three procedures have been described: a curvilinear plantar approach, a transversal dorsal approach, and finally, 2 or 3 longitudinal dorsal incisions. The plantar approach exposes to painful weight bearing on the scar and damages the plantar fat pad (13, 74). Resuming weight bearing is often difficult and painful for the patient.

Dorsal approaches seem more frequently used nowadays. The transversal procedure allows for a better biomechanical visual approach than several longitudinal approaches. Delayed healing always turns to a favourable evolution (50) and possible necrosis is always easier to manage than when using a plantar approach.

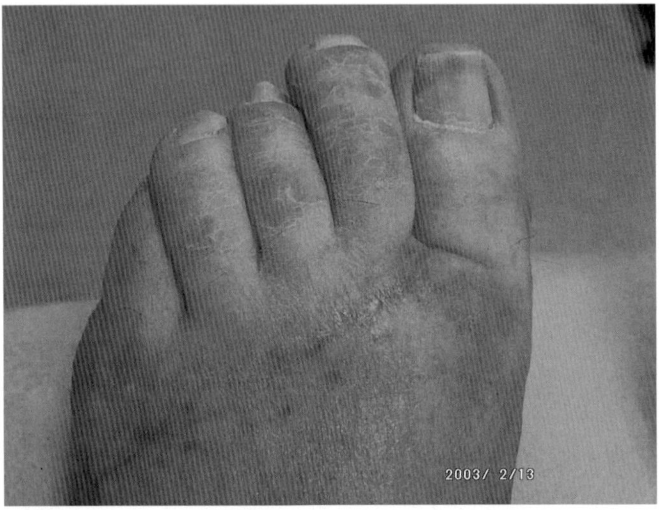

Fig. 9 -

Tendinous surgery

Lengthening extensor tendons is sometimes necessary, despite metatarsal head resection, to prevent metatarso-phalangeal smash up (25, 48, 57).

Resection of the extensor digitorum brevis muscle tendons seems mandatory because its action on extensor tendons is largely responsible for the fibular orientation of the toes.

Stabilization of the metatarsal head alignment-resection

The first descriptions reported by Hoffman then Lipscomb, Fowler, or Lelievre do not mention the temporary state of fixation for metatarso-phalangeal arthroplasties of lateral rays.

Even if Lelievre's biomechanical concepts are taken into account, there is a risk of smash up for the metatarso-phalangeal joint, deprived of its metatarsal head. This would inevitably cause a dorsal relapse of the toe dislocation and of metatarsalgia. Some authors have suggested a temporary metatarso-phalangeal pinning (7, 50), others a trans-nail and pulpar traction anchored on a temporary cast (61, 62). We prefer a surgical syndactyly, using non-absorbable sutures, for 30 days (65).

For us, the fixed point for alignment remains arthrodesis of the great toe which the syndactyly will use to adequately set-up lateral toes, both on the horizontal and cranio-caudal plane.

The Swanson or Gauthier silicone implants also play a role for alignment and to maintain the metatarso-phalangeal gap of lateral rays. Toe syndactyly, from the first to the fifth metatarsal, allows for a controlled healing of the joint capsule, especially if Gauthier's prosthesis on the second ray is combined to a Lelievre resection from the third to the fifth metatarsal. Thus, the prosthesis on the second ray gives the ideal metatarso-phalangeal gap (since it is calculated according to arthrodesis of the first ray), syndactyly between the first and second ray positions the second adequately next to the first and syndactyly, between the second, third and next, aligns the toes adequately in the horizontal plane. It warrants an adequate metatarso-phalangeal gap for the third, fourth, and fifth ray by preventing metatarso-phalangeal smash up.

Post-operative care

Preventing oedema is one of the post-operative therapeutic priorities. It must be medical.

The feet of the bed will be raised. Post-operative bandages must be compressive but must also spare surgical set-ups. Elastic bands are appropriate.

Immediate supine rehabilitation must be first undergone: active and passive mobilization of toes and lymphatic drainage with or without bandages. Elastic bandages should be worn for several weeks to fight against oedema.

Adequate post-operative footwear should be worn. It should let the patient walk easily and in a stable manner, while protecting surgical set-ups.

A second rehabilitation phase is initiated by including the operated foot in a normal gait. Plantar reflexotherapy is useful. Hospitalization in a specialized rehabilitation centre or in a rheumatologic hospital may be interesting for a global management of rheumatoid arthritis.

A temporary interruption of immunosuppressive therapy should be discussed for the perioperative phase so as not to interfere with the cutaneous healing phase.

Indications

Technical references

According to the data from the literature, the ideal surgical strategy is Lelievre's resection- alignment of lateral rays combined with arthrodesis of the first metatarso-phalangeal joint.

Two approaches are recommended: a medial one for arthrodesis of the great toe; a transversal dorsal one for the resection of metatarsal heads. This transversal dorsal approach may be replaced by two longitudinal dorsal approaches (in the second and fourth inter metatarsal space). The plantar arciform approach should no longer be used.

Lelievre's resection-alignment should always come before arthrodesis of the hallux because the level of resection of the first metatarsal depends on that of the second metatarsal head; various metatarso-phalangeal joints can be approached in the space between the extensor digitorum brevis muscle and extensor. Lengthening the extensor tendon will be performed on demand. The extensor digitorum brevis muscle is most often resected because it maintains the lateral deviation of the toes. Clawed toes are most often corrected with external manipulation.

This resection may be completed with the insertion of silicone implant in all or part of the lateral metatarso-phalangeal joints.

Arthrodesis of the first metatarso-phalangeal joint is necessary for the first ray and even more so because valgus deformity and destructive lesions are important. It is used for very specific means. It definitively stabilizes the first ray and provides a harmonious distribution of weight bearing (46, 48, 50). It prevents relapse of deformities on lateral rays. Recurrence of phalangeal valgus after Keller's resection causes relapse of lateral deformities and metatarsalgia in around 50% of the cases (32, 53).

A stable and rigid set-up allows immediate weight bearing and warrants constant fusion in an adequate position for biomechanical constraints. Series in literature are reported as reaching between 77% (32) and 100% of arthrodesis union (20, 50), 90% for Valtin (70). Our technique with a 1/4 tubular screwed plate warrants fusion in 100% of the cases, even when a complementary bone graft is needed to compensate a loss of bone (67, 68). Coughlin (15) chose the screwed plate as the best stabilizing element for arthrodesis, after comparative biomechanical studies.

Particular cases

Does conventional static forefoot surgery have its place in surgical treatment of the rheumatoid forefoot? Some authors (70, 71) suggest using conservative techniques, such as Scarf's, and phalangeal osteotomies for the first ray, combined with Weil's osteotomies for lateral rays. Procedures are logical from the mechanical point of view since when authors suggest using them, lesions are mostly deformities without patent osteo-cartilagineous affections. Could they have an impact on the inflammatory evolution of the disease and on the relapse of deformities?

We do not have enough experience to promote this kind of surgery. Would patients accept to have their forefoot re-operated when they must, for most of them, undergo other surgical interventions?

Surgery on the first ray should be used for an isolated deformity of lateral rays because the gap left by the error of metatarsal heads could cause a hallux valgus deviation. This phenomenon is much less frequent if silicone implants are used for lateral rays because these implants give the second ray enough stability to give stronger support to the first ray.

Results for arthrodesis of the first metatarso-phalangeal joint are poor when there is evolved associated arthritis of the inter-phalangeal great toe joint. In this case, the degenerative inter-phalangeal joint cannot stand the excess weight bearing. This arthritis is a contra-indication for metatarso-phalangeal arthrodesis of the great toe. Keller's resection is indicated in this case, with a careful reconstruction of soft parts and a possible inter-phalangeal arthrodesis or metatarso-phalangeal arthrodesis of the great toe with an interposition implant on the inter-phalangeal joint.

These interposition implants may be used for metatarso-phalangeal joints (32,69) with inter-phalangeal arthrodesis.

Associated lesions

Surgery should be bilateral and performed at the same time for a bilateral forefoot condition (except for particular contra-indications).

One foot should be operated on after the other, and all deformities corrected, for a bilateral condition affecting the fore and hindfoot (5, 63).

A degenerative tibio-fibulotalar joint is not a contra-indication for arthrodesis of the great toe, if an ankle prosthesis is planned.

Forefoot surgery should be the first to be suggested for the lower limb so as to prevent any septic evolution towards a more proximal prosthesis in case of delayed healing or local infection.

Conclusion

Quality surgical management is fundamental for rheumatoid arthritis because functional consequences of foot ailments are severe and frequent in patients.

The fast relief brought to the patient will be completed by trust in the surgeon, and thus in the multidisciplinary healthcare team. This psychological impact on the patient should allow him to face further surgery.

We believe that arthrodesis of the first metatarso-phalangeal combined with surgery for realignment of lateral rays is the best procedure, all clinical conditions included, to face this medical challenge.

References

1. Allieu Y, Claustre J, Simon L (1977) Etude anatomo-pathologique et génèse des déformations du pied dans la polyarthrite rhumatoïde in Le pied inflammatoire. Paris, Maloine, p. 15-33
2. Allieu Y, Ascencio G, Gomis R (1983) Chirurgie de l'avant pied rhumatoïde in Le pied en pratique rhumatologique. Paris, Masson 229-31.
3. Amico JC (1976) The pathomechanics of adult rheumatoid arthritis affecting the foot. J Am Podiatr Assoc 66, p. 227-36
4. Amuso, SJ, Wissinger A, Margolis HM (1971) Metatarsal head resection in the treatment of rheumatoid arthritis. Clin Orthop 74: 94-100
5. Asencio G, Bertin R, Megy B *et al.* (1991) Intrication de l'avant-pied dans la chirurgie de l'avant-pied rhumatoïde. Méd Chir.Pied 74: 185-91

6. Astrom M, Cedell CA (1987) Metatarsal osteotomy in rheumatoid arthritis. Acta Orthop Scand, 58: 398-400.
7. Barton NJ (1973) Arthroplasty of the forefoot in rheumatoid arthritis. J Bone Joint Surg 55: 126-33
8. Beauchamp C, Kirby T Rudge SR, Worthington BS, Nelson J (1984) Fusion of the first metatarsal joint in forefoot arthroplasty. Clin Orthop 38: 107-773
9. Bonnevialle P, Cantagrel A, Gigaud M, Mansat P (2001) Chirurgie de la polyarthrite rhumatoïde. Encycl Méd Chir Paris, Elsevier Appareil locomoteur, 14-222-B-10,
10. Bouysset M (2000) Le pied rhumatoïde in Pathologie ostéo-articulaire du pied et de la cheville sous la direction de M. Bouysset. Paris, Springer-Verlag France. Ed.: 149-67
11. Braun S, Leturia A (1991) Le pied rhumatoïde aurait-il changé? Méd. Chir. Pied. 7(4): 151-7
12. Claustre J (1979) Le pied rhumatoïde. Problèmes podologiques pratiques. Rev. Rhum 46: 673-8
13. Clayton ML (1963) Surgery of the lower extremity in rheumatoid arthritis. J. Bone Joint Surg. 45: 1517-36
14. Clayton ML, Leidholt JD, Clark W (1997) Arthroplasty of rheumatoid metatarsophalangeal joints. Clin Orthop Relat Res., 340: 48-57
15. Coughlin MJ (1990) Arthrodesis of the first metatarsophalangeal joint. Orthop Rev 12: 177-86
16. Cracchiolo A (1982) Management of the arthritis forefoot. Foot Ankle. 3: 17-23
17. Cracchiolo A, Swanson A, Swanson G DeG (1981) The arthritic great toe metatarsophalangeal joint: a review of flexible silicone implant arthroplasty from two medical centers. Clin Orthop 157: 64-9
18. Delagoutte JP, Gagneux E, Peltre G (1986) Etude comparative des voies d'abord dorsale et plantaire dans la chirurgie de l'avant-pied rhumatoïde. Méd Chir Pied n°6, p. 35-7
19. Denis A, Debeyre J, Goutallier D (1981) Chirurgie de l'avant-pied rhumatoïde Rev. Chir. Orthop 67: 747-52
20. Donegan K, Delee JC, Evans JA (1991) Rheumatoid forefoot reconstruction. Presented at the American Orthopaedic Foot and ankle Society. 21st Annual meeting, Anaheim, CA
21. Du Vries HL (1965) Surgery of the feet, 2nd Ed. ST Louis, Mosby-Year Book, Inc
22. Fitzgerald JA (1969) A review of long term results of arthodesis of the first metatarsal joint J Bone Joint Surg 51: 488-93
23. Fowler AW (1959) A method of forefoot reconstruction. J Bone Joint Surg (Br). 41, p. 507-13
24. Gauthier G (1984) Prothèses monobloc en élastomère de silicone mise à l'avant pied. Résultats à la cinquième année. Rev. Chir. Orthop 70(11): 167-169
25. Geppert MJ, Sobel M, Bohne WHO (1992) Foot Fellow's Review. Foot and ankle. Vol 13, n°9, p. 550-8
26. Gordon M, Bullough PG (1982) Synovial and osseous inflammation in failed silicone-rubber prostheses. J. Bone Joint Surg. (Am) 64, p. 574-80
27. Granberry WM, Noble PC, Bishop JO, Tullos HS (1991) Use of hinged silicone prosthesis for replacement arthroplasty of the first metatarsophalangeal joint. J. Bone Joint Surg. 73A, p.1453-9

28. Helal B (1975) Metatarsal ostéotomy for metatarsalgia. J. Bone. Joint. Surg. 57, p. 187-92
29. Henry APJ, Waugh W (1975) The use of footprints in assessing the results of operations for hallux valgus: a comparison of Keller's operation and arthrodesis. J Bone Joint Surg 57, p. 478-82
30. Hoffman P (1912) An operation for severe grades of contracted or clawed toes. Am J Orthop Surg 9: 441-449
31. Huguet D, Bresson C, Decussac JB, Gruber P, Lecouteur P, Letenneur J (1996) La chirurgie de l'avant pied rhumatoïde. Méd Chir Pied. 12(4): 214-6
32. Jarde O, Ruzic JC, Roux O, Trinquier-Lautard JL, Vives P (1998) Intérêt de l'arthrodèse du gros orteil associée à un alignement métatarsien selon Lelievre dans la chirurgie de l'avant-pied rhumatoïde. Rev Chir Orthop 84: 61-6
33. Johnson K (1989) Surgery of the foot and ankle. New York, Raven Press
34. Kates A (1970) Surgery of the rheumatoid foot. Proc. R. Soc. Med., 63: 679-80
35. Kates A, Kessel L, Kay A (1967) Arthroplasty of the forefoot. J Bone Joint Surg, 49: 552-7
36. Keller WL (1904) The surgical treatment of bunions and hallux valgus. N.Y. State J. Med. 80: 741-2
37. Keller WL (1912) Further observations on the surgical treatment of hallux valgus and bunions. N.Y. State J. Med. 95: 696-8
38. Kitaoka HB, Holiday AD, Jr, Chao EYS, Ph D, Cahalan TD (1992) Salvage of failed first metatarsophalangeal joint Implant Arthroplasty by Implant Removal ans Synovectomy: Clinical and Biomecanical Evaluation. Foot and Ankle. Volume 13 n°5: 243-9
39. Leavitt DC (1956) Surgical treatment of arthritic feet. Northwest Med. 55: 1086-8
40. Lelievre J (1968) Mille alignements articulaires métatarso-phalangiens in Podologie Paris, Expansion scientifique française
41. Lipscomb PR (1981) Surgery of the rheumatoid foot. Preferable procedures. Rev. Chir. Orthop. 67: 375-82
42. Mann RA Coughlin MJ (1979) The rheumatoid foot: review of the literature and method of treatment. Orthop Rev 8: 105-12
43. Mann RA Oates JC (1980) Arthrodesis of the first metetarsophalangeal joint. Foot and ankle., 1: 159-66
44. Mann RA (1984) Reconstructing the rheumatoid foot. Strategies in orthop. Surg. 3: 3
45. Mann RA, Thompson FM (1984) Arthrodesis of the first metatarsophalangeal joint for hallux valgus in rheumatoid arthritis. J. Bone Joint Surg. 66A: 687-92
46. Mann RA (1986) Surgery of the foot, 5th Ed. St Louis, C.V. Mosby
47. Mann RA Coughlin MJ (1991) The video Textbook of foot and ankle Surgery. St Louis, medical Video Production
48. Mann RA, Schaekel ME (1995) Surgical correction of rhumatoid forefoot deformities. Foot and Ankle International, 16(1): 1-6
49. Marin GA (1968) Arthrodesis of the metatarsophlangeal joint of the big toe for hallux valgus and hallux rigidis. Int. Surg., 50: 175-80
50. Maynou C, Mestdagh H, Petroff E, Forgeois Ph, Hue E (1997) Traitement chirurgical de l'avant-pied rhumatoïde par alignement par voie dorsale. Rev. Chir. Orthop., 83: 734-8.
51. Mc Garvey Johnson (1996) Keller arthroplasty and resection of metatarsal heads 2-5. Presented at the Mid-American Orthopedic Society Annual Meeting.
52. Morrisson P (1974) Complication of forefoot operations in rheumatoid arthritis. Proc R Soc Med 67: 110-111

53. Piat C, Denis A, Goutallier D, Huber-Levernieux C (1991) Chirurgie de l'avant-pied rhumatoïde: vingt années d'expérience. Méd Chir Pied 7, 4: 165-9.
54. Potter TA, Khus JG (1972) Painful feet. In JL Arthritis and allied Conditions, HollanderJ.L. (ed). Lea and Febiger, Philadelphia,
55. Resnick D (1976) Roentgen features of the rheumatoid mid and hindfoot. J Can Assoc Radiol., 27: 99-107
56. Roger A, Mann, and Mark e Schakel (1995) Surgical correction of rheumatoid forefoot deformities. Foot and ankle international. 16(1): 2-6
57. Saragaglia D, Carpentier E (1985) Le pied rhumatoïde: bases cliniques, indication chirurgicales. Rhumatologie. N°7 Tome XXXVII: 207-12.
58. Simon L, Claustre J, Allieu Y (1980) Le pied rhumatologique. Génèse des déformations. Rev Rhum, 47: 117-22
59. Stokes IAF, Hutton WC, Mech MI, Stott JRR, Lowe LW (1979) Forces under the hallux before and after surgery Clin Orthop, 142: 64-72
60. Swanson AB, Lumsden RM, Swanson, C DeG (1979) Silicone implant arthroplasty of the great toe. Clin Orthop, 142: 30
61. Tillmann K (1979) The rheumatoid foot. Littleton, MA, George Thieme Publishers-Stuffgart PSG Publishing Co: 44-56
62. Tillman K (1979) The rheumatoid foot: diagnosis, pathomechanics and treatment. Littleton, MA, George Thieme Publishers-Stuffgart PSG Publishing Co
63. Tillmann K (1987) The mutual interplay between forefoot and hindfoot affections and deformities in R.A. Rheumatology 11: 97-9
64. Tomeno B, Kaddem SE (1982) L'arthrodèse métatarso-phalangienne du gros orteil. Rev. Chir. Orthop., 68: 379-84
65. Tourné Y, Leroy JM, Maire JP, Saragaglia D (1993) L'arthrodèse métatarso-phalangienne du premier rayon. Méd Chir Pied 9(3): 161-71
66. Tourné Y, Saragaglia D (1995) Prothèse métatarso-phalangienne à glissement edelweiss et chirurgie de premier rayon. Rhumatologie, 47(4): 137-139
67. Tourné Y, Saragaglia D (1995) Résultats de l'arthrodèse métatarso-phalangienne du premier rayon. Rhumatologie, 47(4): 117-21
68. Tourné Y, Saragaglia D, Zattara A *et al.* (1997) Hallux valgus in the Elderly: Metatarsophalangeal arthodesis of the First Ray. Foot and Ankle international., 18(4): 195-8
69. Valtin B (1996) L'avant pied rhumatoïde in Chirurgie de l'avant pied, Cahier d'enseignement de la SOFCOT, collection dirigée par J. DUPARC ED. Paris Expansion Scientifique Francaise 54: 153-62
70. Valtin B, Alnot JY, Houvet P (1990) La chirurgie de l'avant pied rhumatoïde: intérêt de l'arthrodèse métatarso-phalangienne associée à l'alignement des têtes métatarsiennes. Méd Chir Pied 6: 163-9
71. Valtin B, Houvet P, Alnot JY (1991) La chirurgie de l'avant pied rhumatoïde. Méd Chir Pied 7: 177-184
72. Vidal J, Orst J, Boisard JL (1983) Notre expérience du traitement de l'avant pied rhumatoïde in Claustre J, Simon L. Le pied en pratique rhumatologique Paris, Masson: 232-8
73. Viladot A, Viladot R (1983) Biomécanique de l'avant-pied rhumatoïde. In Claustre J, Simon L. Le pied en pratique rhumatologique. Paris, Masson: 28
74. Watson MS (1974) A long-term follow up of forefoot arthroplasty. J. Bone Joint Surg., 56B: 527-33

Additional references

. Clayton ML (1960) Surgery of the forefoot in rheumatoid arthritis. Clin Orthop 16: 136

. Clayton ML (1967) Surgical treatment of the rheumatoid foot. In: Giannestras NJ (ed) Foot and Disorders. Medical and Surgical Management. Philadelphia, Lea and Febiger

. Hamalainen M, Raunio P (1997) Long term followup of rheumatoid forefoot surgery. Clinical Orthopaedics and Related Research. 340: 34-8

. Kerschbaumer F, Von-Salomon D, Lehr F (1996) Der rheumatische Vorfuss. Der Orthopädie. 25 (4): 354-61

. Mulcahy-David, Daniels-Tim-R, Lau-Johnny-Tak-Choy, Boyle-Eleanor, Bogoch-Earl (2003) Rheumatoid forefoot deformity : a comparison study of 2 functional methods of reconstruction J. Rhumatol. 30(7): 1440-50

Hindfoot surgery for rheumatoid arthritis

B. Valtin and Th. Leemrijse

Introduction

Rheumatoid arthritis is a common condition with an incidence ranging from 0.5 to 1.5%. Involvement of the foot and of the ankle depends upon the duration of the disease and will be present in 50% of patients at 10 years and 75% at 20 years (8). Different authors have variably described the frequency of involvement of the subtalar and midtarsal joints during the progressive course of rheumatoid arthritis. These joints were affected in 67% of cases in Vainio's study (11) of 995 cases, while King and Freeman reported a more modest incidence of 30% (4). This difference could be attributed to the relatively mild clinical symptoms or to the relatively common radiological changes in the subtalar joint complex. In fact, these radiological changes are frequently seen in the subtalar, talo-navicular and calcaneo-cuboid joints during the evolution of rheumatoid arthritis although remaining clinically silent for a long time. In fact, Vigidal found radiological disturbances to be twice as frequent as clinical symptoms in the mid-foot and three times more often at the sub-talar joint. In his prospective study of 99 patients that fulfilled the criteria of the American College of Rheumatology, Michelson (8) found involvement of the ankle in 42% of cases, of the forefoot in 28%, of the midfoot in 5% and of the heel in 1%. This wide disparity in results reflects the differences in criteria of appreciation that should be correlated to other criteria such as the functional capacity of the patient and the duration of the disease. Numerous studies have also emphasized the insufficiency of preventive measures employed and of the quality of footwear, which should constitute the primary treatment of the rheumatoid foot.

Articular affections

The extent of articular destruction increases with the prolonged duration of the disease and could affect all the joints of the midfoot and of the hindfoot. According to Bouysset *et al.* (2), the talo-navicular joint is most often involved (31.8%), followed, in the decreasing order of incidence, by the subtalar (23.3%), the naviculo-cuneiform (20.4%) and the cuneo-metatatarsal (14.9%) joints.

As seen in all inflammatory processes of rheumatoid arthritis, the evolution of the rheumatoid foot occurs in two stages:

- *Inflammation stage*: there is a global swelling of the foot with obliteration of the retro-malleolar gutters. The pain is related to the distension of the joints and to the tenosynovitis affecting the fibular and tibialis posterior tendons. The treatment of this stage is primarily medical, eventually associated with corticoid injections and synoviortheses.
- *Articular destruction stage:* the articular cartilage is progressively destroyed. The pain is related to the joint changes and to the eventual deformities of the foot. Surgical treatment is often indicated at this stage.

Disorders of the tarso-metatarsal joints (figs. 1a and 1b), (figs. 2a and 2b)

Clinical manifestations

The involvement of these joints is relatively uncommon with only a few cases being reported in the literature. They are responsible for pain at the midfoot level, which is initially of inflammatory origin and, later, related to the mechanical disturbances produced by the eventual deformities. These bony and articular changes could be partial, predominantly localized to the cuneo-metatarsal joint of the second ray, or global. In the latter case, a sensation of instability, due to the destruction of the plantar capsulo-ligamentous supports and the deformity of the foot, is added to the pain. Although medical treatment and steroid injections could be useful in the localized forms at the inflammatory stage, surgery is indicated in the presence of persistent pain or in the presence of global involvement with extensive articular destruction. Frequently the disease evolues towards a progressive pas plano valgus. The treatment would be a fusion of the affected joints.

Surgical treatment

The localized form of involvement of the second cuneo-metatarsal joint is treated by a limited arthrodesis of the second and third tarso-metatarsal joints. Simultaneous fusion of both these joints is necessary to obtain good contact between the bony surfaces created by excision of the articular cartilage. It also ensures a more rapid and reliable fusion. The joints are exposed via a dorsal incision centred over the second cuneo-metatarsal joint. A judicious excision of the articular surfaces is performed using an osteotome or an oscillating saw. The site of arthrodesis is stabilized using staples. Arthrodesis of all the tarso-metatarsal joints is indicated in

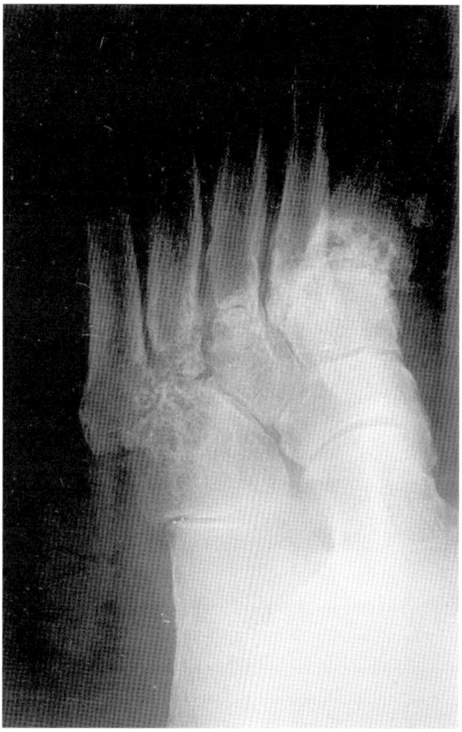

Fig. 1a.

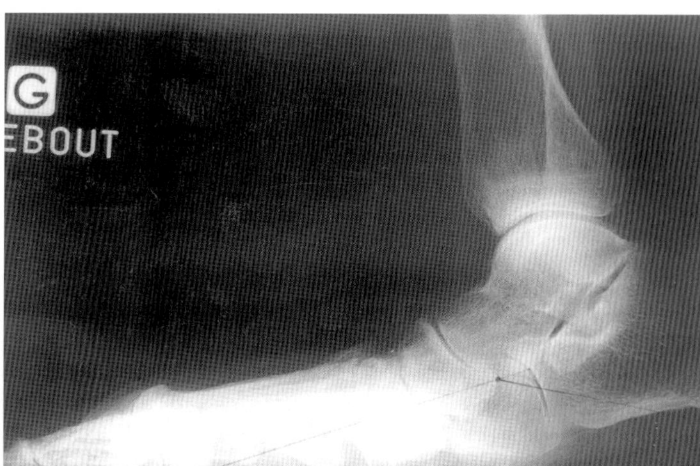

Fig. 1b -

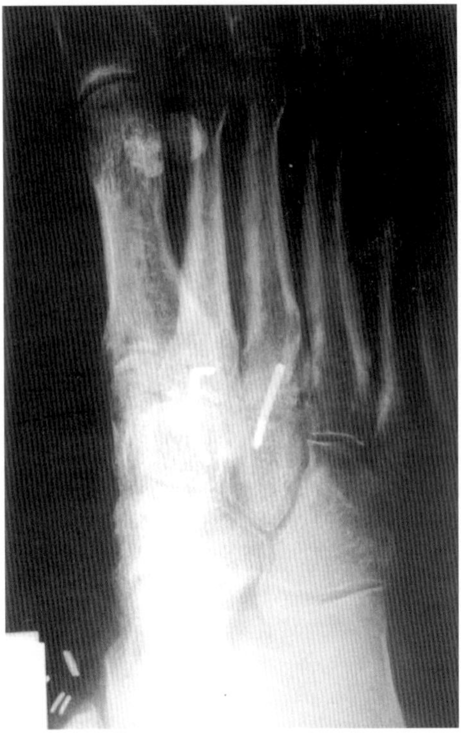

Fig. 2a.

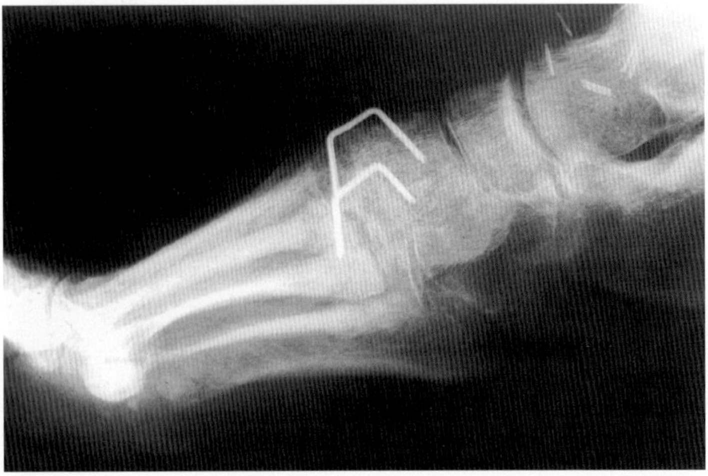

Fig. 2b.

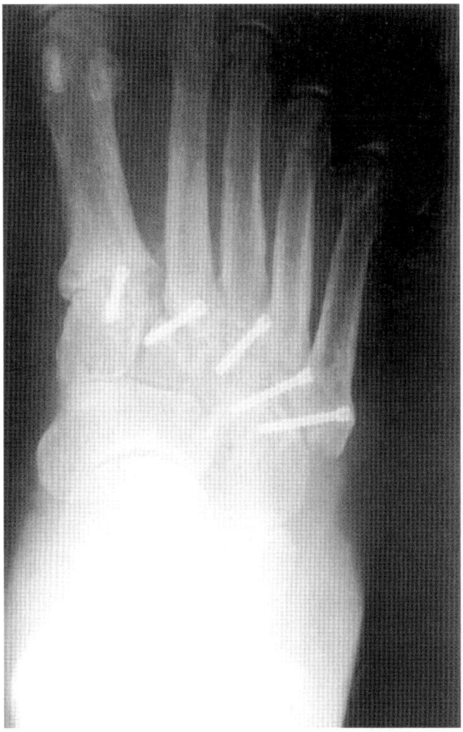

Fig. 3.

the presence of extensive articular destruction (fig. 3) and requires considerable surgical expertise in order to correct the convex deformity of the foot and to restore synchronous loading of the metatarsal heads while walking by re-establishing the proper lengths and heights of the metatarsals. Three separate incisions are necessary: a medial approach over the first cuneo-metatarsal joint and two dorsal incisions over the third cuneo-metatarsal joint, over the medial border of the base of the fifth metatarsal respectively. The extent of excision of the articular surfaces is determined by the necessity of bony contact at the joint that is most severely destroyed by the disease. One starts with the joints of the second and third rays, followed by the first and, finally, the fourth and fifth rays. The articular cartilage is excised using an oscillating saw, the sections being perpendicular to the dorsal bony surfaces of the metatarsals, the cuneiforms and of the cuboid. Further adjustments may be required in order to obtain good bony contact at each of the joints to be fused. The joints are provisionally stabilized using Kirschner wires; one wire is passed through the dorsal cortex of each metatarsal and directed towards the respective cuneiform or the cuboid. The position is confirmed radiographically and definitive fixation is performed using cannulated screws passed over the wires. A second screw or a staple may be required on the medial aspect of the first cuneo-metatarsal joint where it is essential to control the forces in pronation and in supination.

Post-operative course

Patients with good bone quality who have undergone partial tarso-metatarsal fusions may be allowed to bear weight on the affected lower limbs within below-knee casts. On the other hand, total tarso-metatarsal arthrodesis necessitates non weight-bearing immobilisation in a below-knee plaster cast for two months followed, at times, by a weight-bearing cast for one month. This is particularly difficult in patients who have deformities of the hands that interfere with the use of crutches. Hence, these patients have to depend on wheelchairs for ambulation. Proper psychological counselling is necessary so that they can prepare themselves mentally. One must explain the fact that this wheelchair will help them to reduce the load on their upper limbs while their lower limbs are immobilized and that this wheelchair-bound period is strictly temporary. Bony fusion is usually obtained within 2-3 months while complete functional recovery with normal footwear can be anticipated by the end of the fifth month after surgery.

Affection of the innominate line (Naviculo-cuneiform joint) (fig. 4)

Clinical features

Isolated clinical involvement of this joint is relatively rare. It is sometimes associated with involvement of the talo-navicular or tarso-metatarsal joints and can then contribute to the painful symptoms. It can also be observed in association with a valgus flat foot, in which there is an important mechanical stress localized on this joint. Firstly there is mainly a mechanical midfoot pain during walking. Bone scintigraphy often allows to locate isolated involvement of the naviculo-cuneiform

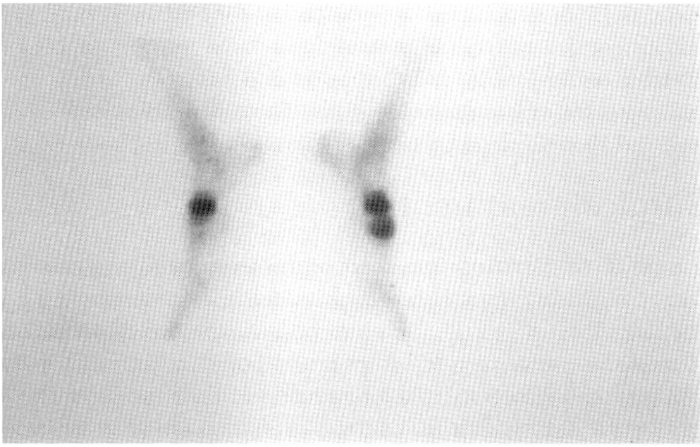

Fig. 4a.

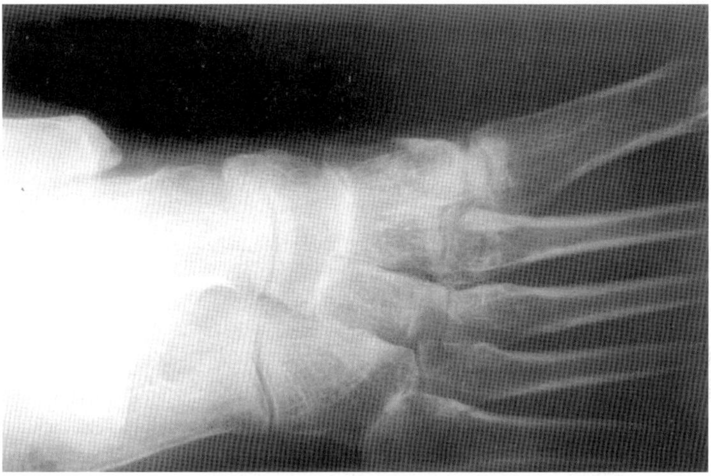

Fig. 4b.

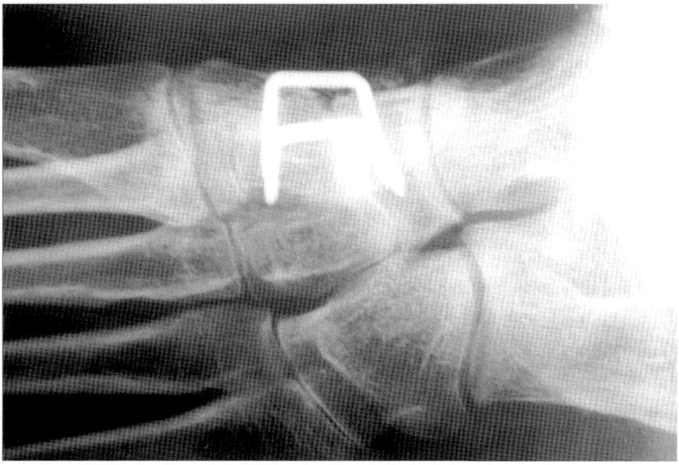

Fig. 4c.

joint and helps to suggest an indication for eventual surgery. Primary treatment usually consists of medical measures to relieve pressure on this joint with the help of suitable orthoses with arch supports and sometimes with intra-articular steroid injections for inflammatory episodes. These help to provide comfort to the patients and also allows different therapeutic options if their relief is transitory.

Surgical treatment

Fusion of the naviculo-cuneiform and inter-cuneiform joints is usually effective in treating this condition. However, it is a technically demanding procedure because of the deep location of the joint and because the defect produced by freshening the joint surfaces may require addition of a bone graft in order to obtain a good bony contact: that allows to avoid an adduction of the forefoot. The joint is approached through a dorsal incision centred over the second cuneiform. Sometimes, two separate incisions are utilized to facilitate access to the third cuneiform that is found pushed laterally by the convexity of the foot. Care is taken to avoid injury to the anterior tibial vessels and nerve. The articular surfaces are excised and the joints are stabilized with staples, with or without addition of cancellous bone grafts. In the presence of more extensive destruction or of associated involvement of the talo-navicular joint, the anterior incision is extended proximally for fusion of this latter joint.

Post-operative course

Surgery of this joint demands as much care and immobilization as that of the tarso-metatarsal joints or of the hindfoot. Complete immobilization for at least six weeks is preferable, particularly if it is necessary to add bone grafts.

Affections of the subtalar joint complex (figs. 4, 5 and 6)

Clinical features

The main clinical features of subtalar joint complex involvement in rheumatoid arthritis include pain aggravated essentially by loading or while walking on uneven ground. The patient can also complain of a sensation of instability in the hindfoot region while walking. The pain is generally antero-medial or lateral. This results in a limp, reduced activities and difficulty in wearing shoes. During inflammatory exacerbations, global swelling of the hindfoot is observed with obliteration of the retro-malleolar gutters, which corresponds anatomically with tenosynovitis of the fibular and tibialis posterior tendons respectively. Exceptionally, the tibialis anterior tendon is also involved. From the articular point of view, the talo-navicular joint is mainly affected, and often progressively destroyed. The condition evolves towards stiffness with the foot remaining aligned with progressively increasing functional disability or towards deviation of the hindfoot, most frequently in valgus, which disturbs the function of the foot with instability, difficulty in footwear and, sometimes, pain of mechanical origin while walking. A varus deformity of the hindfoot may be observed (7%), which usually disturbs function to a greater extent.

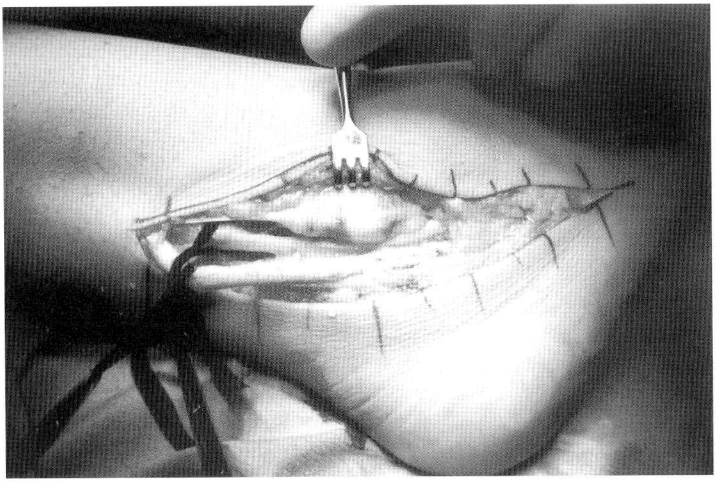

Fig. 5.

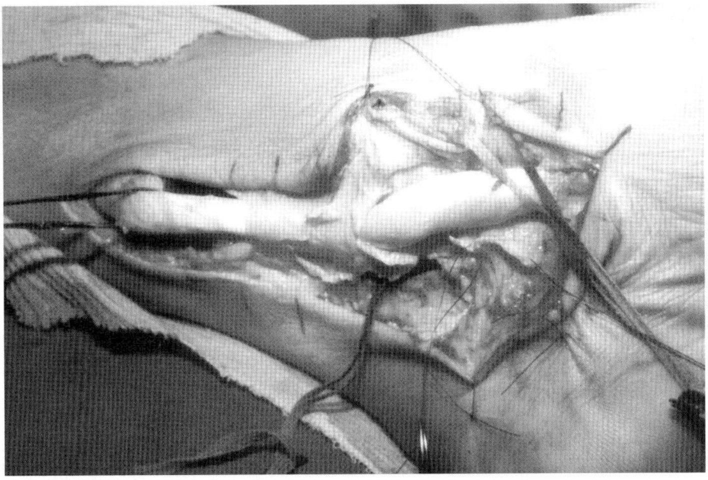

Fig.6a.

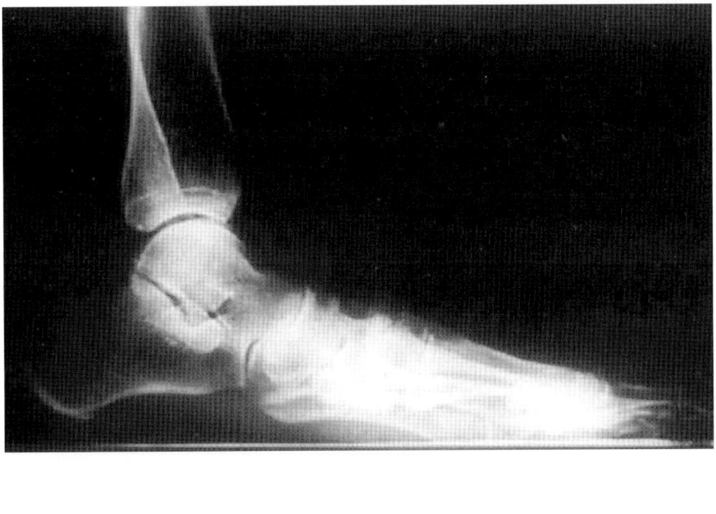

Fig.6b.

Surgical treatment is indicated in the presence of a deformity or there is inefficiency of the medical treatment. A valgus deformity of the hindfoot increases the stress on the forefoot and is a source of residual pain even after surgical correction.

The origin of the deformity is still debated. Keenan *et al.* (10) showed by gait analysis that the deformity is the consequence of pronation of the forefoot and of external rotation of the leg acting on the weakened joints, rather than an insufficiency of the tibialis posterior tendon. This valgus deformation must be corrected quickly in order to prevent troublesome repercussions in the knee and the forefoot.

Anatomo-physiological considerations

Subtalar joint complex

The subtalar, talo-navicular and calcaneo-cuboid joints together constitute a functional unit called the subtalar joint complex, which is the site of complex movements with elements in all three planes in space:

- *varus and valgus of the hindfoot:* these movements occur at the subtalar joint and the mobility of the talus on the calcaneus can be visualized by observation of the divergence (during valgus) and of convergence (during varus) of the axes of these two bones. As a corollary, the axis joining the centre of the anterior surface of the calcaneus to the centre of the anterior articulation of the talus is also modified. This axis becomes more and more vertical with the passage from valgus to varus.
- *pronation and supination of the forefoot:* these movements occur at the midtarsal joint (Chopart) and are linked to the movements of varus and valgus. Convergence of the axes of the talus and of the calcaneus, is automatically associated with a supination of the forefoot due to the changes in the relationship between the anterior surface of the talus and that of the calcaneus, while divergence of these axes produces pronation of the forefoot for the same reason.
- *adduction-abduction of the forefoot:* these movements are also located at the midtarsal joint and are linked to the displacements of the anterior surfaces of the talus and the calcaneus. The associated movements of varus, supination and adduction constitute inversion while those of valgus, pronation and abduction constitute eversion. This pattern of associated movements also determines the pathological deformity of the foot.

The talar and calcaneal columns (fig. 1a)

The different inter-tarsal joints of the foot should be considered to be constituted by two separate columns:

- *the talar column:* formed by the talus, the navicular, the cuneiforms and the medial three metatarsals. It constitutes an anatomical unit that is functionally and physiologically independent of the second column;
- *the calcaneal column:* formed by the calcaneus, the cuboid and the two lateral metatarsals.

Fusion of one polyarticular chain leaves the possibility of some modest movement at the other column. In addition, the fusion of one joint results in compensatory hypermobility at the adjacent joints. Thus, fusion of the talar column could leave some residual mobility due to the movements at the joints in the calcaneal column that could increase progressively with the passage of time.

Pathological conditions

In rheumatoid involvement of the hindfoot, an arthrodesis at this last level could be indicated in different circumstances. Most often, it is a painful element in a plano-valgus foot that produces pain below the lateral malleolus or instability of the foot while walking and, less often, for a varus deformation. An articular disorder in an aligned foot rarely disturbs function to such an extent as to warrant surgery. However, articular destruction in a plantigrade foot can result in severe pain. In such a situation, one has to opt between a fusion of the talonavicular joint, which, as we know from the study conducted by Steinhauser (9), blocks the mobility of the subtalar joint complex hindfoot almost completely and a complete fusion of the subtalar complex that associates, in addition, an arthrodesis of the subtalar and of the midtarsal joint.

Surgical treatment

The technique of fusion of the subtalar joint complex in a plantigrade foot without hindfoot deformity differs considerably from the one required in the presence of a severe deformity of the hindfoot, particularly in valgus.

- *Arthrodesis in a plantigrade foot:* this just entails freshening of the surfaces of the respective joints by excision of the articular cartilage up to the subchondral bone with preservation of the articular morphology.
- *Arthrodesis in the presence of a deformity of the foot:* here, one must consider the effect of correction of the deformity of the hindfoot on the position of the forefoot.

Deviations of the hindfoot: correction of a valgus or varus deformity of the hindfoot during arthrodesis of the subtalar joint complex involves excision of the articular surfaces of the subtalar joint and modification of the relative positions of the two bones reduction of the talo-calcaneal divergence for correction of a valgus deformity and augmentation of this divergence for correction of varus. As a corollary, correction of valgus provokes supination of the forefoot while correction of varus results in pronation of the forefoot. Hence, the secondary deviations have to be corrected by arthrodesis of the midtarsal joint.

Affections of the hindfoot

Each of the three joints of the hindfoot can be affected in the progressive evolution of rheumatoid arthritis of the foot. The incidence of these affections increases with longer duration of the disease. They are sometimes detected accidentally as changes observed during radiological evaluation of a deformed and painful forefoot. However, rheumatoid disease of the subtalar, talo-navicular and calcaneo-cuboid joints exists as a separate entity that can produce pain and disability.

Articular features

Involvement of the talo-navicular joint clearly predominates. It is manifested clinically in the form of pain over the medial aspect of the midtarsal region and restriction of inversion and eversion movements of the hindfoot. The cuneo-navicular joint follow the talo-navicular joint in the frequency of involvement and is often associated with destruction of the latter joint. The clinical features are identical to those described above. Predominant involvement of the subtalar joint is less common and appears clinically in the form of pain that is more often located below the lateral malleolus and, sometimes, over the heel. Valgus-varus movements of the hindfoot aggravate the pain. Clinically, one finds stiffness of variable extent. The calcaneo-cuboid joint can also be involved. This is usually found in association with disease of one or more of the joints mentioned above. It is important to note that isolated involvement of one of these joints is rare. In the presence of clinical and radiological affection of the talo-navicular joint, a CT-scan could reveal changes in one or more joints of the hindfoot, particularly the subtalar joint. Predominant involvement of the talo-navicular joint can be treated surgically in one of the following two ways: isolated arthrodesis of the talo-navicular joint or triple arthrodesis.

Isolated arthrodesis (fig. 7)

Steinhauser's studies (9) have shown that isolated fusion of the talo-navicular joint will block movements of talo-navicular, subtalar and calcaneo-cuboid joints (5, 6). The theoretical indication for this operation is predominant involvement of the talo-navicular joint in the presence of a plantigrade foot without hindfoot deformity or a mobile hindfoot. The joint is approached through an antero-medial incision. Freshening of the articular surfaces is always difficult. Conservative resection in order to preserve the shape of the bones could result in insufficient removal of the subchondral bone with an increased risk of pseudarthrosis. On the other hand, excessive bony resection could produce a defect that would require addition of a bone graft in order to preserve the shape of the foot. Bone grafting inevitably results in a delay in consolidation and could also be responsible for non-union. Hence, it is better to opt for a more secure operation namely triple arthrodesis.

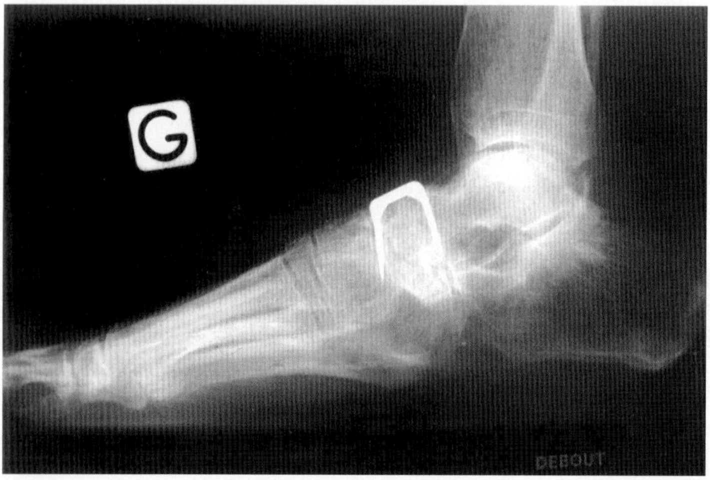

Fig.7.

Triple arthrodesis: (figs. 8a and 8b)

The aim of this operation is to obtain bony consolidation across the subtalar, talo-navicular and calcaneo-cuboid joints by excision of the articular surfaces and correction of the deformity, if necessary.

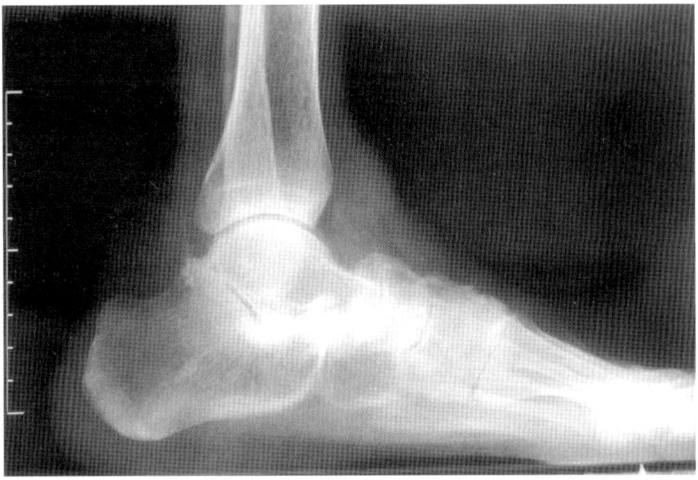

Fig. 8a.

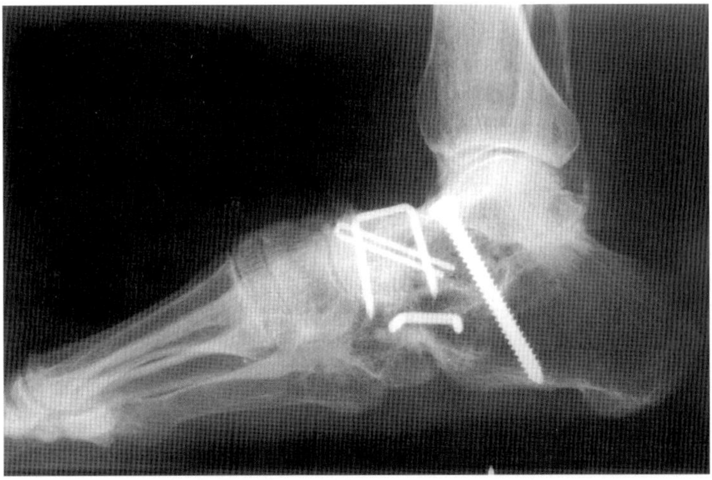

Fig. 8b.

Approach

This surgery can sometimes be performed through a single curved incision extending from the lateral malleolus to the talo-navicular joint. However, it is difficult to freshen the articular surfaces of the talo-navicular joint adequately through this incision and this is the most difficult step in the procedure. In addition, this incision lies obliquely with respect to both sagittal and coronal planes and this makes it even more difficult to visualize the correction of the shape of the foot. Therefore, it is preferable to utilize two approaches. One incision extends from the tip of the lateral malleolus up to the centre of the cuboid or 1 cm proximal to the base of the fifth metatarsal. This incision allows us to approach and excise the articular surfaces of the subtalar and the calcaneo-cuboid joints. The extensor digitorum brevis muscle is retracted dorsally. The Y-shaped ligament is excised and a Hinge retractor is introduced into the sinus tarsi in order to distract the opposing surfaces of the subtalar joint. The articular cartilage is excised using an osteotome and hammer, starting with the anterior joint followed by the posterior one. Care has to be taken to avoid injury to the tendon of the flexor hallucis longus that winds round the posterior aspect of the joint. The articular surfaces of the calcaneo-cuboid joint are removed. The other incision is antero-medial, between the tendons of the tibialis anterior muscle and the extensor hallucis longus muscle. This allows us to deal with the talo-navicular joint. Excision of the talar articular surface usually does not pose a serious problem while the navicular bone is often difficult. It is performed with an osteotome and a hammer and with the help of a Hinge distractor placed in the medial part of the joint for removal of the cartilage from the lateral part and vice versa. The surface is excised at least up to the subchondral bone, taking care to preserve the shape of the joints. Thus, there can be two types of situations:

Plantigrade foot

The opposing bony surfaces are placed in contact with each other and stabilized provisionally using Kirschner wires. The position is confirmed radiologically. Definitive fixation is then performed with the help of a screw passed from the talus into the calcaneus and with staples across the talo-navicular and calcaneo-cuboid joints.

Deviated foot

Pes plano-valgus foot: This problem concerns the correction of the valgus of the hindfoot without creating supination of the forefoot in the presence, most often, of a fixed deformity. At present, it is very important to correct the deviation of the hindfoot because, in cases with progressive disease and eventual involvement of the ankle joint, prosthetic replacement of the latter joint can be performed only if the hindfoot is aligned properly. The valgus deformity of the hindfoot can easily be corrected by re-positioning the talus over the calcaneus. However, this procedure inevitably results in supination of the forefoot. This latter problem can be dealt with in different ways depending upon the presence or absence of abduction of the forefoot in the initial deformity.

hindfoot valgus with abduction of the forefoot

After excision of the adjacent surfaces of the subtalar and calcaneo-cuboid joints, a Hinge distractor is placed in the calcaneo-cuboid joint to separate these two bones.

This step helps to correct the entire deformity in the same way as the Evans operation. At this stage, both aspects of the talo-navicular joint are excised with the help of an oscillating saw at the same levels as the sections in the calcaneo-cuboid joint. The Hinge retractor is removed and the bony surfaces are approximated. A provisional fixation is performed using Kirschner wires, allowing us to evaluate the shape of the foot. If the supination has not been corrected adequately, more bone is excised on the plantar aspect of the talo-navicular joint. The technique of definitive fixation is similar to the one employed in a plantigrade foot.

Hindfoot valgus without abduction of the forefoot

If there is persistent mobility at the midfoot level, excision of the talo-navicular surfaces is performed taking care to preserve the shape of the foot and fixing the freshened surfaces in maximal plantar flexion. If there is practically no residual mobility, which occurs more often, a wedge of bone with a plantar base has to be excised at the level of the talo-navicular and cuneo-navicular joints in order to correct the residual supination of the forefoot. In the presence of a more severe deformation, the excision may have to be extended to the cuneo-metatarsal joint of the first ray.

Hindfoot varus

This is corrected by excising a laterally-based wedge at the subtalar joint, taking care to avoid impingement with the tip of the lateral malleolus. In addition, a small tarsectomy is performed in the presence of an early cavus deformity. The section of the calcaneo-cuboid joint can be extended if there is an adduction of the forefoot. The position is stabilized with the help of a screw across the subtalar joint and staples at the levels of the mistarsal joint.

Post-operative course

The limb is immobilized in a below-knee plaster cast and the patient is not allowed to bear weight on it for two months. Simultaneous affection of the upper limbs could render it impossible to walk with the support of crutches and the patient may have to depend upon a wheelchair for ambulation. Hence, proper psychological counselling may be necessary before surgery. The fact that this wheelchair-bound period is strictly temporary and that the patient can confidently expect better painless ambulation at the end of these two months must be emphasized. The patient is allowed to bear weight on the operated lower limb after removal of the plaster cast. However, the œdema of mechanical origin, which appears after walking, takes time to resolve and delays full functional recovery for 2-3 months more.

The surgery relieves the pain over the midtarsal and hindfoot regions and allows the patient to wear normal, commercially available shoes. It may be necessary to add suitable soles for the correction of slight defects in the balance.

Pathological Associations

The pathological and painful conditions of the hindfoot may be associated with affections of the forefoot or of the ankle joint. The involvement of multiple joints may necessitate several surgical interventions. One must try and reduce the total number of operations without compromising the result. In the presence of combined involvement of the subtalar joint complex and of the forefoot, one must attempt complete correction of the deformity: triple fusion, arthrodesis of the metatarso-phalangeal joint of the great toe and re-alignment of the heads of the metatarsals. For disease affecting the subtalar joint complex and the ankle joint, one has to select between a pantalar fusion (figs. 9a and b) and combination of triple fusion with prosthetic replacement of the ankle joint (figs. 10 and 11). For the latter choice, it may be prudent to perform it in two stages: correction of the hindfoot deformity by triple fusion in the first stage followed, two months later, by total ankle replacement.

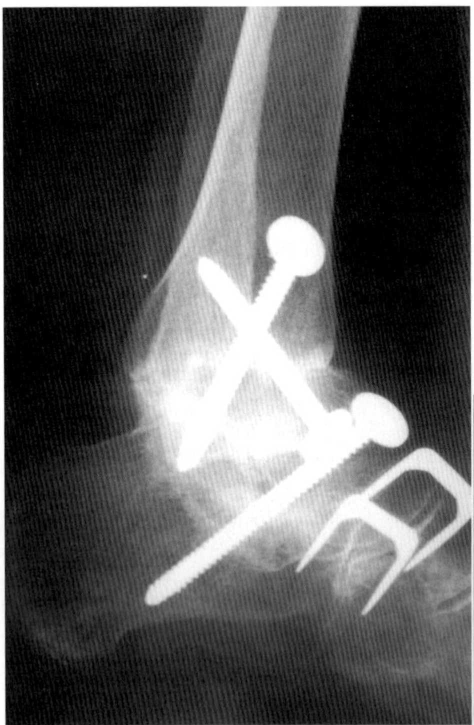

Fig. 9a.

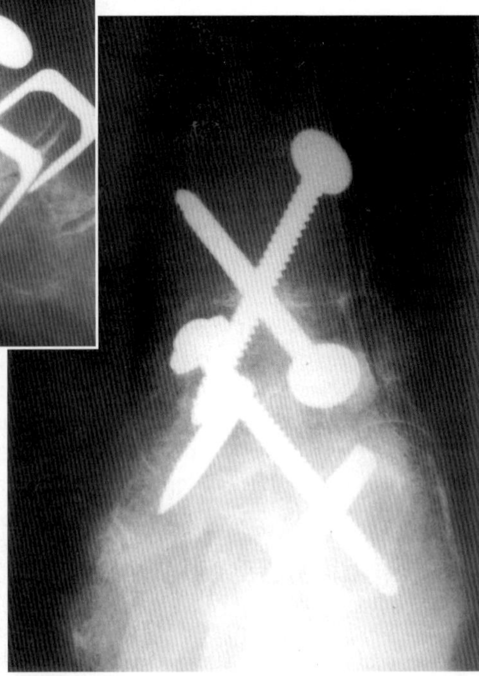

Fig. 9b.

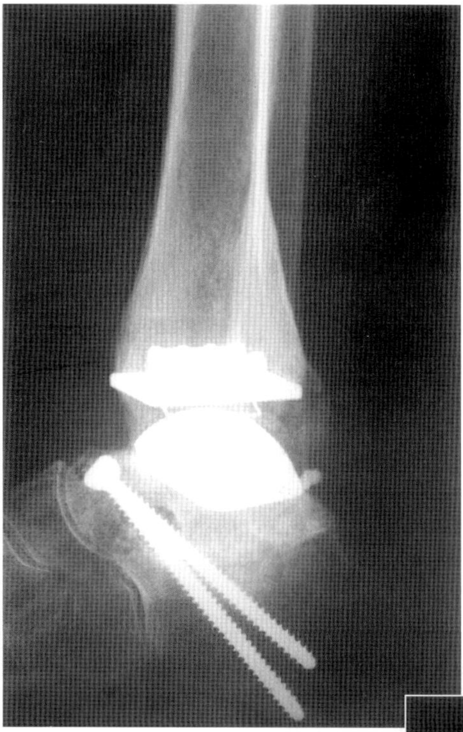

Fig.10.

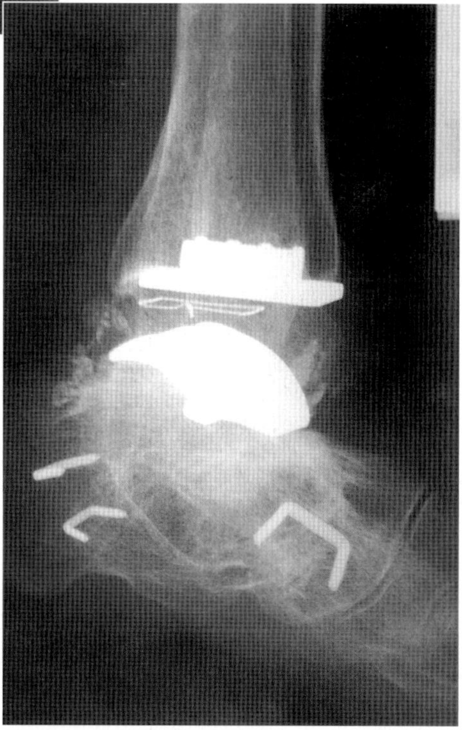

Fig.11.

Conclusion

Rheumatoid arthritis can affect each of the joints of the hindfoot. The articular destruction can result in serious disability: pain while walking and, frequently, deviation of the foot in valgus. These painful mechanical consequences have to be treated by arthrodesis: mainly triple fusion and, sometimes, localized arthrodesis of the affected joints. This treatment has to be integrated in the overall management of the patient so that a combined medical and surgical strategy can be formulated to deal with all the affected joints.

References

1. Adam W, Ranawat C (1976) Arthrodesis of the hindfoot in rheumatoid arthritflis Clin North Am, 7, 827-840
2. Bouysset M, Vianey JC, Tebib JG, *et al.* (1989) Médio-pied rhumatoïde in Monographie de Podologie Masson 10: 198-207
3 Elboar JE, Thomas WH, Weinfeld MS *et al.* (1976) Talonavicular arthrodesis for rheumatoid arthritis of the hindfoot Orthop Clin North Am 7: 821-6
4. King J, Burke D, Freeman M (1978) The incidence of pain in rheumatoid hinfoot and the significance of calcaneo-fibular impigement Int Orthop 2: 255-7
5. Gerard Y, Pierson A, Chelius Ph (1986) Le blocage de l'articulation sous-astragalienne par arthrodèse astragalo-scaphoïdienne Rev Chir Orthop 72,2: 105-8
6. Gerard Y (1994) Les possibilités de l'arthrodèse talonaviculaire dans les atteintes du couple de torsion Podologie Expansion Scientifique Française Edit. 203-10
7. Lowell FL, Perterson, A (1968) Surgery for Rheumatoid Arthritis-Timing and Techniques: The Lower Extremity, JBJS vol50-A, 3,
8. Michelson J, Easley M, Wigeland F, Hellman D (1994) Foot and Ankle Problems in Rheumatoid Arthritis Foot and Ankle International, 15
9. Steinhauser J (1987) Le rôle de l'interligne de Chopart dans la correction chirurgicale des déformations graves du pied de l'adulte. Méd Chir Pied 3 (2): 59-78
10. Stockley, Betts RP, Rowley DI, Getty CJ, Duckworth (1990) The importance of the valgus hindfoot in forefoot surgery in rheumatoid arthritis JBJS vol 72-B, n°4
11. Vainio K (1991) The rheumatoid foot Clin Orthop 165: 4-8
12. Vigidal E, Jakoby RK, Dixion A *et al.* (1975) The foot in chronic rheumatoid arthritis Ann rheum Dis 34: 293

Additional references

. Clayton ML (1960) Surgery of the forefoot in rheumatoid arthritis. Clin Orthop 16: 136
. Clayton ML (1967) Surgigal treatment of the rheumatoid foot. In: Giannestras NJ (ed) Foot and Disorders. Medical and Surgical Management. Philadelphia Lea and Febiger

. Clayton ML (1963) Surgery of the lower extremity in rheumatoid arthritis. J Bone Joint Surg (AM) 45: 1517-36

. Hamalainen M, Raunio P (1997) Long term follow-up of rheumatoid forefoot surgery. Clinical Orthopaedics and Related Research 340: 34-38

. Kerschbaumer F, Von-Salomon D, Lehr F (1996) Der rheumatische Vorfuss. Der Orthopädie 25(4): 354-61

. Miehlke W, Gschwend N, Rippstein P, Simmen BR (1997) Compression arthrodesis of the rheumatoid ankle and hindfoot. Clin Orthop 340: 75-86

. Tillmann K (1979) The rheumatoid foot. G Thieme, Stuttgart, pp 44-56

. Tillmann K (1985) Reconstructive foot surgery. Ann Chir Gynaecol 74: 90-5

. Tillmann K (1987) The mutual interplay between forefoot and hindfoot affections and deformities in RA. Rheumatoid arthritis surgery of the complex foot. Rheumatology 11: 97-9

Points of view about synovectomy of the ankle joint in rheumatoid arthritis

H. Thabe

Introduction

We report of mid- and longterm results of open synovectomy of the ankle joint. Between 1984 and 1999 66 ankle joints in 55 patients with rheumatoid arthritis undervent an open synovectomy. 23 cases needed an additional tenosynovectomy and a supplementary arthrodesis was performed in 30 ankles. The mean age at operation was 52 years, 3 patients died and 5 were lost at time of follow up. The mean follow-up period was 6.4 years, ranging from 2 to 15 years. Clinical examination was based on the Kofoed-ankle-score and all patients undervent a radiological staging orientated on Larsen, Dale and Eek.

At time of follow up pain and swelling was obtained in 72% of patients. In radiological examination we found a mild deterioration. Revision procedures were necessary in 6% of patients. Recurrent synovitis occured in 2% of the ankle joints, a resynovectomy after 34 months after the first operation was done. Progressive destruction was the reason for implantation of endoprosthesis or arthrodeses in 4% of the operated ankle joints. In summary the most benefit of synovectomy results in a good reduction of pain and satisfactory function in midterm follow up. Secundary osteoarthritis with mild deterioration was seen in radiological control studies.

In the course of rheumatoid arthritis most regularly the involvement of the ankle joint occurs. In the literature in 49-55% of cases, an attack on the upper and lower ankle joint takes place and mostly just in early cases the talonavicular joint is affected (13). Just in the early beginning of R.A. you will find, besides articular manifestations, an involvement with retromalleollar tenosynovitis of the peroneal tendons, that of the tibialis posterior and, in few cases, an attack on the extensor tendons (5, 13). The choice of the surgical treatment is influenced by the present state of activity in the lower limb's attack, the radiological stage of destruction according to Larsen, Dale, and Eek's classification (LDE) (6), the spontaneus course of the disease and the prophylactic aspects of our surgical interventions. Under these conditions, the surgical treatment should be done as early as possible to obtain a preventive effect. This determines the prognosis for the effect in the long run and at least the remaining surgical possibilities. A preventive joint surgery is much more important than a joint replacement. The large variety of our conservative tools with adequate supports and correction of the hindfoot with made-to- measure orthopaedic shoe supports as well as the chemical- and radiosynoviortheses should be used prior to any strategic planning of surgical interventions. The benefit of synovectomy results in a good reduction of pain and satisfactory function in midterm follow- up. Secondary osteoarthritis with mild deterioration was seen in radiological control studies.

Pathology of R.A. in ankle joint

A combination of articular and periarticular destruction mechanisms will develop characteristic deformities in the ankle joint. With 87% the main deformity is the pes plano-valgus, in up to 20% with a combination of a varus deformation of the forefoot (13,14). Not that often seen are varus deformations of the hindfoot (9%), mostly associated with valgus positions of the knee joint. The individual appearance of the rheumatoid ankle joint is at least the result of the inflammatory attack on the joint and the surrounding soft tissue and its interactions with congenital and statical factors. The typical pes-planovalgus comes about due to inflammatory attacks to the subtalar and midfoot joints, the asymetric fibular destruction of the upper ankle joint combined with a disturbed soft tissue balancing by the insufficiency of the tibialis posterior tendons. Previous deformities of the foot and countercurrent deformations of the knee axis will worsen this static problem. Starting point of the development of a flatfoot deformity is the tibial joint row with the talo-navicular and cuneo-navicular joint. The crash of the midfoot arc occurs with the insufficiency of the calcaneo-tarsal ligaments and the following destruction of the cuneo-navicular joint. This inflammatory attack of the talo-calcanear and calcaneo-cuboid joint leads to a drop down of the talus head by insufficency of the tarsocalcanear ligament towards plantar and tibial, building up a step in the talo-navicular joint, starting the flatfoot deformity and malalignment of the hindfoot. Asymmetrical fibular destruction mechanisms of the upper ankle joint will additionally support this deformation.

The amount of surgical procedures in the ankle joint was nearly the same compared with those of hip joints in R.A. Between 1986 and 1996, we performed 384 cases of ankle joint surgery, some 16% in our R.A. surgery of the lower limb. According to the stage of deformation we divide R.A. surgery in preventive-joint preserving surgery, mainly with soft tissue surgery and joint replacing or reconstructive surgery. Up to stage 3 of Larsen, Dale, Eek, joint preserving surgery remains possible, beyond this stage only reconstructive surgery is usefull. In our department, 41% of our surgery was a joint preserving procedure, as seen in the table below.

Table I - Ankle joint surgery (Dept. for orthopedics kreuznacher diakonie 1986-1996). 1. Synovectomies; 2 Synovectomies of the tendon sheaths as a single procedure; 3. Arthrodesis of the upper ankle joint; 4. Arthrodesis of the lower ankle joint only; 4. Combined fusion of the lower and upper ankle joint; 5. Ankle replacement.

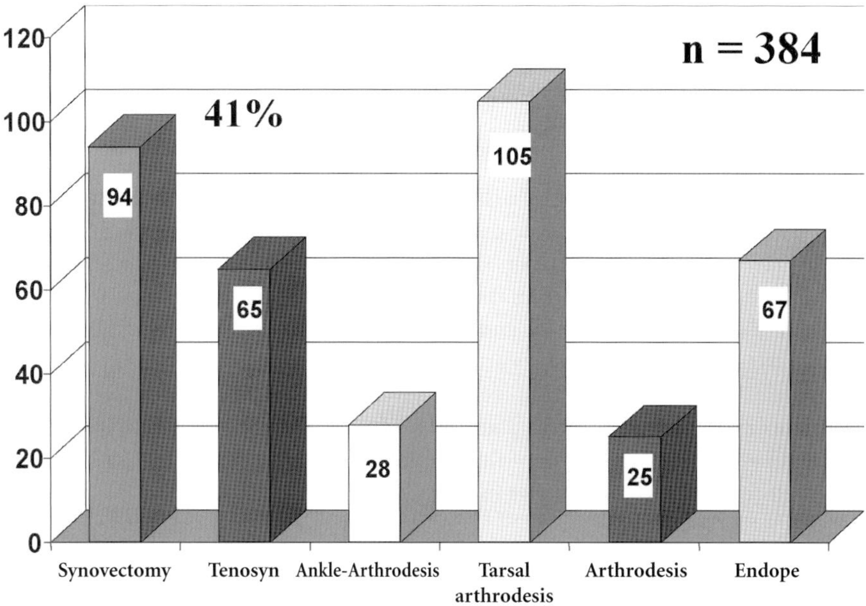

Indication

Synovectomy of the ankle joint is one of the most profitable procedures in R.A. surgery of the lower limb. The onset of indication determines the prognosis of the joint development in the long run and the remaining surgical possibilities. The indication for synovectomy should be done early, to avoid irreparable joint and soft tissue destructions. After visible insufficiency of the stabilizing ligament in the subtalar-tarsal arc, an immediate support is necessary, together with the synovectomy of ankle joints. Synovectomy is therefore indicated, when medical treatment is no longer effective on swelling and pain in early stages of LDE 0-2. Additional local injections may be necessary in cases of combinations of joint and soft tissue attacks, or surgical interventions can solve this problem. Compressions of the tarsal tunnel as well as degenerative osteophytes, mostly signs of long lasting instabilities, can be additionally treated.

In stage 3 of LDE a late synovectomy is often still very effective.

The choice of surgical procedure depends on the current state of activity and destruction of the soft tissue and joints.

Diagnostics

The evaluation of the anamnesis (walking distance, supports, shœs made - to - measured, physical treatment, drug support, intra-articular injections, radioactive injections), clinical exploration, range of motion and radiological examinations are documented together with the Kofoed score. Alignment of the foot in static and dynamic testing, swelling and range of motion are tested in the clinical examination. In severe cases electronical foot prints with the megascan system can lead to an optimal position of the subtalar arthrodesis. Swellings of the synovial tissue are easily varified by ultrasonographic explorations, the standard procedure due to the definitions of the DEGUM will show the extent of the upcoming surgical intervention. In some special cases the MRI gives more information concerning the quality of the important ligament and of the bony structures, developing of necrosis and the extent of the inflammatory attack. Decisions then have to be made to enlarge the surgical procedure with a tenosynovectomy or an arthrodesis of the neighbouring joints. Special X-rays under weight bearing are to be made in cases of malalignment, an axis deviation of the hindfoot or insufficiency of the midfoot arc, cystic deformations might promote further CT scanning investigations.

Operation technique

Arthroscopic synovectomy is chosen in cases of early inflammatory involvement of the ankle joint (LDE 0-2). It is much easier to get into the joint spaces even into the posterior joint space. Small exophytes can be additionally removed with the acromionizer to open the view on the villous hypertrophy of the synovial membrane. These formations can be removed by different shavers and punches, together with a trimming of cartilage degenerations.

Open synovectomy in stage LDE 1-3 is often performed together with additive surgical treatment like tenosynovectomy of the fibular group, subtalar and talo-navicular arthrodesis. The approach is done by vertical skin incision, following the tendon of the extensor hallucis longus muscle. Step by step the retinacula (especially the extensor inferior retinaculum) are explored protecting the superfical and deep branches of the vessels and fibular profundus nerve. The resection of the anterior part of the capsulae allows a very wide approach to the ankle joint. Osteophytes are now removed and, by using spreaders for osteotomies, an exellent view on the whole joint space is guaranted and a subtotal synovectomy can be performed radically. In late cases (LDE 3) sometimes an additional posterior approach via the fibular tendon sheaht is necessary. The borderline between cartilage and bone is treated by electrocoagulation in order to destroy pannus formations.

The lateral approach is done by a retromalleolar skin incision, proximal in the middle of the achilles tendon and the posterior edge of the fibula running down to the os cuboideum and the base of metatarsal 4.

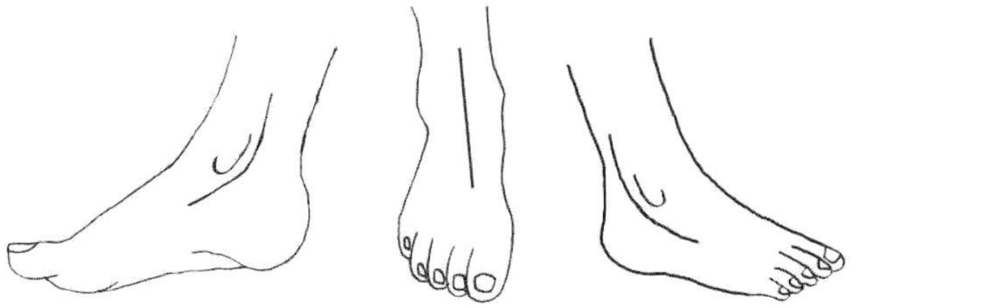

Fig. 1 - Skin incisions at the ankle joint.

Additional treatments

In severe cases of cartilage destruction an interosseous osteotomy of the talus and the tibia according to Benjamin's technique is added; the effect is simular to a sympathectomy with better circulation inside the bony structures and pain relief. Cystic structures are removed and filled up with synthetic bone (biobone o.a.) In most cases supports for conventional shoewear are sufficient in synovectomies. In severe malalignments and arthrodesis, shoes made-to-measure with collateral supports are necessary.

Another important factor is the strength and integrity of the fibular collateral ligament. Laxity and insufficiency will promote further deformations and therefore we often combine our synovectomies in those cases with a ligamentous reconstruction on the principles of Watson-Jones.

In local cartilage destructions a mosaique plastic is possible.

Arthrodesis of the lower ankle joint

Talon-navicular joint

From the same anterior incision an approach to the talo-navicular joint is easily done; a straight incision of the deltoideum ligaments, tibionavicular part and talofibular anterior ligament and subperiostal preparation of the joint cavity. The cartilage is removed with osteotomes and saw blades, cysts are filled up and after reposition and alignment of the axis the position is fixed by Blount staples. The formerly used Shapiro staples are not strong enough and will show fatigue fractures.

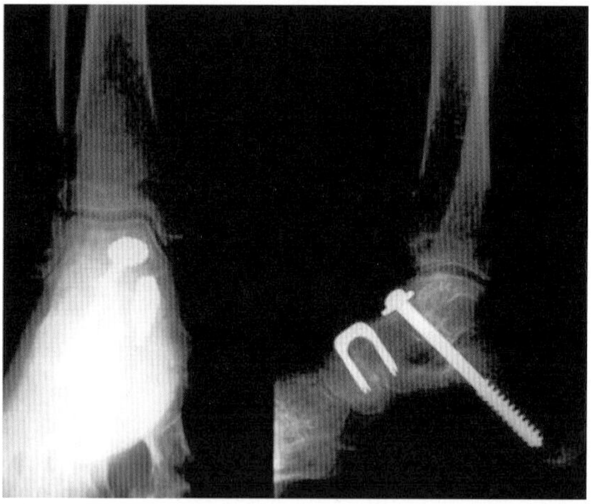

Fig. 2 - Arthrodeses talo-navicular and talo-calcanear (X-ray a.p. and side view).

Talo-calcaneal joint

After subperiosteal clearing of the neck of the talus the reposition of the talus-calcaneus alignment is done and then fixed by an A.O. compression screw driven through the talus and the calcaneus with a perpendicular crossing of the joint line. An approach and opening of the sinus tarsi is only performed in certain cases, if a correction by osteotomy becomes necessary.

Material and methods

Under these guidelines between 1984 and 1998 in 66 ankle joints of 56 patients with R.A. an open synovectomy was performed. Forty-seven patients with 56 operated joints were followed up in 1999 with a responder-rate of 83,3%.

Three patients had passed away at time of follow-up, 5 patients were lost at follow-up.

In 23 cases tenosynovectomies had to be done additionally to the open synovectomy; fibularis tendons in 11 cases; extensor tendons in 4 cases; flexor tendons in 3 cases. In 5 cases a complete involvement of all tendons was present. A supplementary arthrodesis had to be made in 30 cases on the subtalar joint, in 13 joints only talo-navicular, in 7 joints talo-calcaneal and in 10 cases talo-navicular as well as talo-calcaneal.

Women were affected in a relationship of 5/ 2. The follow-up was done after an intervall of 6.4 years on average, with a minimum/maximum follow-up of 1 to 14.8 years. At time of operation patients were 52.1 years old, the onset of the disease was more than 12 years and the ankle attack more than 5 years prior the operation.

The follow up was based on anamnestic, clinical and radiological items, the Kofoed score, known from the ankle replacement scoring, was also used to compare these results with results of reconstructive surgery. This score of 100 points saves 50 points for pain relief with and without weight bearing, 30 points for functional assessment and 20 points for range of motion. Results below 75 points were rated as bad, 76-85 as good and beyond 86 as very good. Beside this pain was evaluated on a visible analogue scale.

Results

In our assessments 16 patients with 21 ankle joints were rated with more than 86 points, 13 patients with 13 joints as good and 18 patients with 23 joints under 75 points. As known in inflammatory diseases, the influence of the polyarticular involvement deteriorates the outcome evaluation severely, due to the malalignment of the affected lower limb (forefoot, gonarthritis, etc.). The score increased from 56.4 points preoperatively to 73.5 points after operation. The benefit of this procedure was at least dedicated to the relief of pain (Tab. II). The preoperative pain in weight bearing and walking on flat ground decreased severely, seen in the analogue-visual score with a drop down from 7.6 to 3.7.

Table II - Pain in Kofoed-ankle-score, VAS: Visual-analogue-scale (maximal 10).

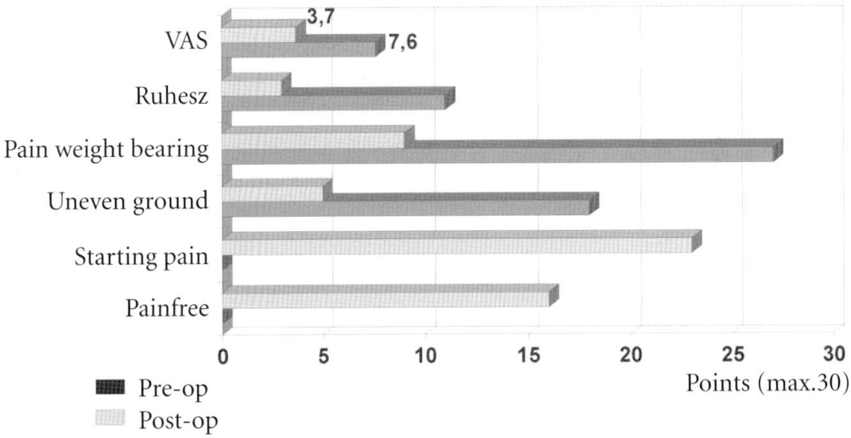

The range of motion in the upper and lower ankle joint worsened during an average of 6 year's intervall in doral/ventral flexion with 3° and in pronation/supination with 5°.

The evaluation of the X-rays was done in the LDE staging. The stages decreased from 1.89 to 2.47 postoperatively after 6 years. These results include 12 joints without any deterioration during the years as well as 24 joints with a decrease of only 0.5 in radiological staging. Eight joints worsened with stages 2 and 3 very early, these joints might have been treated in another way, if preoperative MRI had been done.

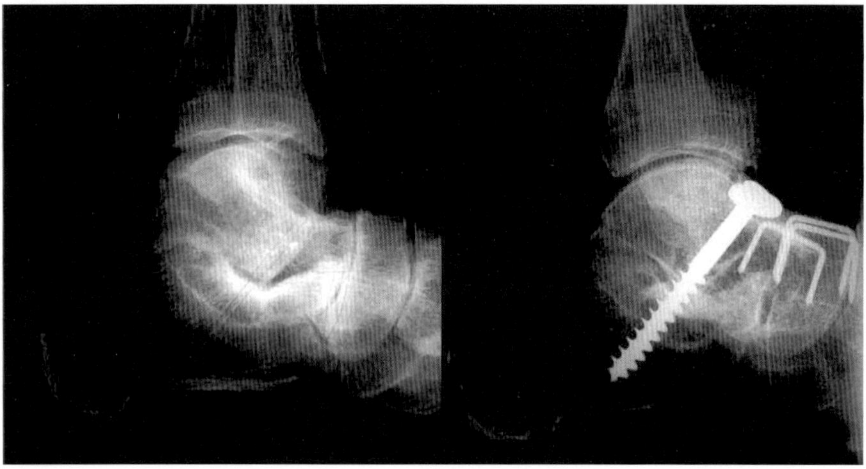

Fig. 3 - Long term radiological results after ankle joint synovectomies.

The necrosis in these joints developed very quickly after operation and was responsible for the bad results. Four joints present a deterioration by only one degree on the scale.

Revisions

Revision rates between 9 and 11% are published. Up to the end of 2000 in our group of 47 patients with 56 synovectomies 3 patients with 3 ankle joint synovectomies hade to be revised, this amounts to 6%. One synovectomy with an additional tenosynovectomy, no later arthrodeses and in 2 cases an ankle joint replacement with a STAR joint were performed. The revisions had to be done on average 34 months postoperatively.

Discussion

To summarize, most of our synovectomies had an excellent relief of pain, shown in the data of the VAS, in contrast to other publications (10,11,12,14). Never the less, pain was seen in all our cases that had to be revised. These revision rates are simular to published ones (1,12,13). (see table of the meta-analysis below).

Over all, the clinical results were good; patients with early synovectomies have better results than late ones. Patients do profit mostly in cases of synovectomies in early LDE stages (11) in spite of low radiological progression, seen in secondary osteoarthritic changes. Patients gain time, before reconstructive surgery has to be considered a real advantage. This causes us to ask and especially to look for the involvement of the ankle joint including ultrasonographic examination, in order to

Table III - Meta-analysis of open synovectomies of the ankle joint.

Author	N°	Follow up	Pain	LDE
Akagi S. (1997)	20	15	-90	75 Progression
Tressel W. (1998)	41	10	-83	?
Tillmann K. (1975)	35	4	-89	?
Biehl C. *et al.* (2001)	56	6	-82	1.9 > 2.5
Schmidt K. (1997)	14	3.2	-70	1.5 > 1.7

avoid early reconstructive surgery or arthrodeses. The new techniques of arthroscopic synovectomies and minimal invasive surgery will better the patient's acceptance for an early surgical intervention. The arthroscopic synovectomies are always combined with a radiosynoviorthesis 6 weeks after surgery. (7, 11). For static significant valid data the number of cases for the results of our arthroscopic surgery is too low and the postoperative time too short.

Nowadays the indication for preventive surgery is done much earlier for hindfoot and subtalar arthrodeses because the insufficiency of the calcaneo tarsal ligaments can never be restored by any synovectomy or injection treatment, and this defect will soon lead to severe malalignment of the hindfoot and axis deviation with all its consequences.

In some cases a synovectomy combined with radioactive injection additionally into the talonavicular joint is effective.

In late stages the open technique allows an easy enlargement of the surgical procedure up to an arthrodeses, tenosynovectomy and, if necessary, a prosthetical replacement.

Conclusion

Even late synovectomies of the ankle joints are still effective and long lasting in R.A. surgery. The open synovectomy, therefore, is a standard procedure, additional surgical treatment can be easily done and if necessary the enlargement up to prosthetic replacement can be performed by the same approach in cases of severe cartilage damage. The open synovectomy in late stages offers good pain relief with astonishing long-lasting effects. Therefore this procedure can be offered as an alternative to early prosthetic replacement. In early involvements of the ankle joint the arthroscopic approach, together with a radioactive injection 6 weeks later, is a real preventive surgical treatment.

References

1. Akagi S, Sugano H, Ogawa R (1997) The long-term results of ankle synovectomy for rheumatoid arthritis. Clin Rheumatol 16: 284 – 90
2. Beck E. (1990) Verletzungen des distalen Schienenbeinendes und des Sprunggelenkes. In Breitner B (Hrsg): Chirurgische Operationslehre, Band XI, Urban & Schwarzenberg, München 174-5
3. Biehl C, Schill S, Thabe H (2001) Mittel- und Langfristige Ergebnisse nach Sprunggelenkssynovektomien. Orthop. Praxis 37: 814 – 7
4. Eyring EJ, Longert A, Bass JC (1971) Synovectomy in juvenile rheumatoid arthritis. Indications and short-term results. J. Bone Joint Surg Am 53: 638 – 49
5. Gschwend N (1977) Die operative Behandlung der chronischen Polyarthritis. Thieme, Stuttgart, New York, S 269 – 72
6. Larsen A, Dahle K, Eek M (1977) Radiographic evaluation of rheumatoid arthritis and related conditions by standard reference films. Acta Radiol 18: 481-91
7. Kerschbaumer F, Kandziora F, Herresthal J *et al.* (1998) Synovektomie und Synoviorthese als Kombinationstherapie bei rheumatoider Arthritis. Der Orthopäde 27: 188 – 96
8. Kerschbaumer F (1995) Alloarthroplastik des Sprunggelenkes. Synovektomie des oberen Sprunggelenkes. In: Bauer R., Kerschbaumer F., Poisel S. (Hrsg.): Orthopädische Operationslehre. Becken und untere Extremität Bd II/2 Thieme, Stuttgart, New York
9. Kofoed H, Danborg L (1995) Biological fixation of total ankle arthroplasty. Food 5 pp. 27-31
10. Mohing W, Köhler G, Colewey J (1982) Synovectomy of the ankle joint. Int. Orthopaedics 6: 117 – 21
11. Rittmeister M, Böhme T, Rehart S, *et al.* (1999) Die Behandlung der rheumatischen oberen Sprunggelenkes mit Synovektomie und Radiosynoviorthese. Der Orthopäde 28: 785 – 91
12. Tressel W Schattenhofer K, Gebhart J (1998): Synovektomie des oberen Sprunggelenkes 10-Jahres-Ergebnisse. Vortrag ARO-Tagung, Zürich
13. Tillmann K (1977): Der rheumatische Fuss und seine Behandlung. In Otte P., Schlegel KF. (Hrsg.): Bücherei des Orthopäden, Bn 18: 77 – 78, Enke, Stuttgart
14. Wolfram U (1997) Die Sprunggelenke. In Thabe H. (Hrsg): Praktische Rheumaorthopädie, Chapman & Hall, Weinheim

Additional references

. Matsumoto Y, Tanaka K, Hirata G, *et al.* (2002) Possible involvement of the VEGF receptor Fit-1-focal adhesion kinase pathway in chemotaxis and the cell proliferation of osteoclasts precursor cells in the arthritic joint. J Immunol 168: 5824-31

Total ankle replacement. History, evolution of concepts, designs and surgical technique

M. Bonnin, T. Judet, T. Siguier and J.A. Colombier

Introduction

In 1977, Evanski and Waugh (13) reviewed the early results of ankle arthroplasty and concluded that they were "clinically comparable" to those of hip replacement.

This initial enthusiasm was soon tempered by the high complication rates and early deterioration of the functional outcome seen with the first-generation implants. The devices used at the time had kinematic patterns that were far removed from the physiological norm, and required extensive bone removal. The failures encountered in those early days delayed the development of total ankle replacement (TAR).

It was not until the second half of the 1980s that interest in TAR was rekindled, as a result of progress made in two important respects: (1) the introduction of a mobile (meniscal) bearing inserted between the tibial and the talar components, which led to a reduction in the mechanical failure rate of the devices; and (2) the use of cementless implants, which allowed more sparing tibial and talar bone resections, involved less risk of implant loosening, and left the option of secondary fusion open.

The history of total ankle replacement. Concepts and designs

The first device: the Lord-Marotte prosthesis

The first attempt at TAR was made by Lord and Marotte, in 1970 (29). The design was a ball-and-socket joint, patterned on total hip replacements. A cup-shaped polyethylene (PE) component was cemented into the calcaneus and into the head of the talus, while a metal ball component with an anteriorly bowed intramedullary stem was cemented into the tibia. The design was fully congruent (figs. 1a and b).

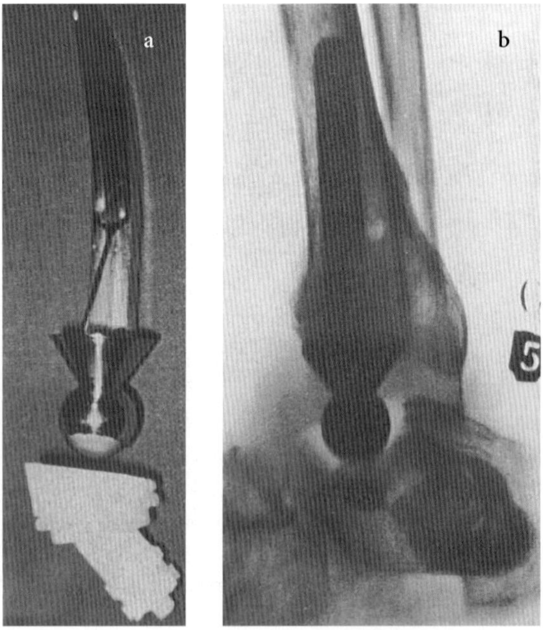

Fig. 1 - The Lord-Marotte prosthesis (from (28, 29), with permission). **a)** The two implant components; **b)** Lateral check radiograph.

Results were poor, with a high rate of secondary varus instability (28, 29), and the design was short-lived.

The Roy-Camille prosthesis was based upon the same principle, and equally fraught with a high rate of early implant failures. With this pattern, too, the main problem was hindfoot tilt into varus (38).

Two-component sliding TARs – the second generation

In 1972, Toméno and Cornic (47) described a sliding cylinder-type device, without mortise extensions; the talar component was made of metal, and the tibial component of PE. In the same year, Freeman proposed a more constrained cylindrical pattern, with flanges (39). A third pattern, with a spherical component, was proposed by Smith *et al.*, in 1972. (9, 14, 40)

Since those early designs, many cylindrical and spherical patterns have been devised. The different devices may be classified in terms of their degree of congruency and their geometry.

Incongruent surface types – the Newton prosthesis

In this pattern, the PE tibial component is a section of a cylinder, while the Vitallium talar component is a section of a sphere with a slightly smaller radius (33). Because of the relative incongruency of the articulating surfaces, movement is not confined to flexion/extension.

In his paper on the outcome of 50 incongruent arthroplasties, Newton (34) reported a rate of satisfactory results of only 50%. The most frequently encountered cause of failure was loosening, with most of the instances involving the tibial component. A non-progressive lucency at the cement-bone interface was observed in 40% of the cases.

Congruent surface types

Spherical type

The principle adopted in the design of these devices is the reproduction of the ball-and-socket ankle seen in cases of major talocalcaneal synostosis. The implant geometry allows flexion/extension, as well as varus/valgus movements. The Smith prosthesis and, later, the Bath & Wessex prosthesis, were designed along those lines (6, 9, 15).

The main complications reported were loosening (observed in up to 50% of the 52 cases in the study by Carlsson *et al.* (6)); hindfoot tilt into valgus, with calcaneofibular impingement; and persistent pain, which, in some cases, necessitated removal of the implant. In the study by Carlsson *et al.*, (6) the rate of implant removal was 15% (fig. 2).

Toroidal type

In this pattern, flexion/extension and varus/valgus movements are similar in range to those permitted by spherical types. However, axial rotational movement is limited by the increasing restraint of the components during rotation. The only device incorporating this principle was the IAA (Irvine Ankle Arthroplasty) designed by Waugh. Results were poor, with a high rate of complications (13, 50).

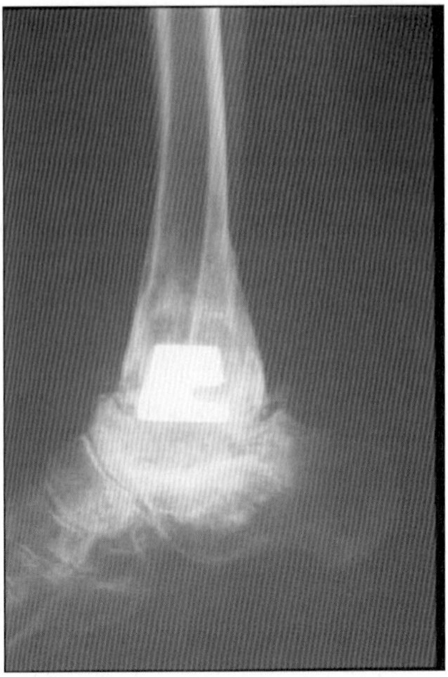

Fig. 2 - Loosening of a spherical prosthesis.

Cylindrical type

Semi-constrained cylindrical prostheses

These devices do not include any flanges, and do not, therefore, have inherent transverse stability. The Toméno prosthesis is a typical example. Results were poor, with a 50% rate of secondary fusion in a series of eight cases (47).

Constrained cylindrical prostheses

In this pattern, the talar component has only one degree of freedom (flexion/extension), since the flanges prevent movement in the coronal and in the axial plane. The Mayo Clinic prosthesis is a typical example. It is a cemented device, with a metal talar component that articulates with a tibial component made of PE. Several studies have been published (8, 28, 43, 44, 48). The largest studies to date have been the ones by Kitaoka *et al.* (21, 22), in which 204 prostheses were implanted in 1974 through to 1988. Results were poor, with implant removal required in 27.9% of the cases, on average four and a half years after the index arthroplasty. Risk factors for failure were previous operative procedures on the ipsilateral foot or ankle, and an age of 57 years or less. However, the nature of the underlying disease – rheumatoid arthritis (RA) or post-traumatic osteoarthritis (OA) – did not affect implant survival; neither did gender or body weight.

In the light of these results, Kitaoka *et al.* advised against the use of the constrained Mayo implant, in either RA or post-traumatic OA of the ankle (22).

The ICLH (Imperial College London Hospital) prosthesis was designed along the same lines. It had large flanges forming what amounted to medial and lateral talomalleolar joints. This device, too, had a high rate of loosening, documented in a number of studies (1, 12, 17).

The other devices incorporating this concept (16, 35) had high failure rates. Some of the uniaxial cylindrical patterns were particularly constrained, because of the geometry of the components. This was true of the Kofoed prosthesis, in its original two-component form. The results reported by the author (23) in a series of 28 prostheses implanted between 1981 and 1985 were poor, with a failure rate of 30%.

The highly constrained C.T.A.R. (Conaxial Total Ankle Replacement) designed by Beck and Steffee also had a high rate of loosening (27% at two years, 60% at five years, and 90% at ten years) (52).

To summarize, the second-generation two-component TARs suffered from mechanical loosening, which was a particular problem with the highly constrained cylindrical types, (1, 12, 17, 52) and constituted the prime cause of failure of this type of arthroplasty. While the spherical and toroidal types were less constrained, they, too, were fraught with this complication. Also, secondary hindfoot deformity was a risk because of these patterns'lack of inherent stability.

The frequency of failures appears to have been largely related to the use of implants with a kinematic pattern far removed from the physiological norm of ankle movement. Implant loosening was encouraged by the small fixation surfaces in contact with the host bone, poor cementing technique, component malpositioning, and the use of inappropriate component sizes.

The functional outcomes reported vary with the reporting period, the implant pattern, and the criteria employed in the assessment of the functional outcome.

Overall, the studies published prior to the mid-1980s showed poor functional outcomes, regardless of whether the devices used were of the spherical or the cylindrical type. The poor functional outcome was due either to mechanical failure (implant loosening) or to persistent pain. The most frequently observed cause of persistent pain appears to have been malleolar impingement, which was reported by a number of authors. (1, 6, 28, 43, 44, 48, 52).

A small number of authors (35, 49) reported better functional results during the same period. However, these were small series with limited follow-up; to the best of our knowledge, the outcomes reported were not confirmed at longer follow-up.

Other authors (37) have recommended arthrodesis of the tibiofibular syndesmosis plus arthroplasty, so as to obtain a larger surface area for bone growth into the tibial component. It was thought that this procedure would produce increased stability of the components. However, the arthrodesis increases the magnitude of the procedure, and union of the syndesmosis is not reliably obtained in all cases.

Three-component sliding TARs – third-generation implants

Over the last decade, cementless TARs (4, 5, 39, 45) with a mobile bearing (4, 5) and requiring minimal bone resection have been introduced. The benefits of cementless fixation were stressed by Scholz, in 1987 (39), Takakura *et al.*, in 1990 (45), and

Kofoed, in 1998 (26). A mobile bearing placed between the tibial and the talar component reduces the stress on the fixation of the implants (fig. 3). Bone resection is reduced to the amount required for resurfacing; this means less risk of talar component subsidence, and leaves secondary fusion as an option in the event of implant failure (fig. 4).

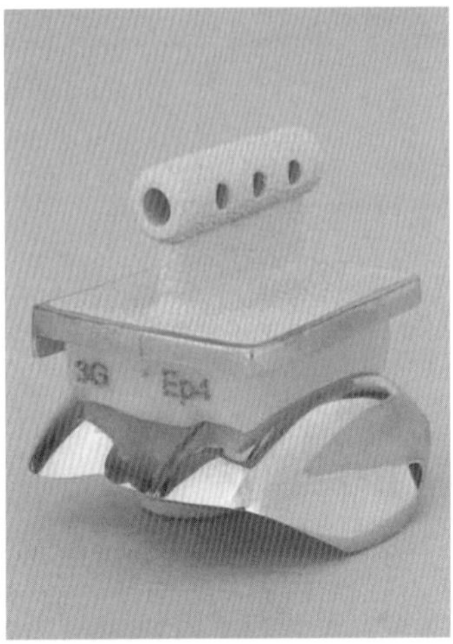

Fig. 3 - Cementless three-piece prosthesis. The PE mobile bearing is free to move in all planes. (Salto prosthesis).

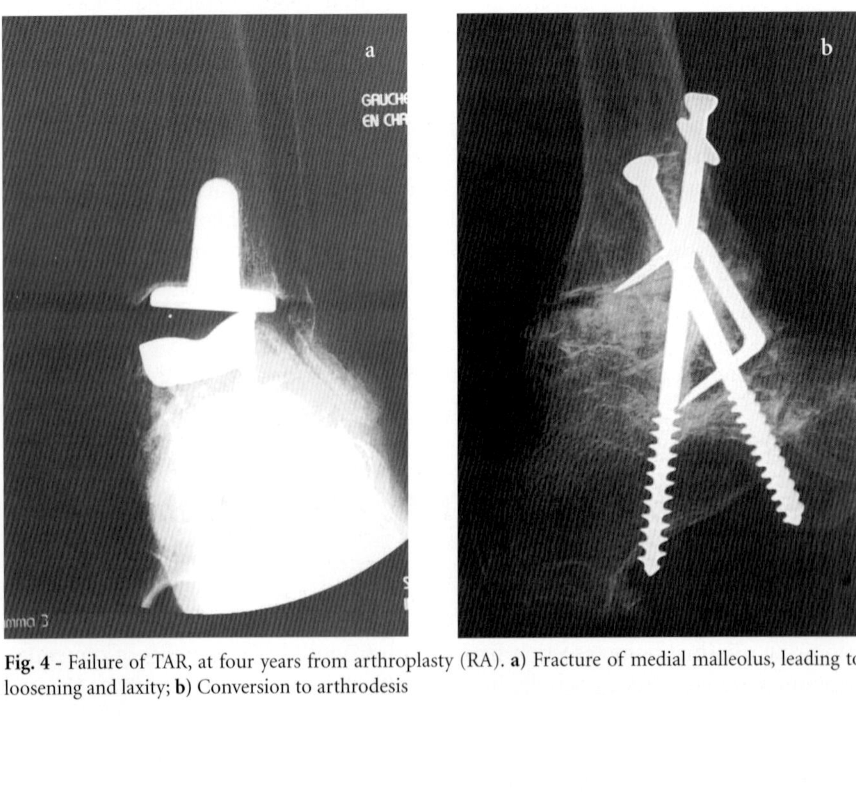

Fig. 4 - Failure of TAR, at four years from arthroplasty (RA). **a)** Fracture of medial malleolus, leading to loosening and laxity; **b)** Conversion to arthrodesis

The studies published after the mid-1980s concerning this new TAR concept have shown good functional outcomes. (4, 5, 10, 20, 24, 40, 51). The rate of mechanical failure has been reduced, and revision surgery after implant failure has become a rare event. Buechel *et al.* (4) were the first, in 1988, to report a series of three-component implants with a PE mobile bearing inserted between the tibial and talar components. Kofoed (26, 27), Kofoed and Danborg (24), and Kofoed and Sørensen (25) also reported good outcomes following the use of the STAR prosthesis, a cylindrical cementless device with a mobile bearing. Unlike the New Jersey TAR, the STAR does not require an anterior cortical window for its insertion.

A failed cemented TAR is difficult to convert to an arthrodesis. The time to fusion will be much longer than in the case of a primary arthrodesis (17), and talar collapse may cause major technical difficulties. These problems appear to be reduced with the third-generation, minimal-resection TARs.

Remaining problems, and future directions

Malleolar impingement

Post-TAR perimalleolar pain has been reported by a large number of authors (1, 6, 28, 33, 34, 48, 52), regardless of the implant type used.

This peri- and inframalleolar pain is probably multifactorial in origin. (1) It may be due to persistence of osteoarthritic pain in the talar and malleolar surfaces that have not been replaced. This seems to be the leading cause of malleolar or perimalleolar pain following TAR. (2) Excessive removal of tibial or talar bone stock may have altered the anatomical relationships, and caused talomalleolar or even calcaneomalleolar impingement. (3) The mobile bearing may be too thin. (4) The mobile bearing may be involved in medial or lateral impingement. (5) Subsidence of the talar component may have altered the anatomical relationships of the ankle mortise.

Implant fixation

Talar component subsidence

This complication was very frequently reported in first-generation TARs.

Carlsson *et al.* (6) felt that subsidence was mainly due to suboptimal cementing conditions in the dense trabecular structure of the talus. Also, the limited support surfaces (less than 10 cm^2) will be exposed to high compressive loading.

The risk of subsidence has been controlled, thanks to the use of cementless implants anchored in sound subchondral bone, and to sparing bone resection.

Tibial component migration is less frequently observed, regardless of the geometry and the manner of fixation of the implant. This is probably due to the fact that the tibial component has wider support in the host bone, with cortical seating of the implant, whereas the talar component has a smaller support area and is housed mainly in cancellous bone.

Implant-bone interface

The radiographic analysis of the interface between cementless implant components and the host bone is fraught with the same problems as interface analyses of cementless total hip or total knee replacements.

A periprosthetic lucency around the tibial component has been interpreted by Buechel *et al.* (4, 5) as evidence of "fibrous fixation". This radiographic finding does not appear to be a harbinger of trouble (4, 41), nor does it seem to be associated with an increased risk of radiological loosening of the implant.

In all the reported series, cement-bone interface lucencies (in the case of cemented devices), or implant-bone interface lucencies (in the case of cementless prostheses) appeared to occur chiefly around the tibial component. The lesser rate of talar periprosthetic lucencies would appear to be related to the fact that talar component subsidence may hide what would otherwise appear as a lucency.

Kinematics

Implant longevity is predicated upon a reduction in component stress levels. The most recent TARs – cylindrical patterns with a mobile bearing between the tibial and talar components – produce lower levels of implant stress, especially in rotation and translation.

However, they do not automatically restore physiological ankle joint movement; this movement remains governed by the design of the implant components. Thus, cylindrical TARs, even those with a mobile bearing, do not take account of talar asymmetry in the coronal plane or the truncated-cone pattern of the bone in the axial plane.

As a result of their design, the axis of ankle motion in these TARs is exclusively in a transverse plane, and the design does not reproduce the threefold obliquity, in space, of the physiological ankle joint axis.

Since physiological ankle joint kinematics are not replicated, more stress is placed on the implant components, even though the stress levels in contemporary TARs are very much lower than those in the more constrained uniaxial patterns.

Non-physiological ankle joint movement may also interfere with the harmonious interaction of the ankle joint complex and the torsion mechanism (subtalar and mid tarsal joint).

Surgical technique

Specific problems in patients with rheumatoid arthritis (RA)

While TAR is mainly carried out for RA, it should be remembered that the condition may pose specific problems when it comes to surgery.

Ankle – hindfoot malalignment

The normal ankle joint line is perpendicular to the mechanical axis of the tibia, and the hindfoot axis is in slight (5°– 10°) valgus in relation to the tibial axis. In the interest of implant longevity, a physiological alignment will need to be restored. Inserting a TAR into a malaligned tibia or hindfoot is a recipe for early loosening. The chief problem in RA ankle surgery is hindfoot deformity, usually in valgus, associated with subtalar joint disease, which may be made worse by tibialis posterior tenosynovitis. This deformity will need to be corrected by a separate procedure, with subtalar and midtarsal arthrodesis (2, 3); lateral malleolar osteotomy may be required if there has been malleolar malunion.

Available bone stock

Implant fixation requires sufficient bone stock in the talus and in the tibia, and an intact ankle mortise. In RA patients, there may be major bone loss, and defects may have to be grafted. In particularly severe cases, TAR may be ruled out altogether.

Surrounding joints

The surrounding (subtalar or talonavicular) joints may be arthritic and require fusion, even in the absence of deformity. Their condition must not be overlooked. They must be carefully studied with meticulous clinical examination, radiography, and, often, CT or MRI.

Stability

Instability associated with a major and long-standing valgus (less often varus) deformity will usually be corrected by a TAR that allows the laxity to be corrected, and by the pre-arthroplasty fusion of the subtalar and midtarsal joints, which restores hindfoot alignment. Where laxity is severe, TAR may not be feasible (fig. 5).

Ankle stiffness

Ankle stiffness in equinus is comparatively rare in RA; more often, the problem is laxity. However, stiffness may be severe, and cases of spontaneous fusion of the ankle joint are not unknown. In such situations, releases will need to be performed, with excision of anterior ossifications, take-down of talomalleolar adhesions, posterior capsulectomy, and Achilles tendon lengthening.

Preoperative work-up

The preoperative work-up must provide a picture of the extent of bone and ligament involvement around the ankle joint, and of any deformities or lesions at more distant sites.

Investigations comprise a clinical examination, AP and lateral weight-bearing radiographs, as well as a mortise view to show the lateral talomalleolar joint. Long films and CT scans of the ankle and hindfoot, with coronal sections, should be done in all the patients.

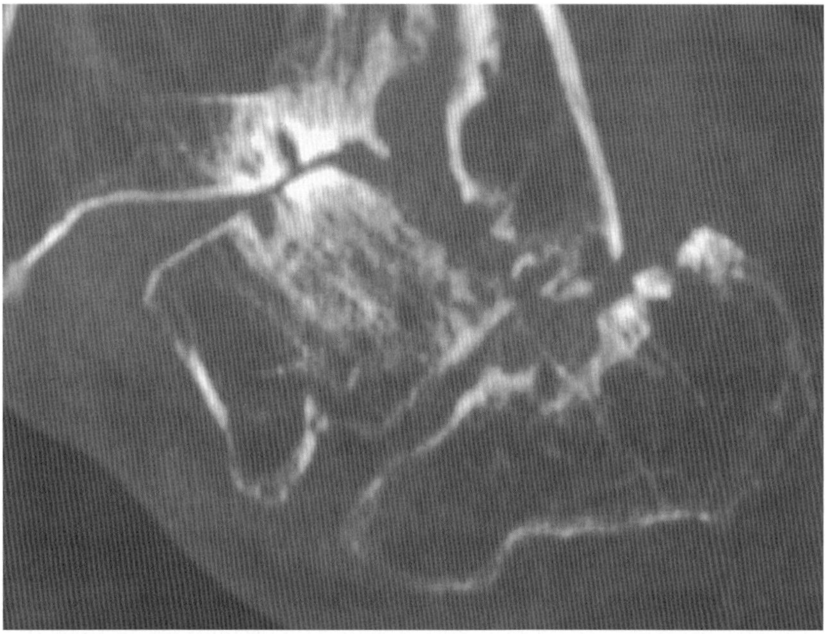

Fig. 5 - Juvenile rheumatoid arthritis. Major destruction of ankle joint, with laxity ruling out TAR.

This work-up will allow the surgeon to:

- choose the optimal implant size, using templates. An oversized prosthesis will alter the centres of rotation, and may give rise to pain and stiffness. If the talus is excessively deformed, the template should be applied to the contralateral, unaffected ankle;
- determine the reference for establishing the tibial resection level, taking into account the extent of wear;
- analyse the alignment of the tibiotalar joint line in relation to the tibial shaft axis. Asymmetrical wear of the tibial pilon, or osseous deformity, will need to be corrected by bone cuts that must be determined preoperatively;
- analyse the morphological pattern of the body of the talus, to see if there has been asymmetrical loss of bone stock. Any asymmetry found will need to be taken into account in the resection of the talus;
- analyse the subtalar joint, which should be fused prior to arthroplasty if it is found to be deformed or destroyed.

General principles

Restoration of a physiological tibiocalcaneal axis

The implant should be placed in such a way as to produce a joint line at right angles to the mechanical tibial axis, and to reproduce the physiological 7° posterior slope.

An extramedullary guide is mandatory. The guide must reference off the anterior tibial border or a line joining the knee and a point midway across the distal tibial surface.

Establishing a correct joint line

The final level of the implant joint line will depend upon the level of the tibial cut. The level is determined in the light of the preoperative radiographs. Depending on the status of the tibial pilon, the anatomy of the malleoli, and lateral talomalleolar congruency, four different patterns may be encountered (fig. 6):

- the ankle mortise is intact, and there is no asymmetrical wear of the tibial pilon. The choice of resection level will be guided by the bulk of the implant, the aim being a "size-for-size" replacement of resected bone by the implant;
- the ankle mortise is intact, but the tibial pilon is asymmetrically worn. This pattern is seen in advanced RA, especially in the wake of long-term steroid therapy. In this case, a sound zone on the distal tibia will have to be found during preoperative planning, to serve as a reference for bone resection;
- the malleoli are deformed, but the tibial pilon is intact. Usually, the deformity involves the lateral malleolus. This pattern is seen in RA with severe hindfoot valgus that has resulted in a fatigue fracture of the fibula. In this case, the lateral malleolus will need to be addressed in the first instance, with malleolar osteotomy and plating;
- the malleoli are deformed and the tibial pilon is worn or depressed. These cases will need to be managed with a combination of the principles discussed above: first, a normal ankle mortise pattern will have to be created, and then a resection level will need to be determined taking into account the extent of loss of tibial bone stock.

Surgical technique

Patient positioning

The patient is positioned supine, with a pad under the ipsilateral buttock, to position the foot pointing to the ceiling. A tourniquet is applied high on the limb. A pillow placed behind the knee will allow the Achilles tendon to relax, and may improve exposure. The foot should be right against the edge of the table, without overhanging. Placing a rolled towel under the ankle makes mobilization easier. The towel should be behind the calcaneus during distal tibial resection, so as to let the posterior soft tissues "escape" from under the saw. The knee must be included in the sterile field, so as to provide access to the bony landmarks (patella, tibial tubercle) and to allow mobilization.

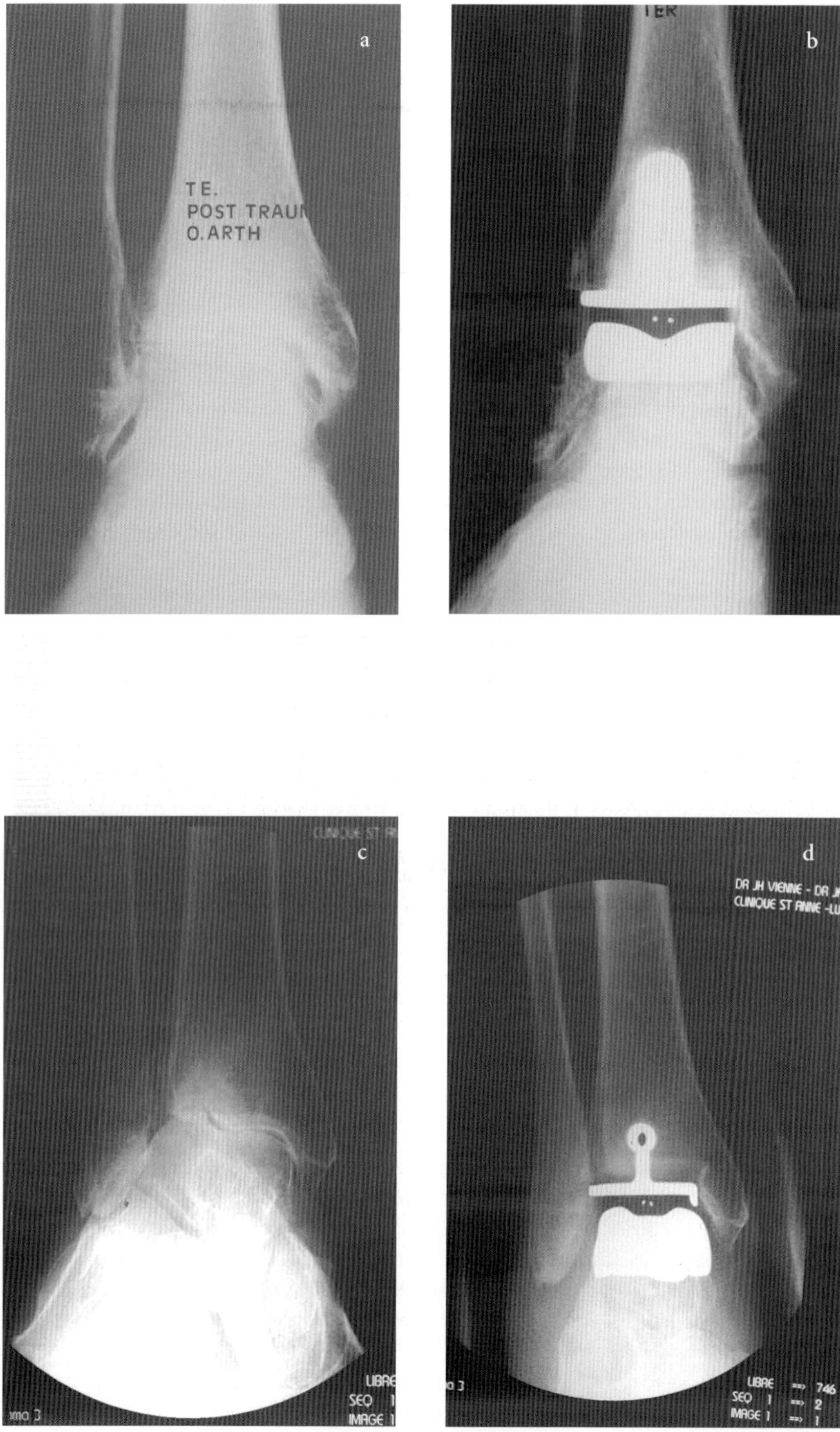
a
T E.
O.ARTH
b
c
d
LIBRE ==> 746
SEQ 1 ==> 2
IMAGE 1 ==> 1

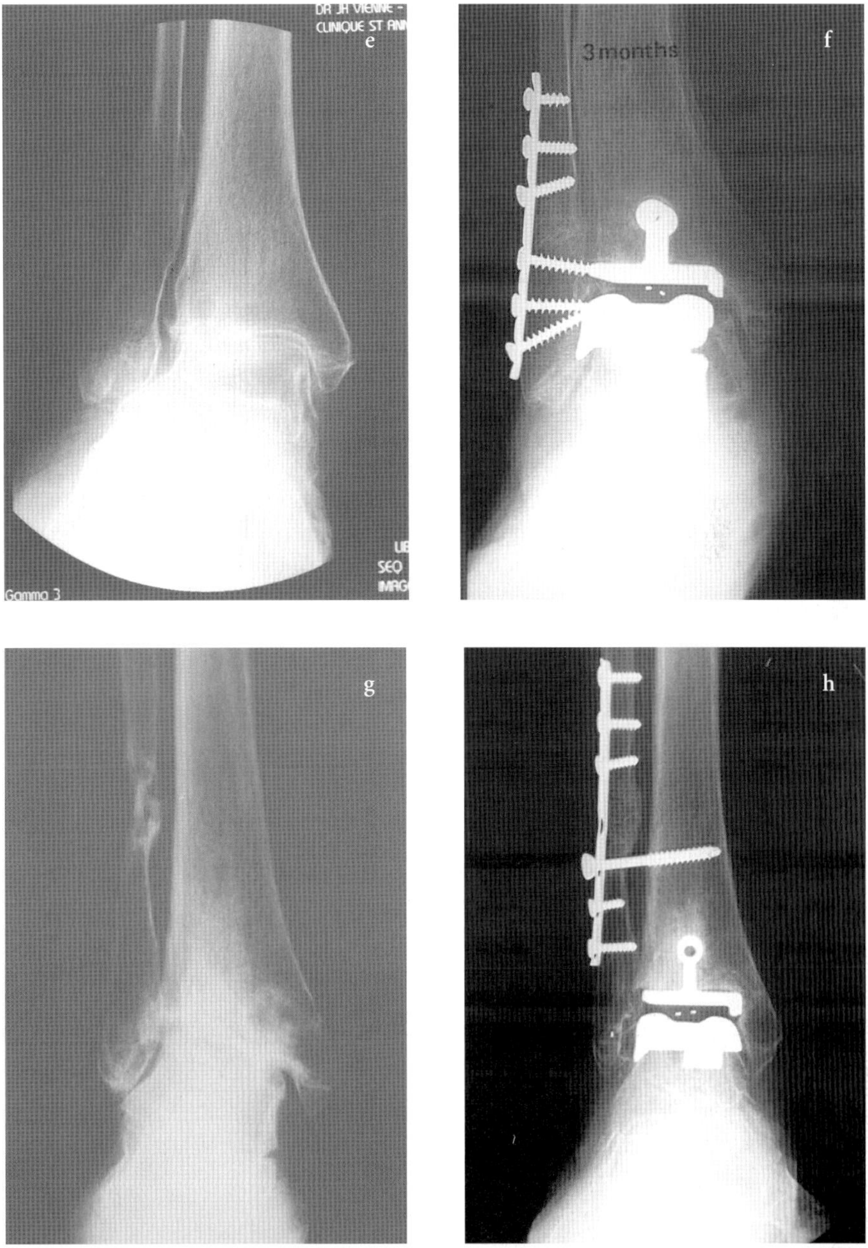

Fig. 6 - Determination of joint line. **a**) Intact ankle mortise. No asymmetrical wear of tibial pilon. The resection level is measured from the tibial plafond, to obtain "size-for-size" replacement of bone by implant; **b**) Postoperative view; **c**) Intact ankle mortise. Asymmetrical wear of tibial pilon. The cut should be referenced off a sound zone in the plafond as seen on radiographs or CT images; **d**) Postoperative view; **e**) Deformed ankle mortise. No asymmetrical wear of the tibial pilon. The malleolar deformity will need to be corrected prior to the actual arthroplasty; **f**) Postoperative view; **g**) Deformed ankle mortise. Asymmetrical wear of tibial pilon. This condition will need to be managed by a combination of the techniques referred to in c and e above; **h**) Postoperative view.

The surgeon stands at the foot of the table, with the assistant at the lateral side of the patient's leg.

Surgical approach

The joint is approached through an anterior midline incision extending from a point 10 cm proximal to the joint line to the midfoot. The skin over the front of the ankle has a very precarious blood supply, and should be undermined as sparingly as possible. The skin incision must be long enough to avoid undue tension on the skin edges, which may give rise to necrosis, especially in patients who have been treated with steroids.

Haemostasis of the loose subcutaneous tissue must be meticulous; however, electrocautery should be used sparingly, so as not to cause skin burns. Wherever possible, vessels should be ligated rather than coagulated.

The crural fascia and the retinacula are incised along the lateral border of the tibialis anterior tendon; the tendon itself must remain covered with fascia so as to remain separate from the incision after closure of the wound.

Next, the incision is deepened between the tibialis anterior tendon and the extensor hallucis longus tendon. The tendons are held out of the way with Farabeuf angled retractors, and the anterior tibial artery is identified in the proximal part of the incision, between the two tendons. The vessel is reflected laterally. The anterior periosteum is incised with electrocautery, as far distally as the joint line, following which it is stripped up with an elevator on the medial aspect of the lower end of the tibia, and the angled retractor is exchanged for a double-angled one. Laterally, the tibial periosteum is stripped up all the way to the lateral aspect against the fibular malleolus. A double-angled retractor is inserted at this site. This provides exposure of the anterior region of the ankle, and allows anterior arthrotomy to be performed. The joint is approached step by step, with the capsule and tendons being reflected distally. A lateral retractor is placed against the lateral malleolus, and a medial one against the upper part of the medial malleolus. Any anterior osteophytes are removed with an osteotome, and the talar facets are cleared with a rongeur. At this stage, care should be taken to ensure that the tips of the malleoli are properly debrided, by removing any osteophytes, ossifications, and loose bodies with rongeurs. Once these steps have been completed, it should be possible to mobilize the talus, and the medial and lateral gutters should be fully exposed.

Tibial resection

Resection level

The only reliable landmark is the plafond of the tibial pilon. The anterior margin of the pilon is resected using an osteotome. This will provide exposure of the joint surface. From this reference, the required cut is determined, taking into account the type of implant to be used, and aiming to remove as little bone as possible (fig. 7).

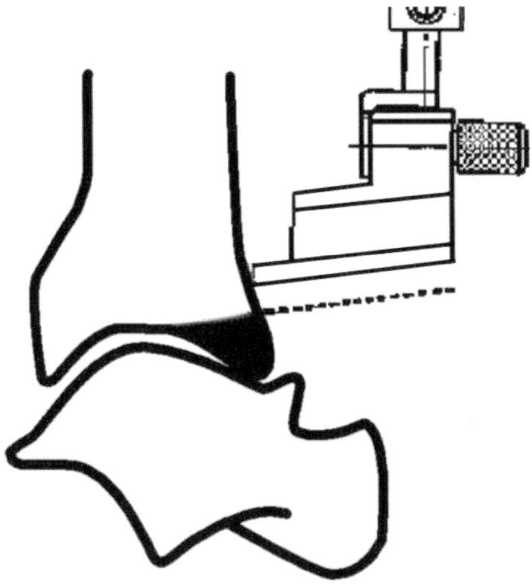

Fig. 7 - The tibial cut is made with an oscillating saw, using a jig aligned on the anterior tibial border.

Orientation of the cut

In the coronal plane, the tibial cut must be at right angles to the mechanical tibial axis. Resection is performed using an extramedullary guide referencing off the anterior tibial border (fig. 8). None of the systems available has automatic positioning, and the surgeon will need to take into account the preoperative radiographs of the involved and sometimes of the uninvolved ankle, and any associated deformities that may be present.

The orientation of the cut in rotation will be a function of the local anatomical pattern. Ideally, the implant should be centred on the line bisecting the space between the medial and lateral margins (fig. 9).

In the sagittal plane, jigs provided with the different prostheses are used to establish the posterior slope (usually of 7°) referenced on the anterior tibial cortex. This orientation is vital. Regardless of the implant system used, the resection guide must be placed against the tibis in order to ensure correct angulation of the cut.

Making the cut

The jig guides the saw blade, to achieve a cut of the desired orientation. The cut must be taken all the way to and through the posterior edge of the tibial pilon.

During resection, the malleoli – and the medial malleolus in particular – must be adequately protected. A short saw blade with limited excursions is advisable, as are protective pins that act as stops on the sides of the resection surface (fig. 10).

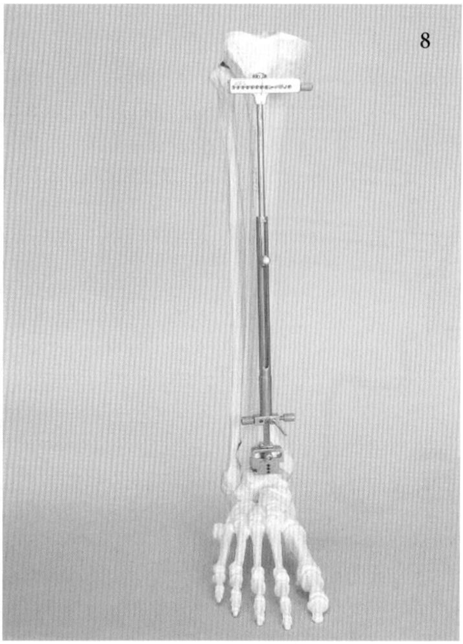

Fig. 8 - An extra medullary-guide is aligned with the anterior tibial crest.

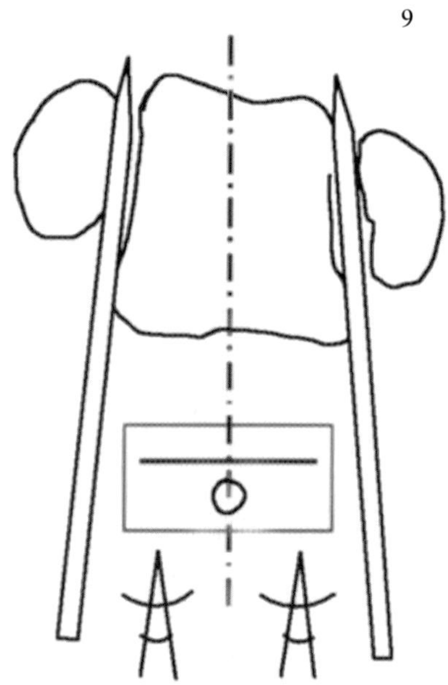

Fig. 9 - The rotational alignment of the talar cut is based on the line bissecting the talo-malleolar gutters.

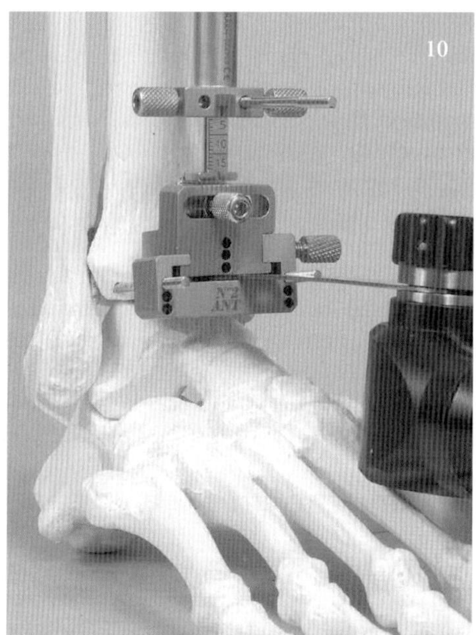

Fig. 10 - The distal tibial cut is done with an oscillating saw.

Removing the resected bone

The resected bone wafer has to be removed. Abrupt mobilization at this stage may result in a fracture of the medial malleolus, if the cut is not complete, especially in an ankle that has stiffened in equinus. This problem can be obviated by marking the edges of the resection surface with a drill bit, or by "nicking" them with an osteotome.

The removal of the distal tibial section is rarely done in one piece; usually, piecemeal removal will be required. First, the anterior half is removed, followed by the posterior portion.

A self-retaining retractor will improve exposure; however, it must be inserted gradually and with due care. If distraction is unduly forceful, the tibial resection surface may be depressed and the medial malleolus avulsed.

Talar preparation

Next, the talus needs to be mobilized, and the ankle placed at an angle of 90°. This angle is almost always obtained at this stage, since the removal of bone from the tibia will have created more space, even in a stiff ankle. Posterior capsulectomy may have to be performed through the anterior tibiotalar space, if there is major ankle stiffness.

Depending on the implant system to be used, talar preparation will involve simple resurfacing with a power reamer, or bone cuts guided by a jig.

Resection level

The talar resection level will essentially depend upon the local anatomical pattern, the object being to have sound fixation of the implant in healthy bone, whilst resecting sparingly in order to preserve as much bone stock as possible.

With simple resurfacing, preparation proceeds step by step, using a reamer and an osteotome so as to obtain optimal seating of the talar component on the implant bed.

Where bone cuts have to be made, the saw blade is guided by a jig. The pattern of the proximal cut varies with the implant design used: the STAR prosthesis requires a horizontal cut with an anterior and a posterior chamfer; the Salto, a cut sloping 20° posteriorly and an anterior chamfer.

The lateral cut removes the lateral side of the talus. A medial cut is required only for the STAR prosthesis.

Orientation in the sagittal plane

The talar component should be placed horizontally on the talar dome. If the cuts are made with an oscillating saw, the reference cut produced by the instruments supplied with the implant determines the sagittal positionning. Regardless of the system used, the orientation of the reference cut must be obtained with the foot in strictly neutral position between flexion and extension. Too much dorsiflexion at this stage would lead to talar component placement with a forward tilt, while too much plantar flexion would tilt the implant backwards.

With simple resurfacing prostheses, positioning is controlled by the preparation of the joint surface, without any jig to assist in the process.

Rotational positioning

Rotational malpositioning of the talar component will result in increased stress being placed on the fixation system, and may interfere with the kinematics of the joint replacement. Implants with mobile bearings are more forgiving, and may compensate for a certain degree of malpositioning. However, even with these implants, every effort should be made to obtain anatomically correct placement, with the implant centred with regard to the line bisecting the space between the lateral and medial talar facets.

Orienting the implant in relation to the forefoot may be useful; however, this may introduce errors, if there is midfoot or forefoot deformity.

Cutting the lateral and medial talar facets

These cuts are made with the aid of a cutting jig, using an oscillating saw. The position of the talar component in rotation will, to some extent, depend upon these cuts. This is why great care should be taken to ensure that the jig is correctly placed.

Insertion of trials

Tibial and talar trials of the chosen size are inserted. The aim should be to have maximum coverage of the tibial cut surface, and to avoid oversizing of the talar component. The use of a mobile bearing allows different sizes to be employed in the tibia and in the talus; where this option is being used, the choice of bearing size should be guided by the size of the talar component.

The mobile bearing is inserted. Bearing thickness is crucial to the stability of the implant. A bearing of correct thickness will need to be pushed rather than slipped into the joint.

The joint is ranged, and stability is checked. The implant should be stable in the coronal plane, without any residual laxity; dorsiflexion of greater than 10° should be readily obtained.

At this stage, a variety of problems may be encountered.

- It may prove impossible to insert even the thinnest bearing. In this case, the tibial side will need to be re-resected.
- Dorsiflexion may be unobtainable. This may be due to such causes as insufficient bone resection, an insufficient tibial slope, too large a talar component, forward translation of the talar component, or contracture of the Achilles tendon and/or the posterior capsular structures. Where such problems are encountered, it will be necessary, firstly, to check the size and the positioning of the talar component; secondly, to perform percutaneous lengthening of the Achilles tendon; thirdly, to check that the posterior capsular structures and the medial and lateral talar margins have been adequately cleared; and, fourthly, to re-resect the tibia.

- There may be asymmetrical laxity. Such laxity is unacceptable, since it may lead to implant loosening or early component wear. A release on the concave side may be performed, so as to allow a thicker PE component to be used. If there is overall residual laxity, or instability of the thickest bearing available, the joint will have to be fused.

Insertion of the definitive components

The definitive components are inserted. The prosthesis must have sound initial stability. Prior to the impaction of the components, any tibial or talar subchondral cysts or other bone defects may be filled.

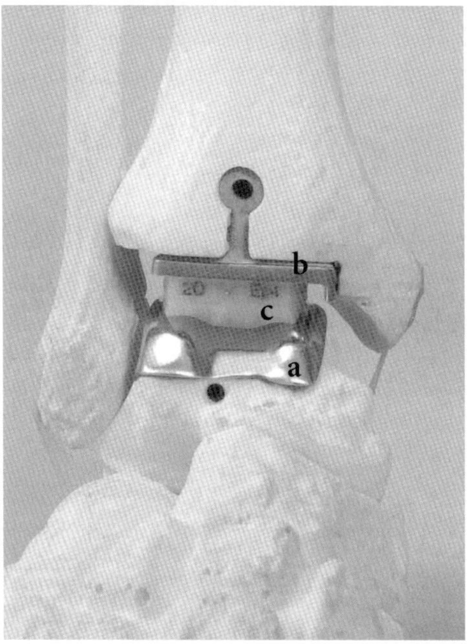

Fig. 11 - Definitive components in place: a) talar component, b) tibial component, c) mobile bearing.

Closure of incision

Since the skin over the ankle is very delicate, skin closure must be meticulous. The wound is closed over an intra-articular drain. The fascia and the retinacula are sutured. The toe extensor tendons, and, particularly, the tibialis anterior tendon, must be kept well away from the fascial suture line. The loose subcutaneous tissue and the skin are closed with interrupted sutures.

A below-knee plaster cast is applied, with the ankle in maximum dorsiflexion.

Postoperative management

The drain is removed the day after the operation. Once the swelling has subsided, a below-knee circular resin cast is applied.

As a general rule, weight-bearing may be resumed once the resin cast has been applied.

Patients who have undergone Achilles tendon lengthening will be kept off weight-bearing for a period of three weeks; where a tibial window has been performed (Buechel-Pappas prosthesis), or where there has been a malleolar fracture, the period off weight-bearing will be 45 days.

The cast is removed after 45 days to prevent skin problems, and physiotherapy is commenced.

References

1. Bolton-Maggs BG, Sudlow RA, Freeman MAR (1985) Total ankle arthroplasty. A long-term review of the London Hospital experience. J. Bone Joint Surg 67-B: 785-90
2. Bonnin M, Bouysset M, Tebib J *et al.* 1999 Triple arthrodesis associated with total ankle arthroplasty in rheumatoid arthritis. American Orthopaedic Foot and Ankle Society, 29th meeting, Anaheim, California
3. Bouysset M, Tavernier T, Tebib J *et al.* 1995 CT and MRI evaluation of tenosynovitis of the rheumatoid hind foot. Clin Rheumatol 14: 303-7
4. Buechel FF, Pappas MJ, Iorio LJ 1988 New Jersey low contact stress total ankle replacement: biomechanical rationale and review of 23 cementless cases. Foot Ankle 8: 279-80
5. Buechel FF, Pappas MF, Ioro JL 1992 Survivorship and clinical evaluation of cementless, meniscal bearing total ankle replacement. Semin. Arthroplasty 3: 43-50
6. Carlsson ÅS, Henricson A, Linder L, *et al.* 1994 A survival analysis of 52 Bath & Wessex ankle replacements. A clinical and radiographic study in patients with rheumatoid arthritis and a critical review of the literature. The Foot 4: 34-40
7. Cypres A 1990 La prothèse de cheville. À propos de 23 arthroplasties par resurfaçage tibio-astragalienne. Saint Etienne, Thesis, 130 p.
8. Demottaz JD, Mazur JM, Thomas WH, *et al.* (1979) Clinical study of total ankle replacement with gait analysis. A preliminary report. J. Bone Joint Surg.,,61-A, 7: 976-88
9. Dini AA, Basset FH (1990) Evaluation of the early result of Smith total ankle replacement. Clin. Orthop., 146: 228-30
10. Doets HC (1997) Ankle arthroplasty for rheumatoid arthritis (New Jersey Ankle). First International Congress on Ankle Arthroplasty, Copenhagen, 20-21 June

11. Drzala M, Lin SS, Eng KO (1991) Independent evaluation of Buechel-Pappas 2nd generation cementless total ankle arthroplasty. American Orthopaedic Foot and Ankle Society, 28th meeting, New Orleans, Louisiana

12. Endrich B, Terbruggen D (1991) Endoprosthesis of the ankle joint. Indications and long-term results. Unfallchirurg 94: 525-30

13. Evanski PM, Waugh TR (1977) Management of arthritis of the ankle. An alternative to arthrodesis. Clin. Orthop., 122: 110-5

14. Freeman MAR (1976) Current state of total joint replacement. Br Med J, 2: 1301-4

15. Hay SM, Smith TWD, Elson RA, Hay SM (1993) Long term follow-up of total ankle arthroplasty: the Sheffield experience. J Bone Joint Surg. 75-B, Supp III: 297

16. Hay SM, Smith TWD (1994) Total ankle arthroplasty: a long-term review. The Foot, 4: 1-5

17. Herberts P, Goldie IF, Körner L, (1982) Endoprosthetic arthroplasty of the ankle joint. A clinical and radiological follow-up. Acta Orthop. Scand., 53: 687-96

18. Jakubowski S, Mohing W, Richter R. Operationen am rheumatischen Fuss. Therapiewoche, 1970,20: 762-68

19. Johnson K (1989) Replacement arthroplasty of the foot and ankle: total ankle arthroplasty. In Surgery of the foot and ankle arthroplasty. K.A. Johnson, New York Raven Press: 265-80

20. Keblish PA, Buechel FF, Fenning J (1998) Cementless meniscal bearing (shallow sulcus) T.A.R.: multicenter clinical trial results of 237 cases. Communication at Journées Orthopédiques de Fort de France, February

21. Kitaoka HB, Patzer GL, Ilstrup DM, (1994) Wallrichs S.L. Survivorship analysis of the Mayo total ankle arthroplasty. J. Bone Joint Surg. 76-A: 974-9

22. Kitaoka HB, Gary L, Patzer RN (1996) Clinical results of the Mayo total ankle arthroplasty. J. Bone Joint Surg. 78-A: 1658-64

23. Kofoed H (1995) Cylindrical cemented ankle arthroplasty: a prospective series with long-term follow-up. Foot and Ankle Int., 16: 474-9

24. Kofoed H, Danborg L (1995) Biological fixation of ankle arthroplasty. A sequential consecutive prospective clinico-radiographic series of 20 ankles with arthrodesis followed for 1 – 4 years. The Foot, 5: 27-31

25. Kofoed H, Sørensen TS (1998) Ankle arthroplasty for rheumatoid arthritis and osteoarthritis. Prospective long-term study of cemented replacements. J. Bone Joint Surg. 80-B: 328-32

26. Kofoed H (1998) Comparison of cemented and cementless ankle arthroplasty. In Kofoed current status of ankle arthroplasty, Berlin, Heidelberg, New-York: Springer-Verlag: 47-49

27. Kofoed H (1998) Medium-term results of cementless Scandinavian total ankle replacement prosthesis for osteoarthritis. In Current status of ankle arthroplasty, Berlin, Heidelberg, New-York: Springer-Verlag,: 116-21

28. Lachiewicz PF, Inglis AE, Ranawat CS (1984) Total ankle replacement in rheumatoid arthritis. J. Bone Joint Surg. 66-A: 340-3

29. Lord G, Marotte JH (1973) Prothèse totale de cheville: technique et premiers résultats. A propos de 12 observations. Rev. Chir. Orthop. 59: 139-51

30. Lord G, Marotte JH (1980) L'arthroplastie totale de cheville. Expérience sur 10 ans, à propos de 25 observations personnelles. Rev. Chir. Orthop. 66: 527-30

31. McGuire M.R., Kyle R.F., Gustilo R.B. *et al.* (1988) Comparative analysis of ankle arthroplasty versus ankle arthrodesis. Clin. Orthop. 226: 174-81

32. Nelissen RGHH, Doets HC, Meskers C (1998) The value of ankle prostheses. A gait analysis approach. In Kofoed H. Current status of ankle arthroplasty. Berlin: Springer: 72-8

33. Newton S.E. (1979) An artificial ankle joint. Clin. Orthop. 142: 141-5

34. Newton S.E. (1982) Total ankle arthroplasty. Clinical study of fifty cases. J. Bone Joint Surg. 64-A: 104-11

35. Pipino F., Calderale P.M. (1983) PC ankle prosthesis. Five year follow-up. Acta Orthop. Belg. 49: 725-35

36. Piriou P, Tremoulet J, Garreau de Loubresse C *et al.* (2000) Tenotomie d'Achille percutanée dans les raideurs de cheville de l'adulte. A propos de 80 cas. Rev. Chir. Orthop. 86: 38-45

37. Pyevich MT, Saltzman CL, Callaghan JJ *et al.* (1998) Total ankle arthroplasty: a unique design. Two to twelve-year follow-up. J. Bone Joint Surg., 80-A: 1410-20

38. Saillant G, Catonne Y (1980) Les prothèses totales de cheville. Pathologie traumatique de la cheville et du pied. Paris: Masson, 170-7

39. Samuelson KM, Freeman MAR, Tuke MA (1982) Developpment and evolution of the ICLH ankle replacement. Foot Ankle, 3: 32-6

40. Scholz KC (1987) Total ankle arthroplasty using biological fixation components compared to ankle arthrodesis. Orthopedics 10: 125-31

41. Siguier T (1996) Prothèse totale de cheville: révision d'une série continue de 22 cas. Thesis, Paris

42. Spector EE (1984) Ankle implants. Clin Podiatry, 1: 225-35

43. Stauffer RN (1979) Total joint arthroplasty. The ankle. Mayo Clin. Proc., 54: 570-5

44. Stauffer RN, Segal NM (1981) Total ankle arthroplasty: four years'experience. Clin Orthop, 160: 217-21

45. Takakura Y, Tanaka Y, Sugimoto K, *et al.* (1990) Ankle arthroplasty. A comparative study of cemented metal and uncemented ceramic prostheses. Clin. Orthop. 252: 209-16

46. Tillmann K (1990) Recent advances in the surgical treatment of rheumatoid arthritis. Clin. Orthop. 258: 62-72

47. Tomeno B., Cornic M. (1981) Que faut-il penser de l'arthroplastie de cheville? Rev. Chir. Orthop. 67: 141-5

48. Unger AS, Inglis AE, Now CS, *et al.* (1988) Total ankle arthroplasty in rheumatoid arthritis: a long-term follow-up study. Foot Ankle 8,4: 173-9

49. Viladot A (1982) À propos des arthroplasties de la cheville. Cheville et médecine de rééducation. Paris Masson 237-43

50. Waugh TR, Evanski PM, McMaster WC (1976) Irvine ankle arthroplasty. Prosthetic design and surgical technique. Clin Orthop 114: 180-4

51. Wood P (1997) Total ankle replacement (STAR-Link) for rheumatoid arthritis. First International Congress on Ankle Arthroplasty. Copenhagen

52. Wynn A.H., Wilde A.H. (1992) Long-term follow-up of the Conaxial (Beck-Steffee) total ankle arthroplasty. Foot Ankle 13, (6): 303-6

Some reflections about the evolution of ankle prosthesis

H. Kofoed

Introduction

The aim with an ankle arthroplasty is to give freedom from pain, to retain or improve function and mobility. To achieve these goals it is necessary to know:
- underlying pathology of the degenerated ankle joint;
- the possibilities for a safe access to the ankle joint;
- fixation of the prosthetic components, and;
- the biological, biomechanical and kinematic behaviour of the hindfoot complex.

A successful result of an ankle arthroplasty will depend on all these features. The different arthroplastic designs seen since the seventies have more or less neglected vital parts of these goals. The results have been disappointing compared to the results of hip and knee arthroplasties. The reason is obviously that the ankle joint is a much more complex joint than the simple hip and the rather simple knee and the influence of the neighbouring joints. Thorough knowledge of the inside anatomy of the ankle joint is mandatory when considering an ankle arthroplasty. The shape of the talus, the possibility for talus rotation inside the ankle mortise, the rotation of the fibula, and the weight-bearing of not only the upper part of the talus but also the joints between the malleoli and the talus facets must be considered (14). Furthermore, the access to the ankle joint is difficult, and especially fixation with cement is a difficult task provided only limited bone resections are needed. The influence of the soft tissue structures is of utmost importance as these guide the mobility, and allow function and stability. Thus the lateral ligaments are major players in this aspect. Let it be said initially, the task with the painful degenerated ankle joint is to restore alignment, mobility and stability before considering to insert a prosthesis. To simply insert any prosthetic device will not do the job. As rheumatoid arthritis is the subject for this paper the specific features that relates to that entity will be the focus of this paper. It has often been said that ankle arthroplasties in rheumatoid arthritis function better than in osteoarthritric cases. This is a superficial statement. The tolerance of pain and diminished function is well known in patients with rheumatoid arthritis, and this causes this apparent difference. In fact osteoarthritic patients are having better mobility and function, but they may not have the same degree of satisfaction as they are usually not multi-joint disabled.

The normal kinematics of the ankle and hindfoot

In a normal ankle joint there is gliding during motion between the talus and the tibia (3, 23). The talus rotates between the malleoli during the arc of motion (18). The joints between talus and the calcaneus allows for some plantar flexion and some extension apart from the main movements in eversion and inversion. The talo-navicular joint allows for extension-flexion apart from its main rotation movement. During the arc of motion in the ankle joint the wider anterior part of the talus must have space in the ankle fork in order to get extension. It is still debated how this mechanism is possible when the ankle joint should be congruent during the arc of motion. Is there a widening of the ankle mortise or is the congruency established by adaptive rotation of the lateral mallolus? The last solution seems the more plausible (6).

The main trouble with rheumatoid arthritic ankle is that the kinematics are distorted. This should to the greatest possible extent be corrected during surgery before the ankle is suited for an ankle arthroplasty. The problems with the rheumatoid ankle are related to:

- valgus or varus hindfoot;
- osteoporosis;
- deteriorated and stiff neighbouring joints, and;
- getting the patients at a too far gone stage.

The ankle joint is absolutely vital for a plantigrade foot function. Fuse all other joints in the foot and it can still be used for walking provided that the ankle joint is functioning. Fuse the ankle joint in such cases and walking will be extremely difficult and function worse than with a below knee amputation and a prosthesis (16).

The hindfoot pathology in rheumatoid arthritis

In juvenile rheumatoid arthritis the hindfoot is most often in varus whereas in adult rheumatoid arthritis the hindfoot is in valgus. The ankle joint may be in varus or valgus, and there may be bone destructions either in the distal tibial plafond or a flattening of the talus. Subchondral synovial cysts may have created severe bone deficits. A special entitity, that is not easily recognised on radiographs is the engravement of the talus into the medial malleolus. This not only limits the mobility but it may lead to breakage of the medial mallolus if one tries to force movements in the ankle joint. Ankylosis of the joints between the malleoli and the talus may produce malleolar fractures if the ankle joint is forcefully moved. Usually the ligaments are slack in rheumatoid arthritis. This means that bone resections should be extremely moderate if too much spacing by the prosthetic components should be avoided.

The bone of rheumatoid arthritis

Osteoporosis is the normal feature. This is provided either by the medication the patients are receiving or most properly by disease osteoporosis. The bone should therefore be handled with utmost care as saws or chisels will easily destruct the soft bone. Sometimes the bone will be too osteoporotic to carry an endo-prosthesis. Large synovial cysts must be eradicated and transplanted in order to retain as much bone as possible.

The valgus/varus hindfoot complex and alignment

A valgus or a varus deformity could be in the ankle or in the subtalar joints. It is not easily correctable with the prosthesis alone. Most devices can at the most correct 10° of valgus and 5° of varus. When the deformity is larger than these limits other measures must be taken in order to align the ankle-hindfoot-complex. It is vital that correct alignment is obtained as the load distribution to both the prosthetic parts and to the bone will otherwise lead to loosening of the prosthesis components. If the deformity is in the subtalar joints some prefer to perform a correction arthrodesis before considering the ankle arthroplasty. Others will perform both operations as a one-stage procedure.

Prosthetic devices

Since the beginning of the 1970s several ankle arthroplastic designs have been introduced. Only a limited number of them have considered the above mentioned features of the degenerated rheumatoid ankle joint, and whether this could be fitted with a prosthesis or not. Studying the different designs several general mistakes have been encountered.

- Replacing only the top of the talus will not help provided the talus facet joints are obliterated, and it will not be helpful if a protrusion of the medial talus facet into the medial malleolus is present.
- A straight horizontal cut of the talus dome often leads to loosening of the talus component as this has a tendency to slide off (2).
- Only the lower 1 cm of the tibia has sufficient strong bone to carry a prosthesis. There is only fatty bone marrow above that level. Working above the 1 cm level is unsuitable for the prosthesis insertion and fixation whether fixation is tried with cement or without cement. Most of the experience with ankle prostheses relates to the cemented devices that were used during the 1970s and 1980s.

The experience shows that :

- non-congruent prosthetic devices have a great loosening rate (7, 19).
- Congruent and internally stabilized devices have likewise shown great loosening rates (5, 22, 24).
- Spherical devices, meant to give eversion/inversion simultaneously with flexion/extension do not have the kinematics of a normal ankle and they have seriously failed (2, 8).

None of these devices could solve the problem with valgus/varus and alignment of the hindfoot if the deformity was more than 10°. Inability to correct deformities and alignment obviously means abnormal load distribution through the below knee-ankle-hindfoot axis. That in it self may very well be one of the major reasons for the loosening tendency of the devices. The cementing technique of especially the tibial component in the ankle is difficult. There is minimal space and compression and even distribution of the cement in the bone bed is troublesome. This is another reason for loosening. Furthermore, too high cutting of the tibia, in order to get space, leaves no solid bone bed to receive the cement. On the other hand, taking too much off the talus dome may deteriorate the vessels to the talus which could lead to a talus collapse. The internal arrangement of the bone trabeculae is also destroyed by such a technique and that will weaken the bearing possibilities in the talus bone.

To find the right level of rotation level in the ankle seems vital. This was initially investigated by Pappas, Pipino, Calderale (20, 21) and they designed their prostheses accordingly. They also tried to make the prostheses as anatomical as possible. Only the top of the talus was resurfaced. In order to have minimal bone resection for the two-part devices they both used stemmed tibial components to be pushed in from the front. Stemmed tibial components normally fared badly (8, 17, 19, 21). Later on it was demonstrated that the right tension in the lateral ligaments is vital for function and mobility (15). This can only be achieved if the right level of resection of both the tibia and the talus is chosen. The introduction of a mobile meniscus in knee prosthesis (4) started a new era. This also occurred with the ankle prostheses when this principle was used by splitting the tibial component into a metal gliding component and a polyethylene insert between the talus and the tibial component (1, 10). This also facilitated uncemented use of the prostheses. The biomechanics of these constructions allowed only compressive forces to act on the prosthetic components as the rotation and gliding of the meniscus against the flat tibial component took away the shear stresses from the bone-prosthesis interface. The replacement of the talus facet joints is only used by the STAR prosthesis (9). The option of this construction allows major regulation of valgus and varus deformities of the entire hindfoot. This is performed by using a sculpturing technique on the talus within the cartilage covered parts inside the ankle fork. Thus, before inserting the prosthetic parts the entire hindfoot complex is rotated into normal alignment by guided cuts, and the prosthesis components are not inserted until normal alignments have been achieved. The technique has been described in detail elsewhere (11). The uncemented meniscal-bearing ankle prostheses respecting biomechanics and kinematics of the ankle joint have shown mid-term and 10 years survival rates compatible to those of knee arthroplasties (1, 12). It has also been shown that they give excellent mobility and imitation of ankle kinematics (13) and biologically behave very soundly (25). Cases with rheumatoid arthritis and other forms of osteoporosis gain mostly in bone mineral content adjacent to the prosthesis.

The future

There is no doubt that the current results with uncemented and meniscal bearing ankle prostheses have revived the interest in ankle arthroplasty. At the Millennium Course 2000 of the European Rheumatoid Arthritis Surgical Society ankle arthroplasty was judged the first choice for painful degenerated rheumatoid ankles. This does not mean that all the problems with ankle prosthesis have been solved and that there is not space for further investigations and search for better devices. We still need to find out whether better materials and better constructions can optimise the present results. These should of course be along the lines scheduled here: achieve normal alignment, normal kinematics, normal mobility, good biomechanics, and excellent biological behaviour. Still, ankle arthroplasty is a demanding surgical procedure, and it is not foremost the prosthesis that makes the success but the surgical work before it is inserted. Furthermore, the contraindications as they have been elucidated throughout the years, should be respected. That means foremost talus necrosis, Charcot joints, very aggressive arthritis, mental and neuro-motor disturbancies, and severe arteriosclerosis.

References

1. Buechel FF, Pappas MJ (1992) Survivorship and clinical evaluation of cementless, miniscal-bearing total ankle replacements. Semin Arthroplasty 3: 43-50
2. Carlsson ÅS, Henricson A, Linder L, Nilsson J-A, Redlund-Johnell I (1994). A survival analysis of 52 Bath & Wessex ankle replacements. Foot 4: 34-40
3. Demottaz JD, Mazur JN, Thomas WH, Sledge CB, Simon SR (1979) Clinical study of total ankle replacement with gait analysis: preliminary report. J Bone Surg (Am) 61: 976
4. Goodfellow J, O'Connor J (1978) The mechanics of the knee and prosthetic design. J Bone Joint Surg (Br) 60-B: 358-69
5. Groth HE, Fitch HF (1987) Salvage procedures for complications of total ankle arthroplasty. Clin Orthop 224: 245-249
6. Helweg J, Kofoed H (1998) The fibula rotates during motion in the ankle joint. In Current status of ankle arthroplasty. Ed. H. Kofoed, 61-63, Springer-Verlag
7. Jensen NC, Kroener K (1992) Total joint replacement. A clinical follow-up. Orthopedics 15: 236-9
8. Kirkup J (1985) Richard Smith ankle arthroplasty. J R Soc med 78: 301-4
9. Kofoed H (1986) A new total ankle prosthesis, in Material Sciences and Implant Orthopaedic Surgery. Eds R. Kossowsky, N Kossowsky. Nato Asi series E 116: 75-84. Martinus Nijhoff Publ
10. Kofoed H, Danborg L (1995) Biological fixation of ankle arthroplasty. Foot 5: 27-31
11. Kofoed H (2000) Total replacement of the ankle joint in: Surgical Techniques in Orthopaedics and Traumatology, 55-630-D-10, Ed. DuParc *et al.*, Elsevier SAS, Paris
12. Kofoed H (2001) Unanswered questions and unquestioned answers. The STAR prosthesis. AAOS 68 meeting. San Francisco, USA

13. Komistek RD, Stiehl JB, Buechel FF, Northeut EJ, Hajner ME (2000) A determination of ankle kinematics using fluoroscopy. Foot Ankle Int 21 (4): 343-50
14. Lambert KL (1971) The weight-bearing function of the fibula. J Bone Joint Surg (Am) 51: 146-58
15. Leardini A, O'Connor JJ, Catani F, Gianinni S (1999) A geometrical model for the human ankle joint. J Biomechanics 32: 585-91
16. Leicht P, Kofoed H (1992) Subtalar arthrosis following ankle arthrodesis. Foot 2: 89-92
17. LordG, Marotte JH. (1980) Total ankle replacement. Rev Chir Orthop 66: 5227-530
18. Lundberg A (1989) Kinematics of the ankle and foot. Stereophotogranmmetric analysis. Acta Orthop Scand 50: Suppl 223: 1-23
19. Newton SE 3rd (1982) Total ankle arthroplasty. Clinical study of 50 cases. J Bone Joint Surg (Am) 64: 104-11
20. Pappas MJ, Buechel FF, DePalma AF (1976) Cylindrical total ankle joint replacement: Surgical and biomechanical rationale. Clin Orthop 118: 82-92
21. Pipino F, Calderale PM (1976) An ankle prosthesis of new design. II policlino Lez chir. 83: 559-63
22. Scholtz KC (1987) Total ankle arthroplasty using biological fixation components compared to ankle arthrodesis. Orthopedics 10: 125-31
23. Stauffer RN, Chao EYS, Brewster RC (1977) Force and motion analysis of the normal, diseased nd prosthetic ankle joint. Clin Orthop 127: 189-96
24. Wynn AH, Wilde AH (1992) Long-term follow-up of the Conaxial (Beck-Steefee) total ankle arthroplasty. Foot Ankle 13: 303-6
25. Zerahn B, Kofoed H, Borgwardt A (2000) Increased bone mineral density adjacent to hydroxyapatite-coated ankle arthroplasty. Foot Ankle Int 21 (4): 285-9

Total ankle replacement in rheumatoid arthritis: treatment strategy

M. Bonnin, M. Bouysset, J. Tebib and E. Noël

Rheumatoid arthritis (RA) of the ankle poses specific problems, since the tibiotalar joint is rarely affected in isolation, and treatment will need to be designed so as to manage all the aspects of the disease in the particular patient. Some management aspects are of particular importance.

Tibiotalar and subtalar joint involvement

Compared with the large joints of the lower limb, the ankle joint is comparatively rarely affected by RA. However, there is no consensus on the actual rate of ankle joint involvement in RA patients, with figures ranging from 9% in the study by Vainio (28), in which clinical criteria were used, to 40% in the study by Jakubowski *et al.*, (14) which employed radiographic criteria. Also, ankle joint involvement tends to occur late in the disease process, with symptoms not occurring until after a mean disease duration of between 17 and 19 years (1, 3). By then, other joints will, as a rule, have been affected.

The pattern observed in the hindfoot joints is different. The subtalar, talonavicular, and calcaneocuboid joints are very frequently affected. Between 30% and 67% of RA patients will experience involvement of these joints (28, 29). The rate of hindfoot joint involvement increases over time, from 8% after a disease duration of less than five years, to 52% after more than nine years (13, 22). Subtalar RA results in a pes planovalgus deformity, which may cause or accelerate ankle joint destruction. Any associated tibialis posterior tenosynovitis will make matters even worse (5).

For these reasons (disproportionately higher rate of involvement of the subtalar, as compared with the tibiotalar, articulation; and repercussions of subtalar disease on the condition of the ankle joint), there will often be lesions in both these articulations, which will need to be managed jointly. The association of subtalar and ankle joint disease has been stressed by a number of authors, (7, 8, 12, 22) with reported rates of associated hindfoot involvement ranging from 56% to 92% in patients whose tibiotalar RA had advanced to the stage where surgery was required.

In patients with tibiotalar RA and subtalar RA with a hindfoot valgus deformity, management options are limited. Pantalar arthrodesis (fusing the tibiotalar, subtalar, and midtarsal joints) may accelerate the destruction of the surrounding joints (24, 25) and produce a poor functional outcome. Isolated total ankle replacement (TAR) will not correct hindfoot malalignment, and may therefore fail rapidly as a result of asymmetrical stress distribution (fig. 1a – c).

It follows that, in such cases, both joints will need to be addressed in order to obtain a sound and lasting result.

Involvement of other joints in the lower limb

Usually, by the time tibiotalar RA has developed, other joints in the lower limb will have been affected; in some cases, surgery of these joints will have been performed (7). In these patients, the additional stress placed on the other joints by blocking the ankle joint could have even worse effects than would fusion of an ankle joint affected by isolated osteoarthritis (OA) (7, 13, 20, 24, 25). This prospect of a poor outcome would be even greater in patients whose RA of the hindfoot joints necessitates fusion of the subtalar and midtarsal as well as of the tibiotalar joints. There have been very few specific studies of the functional outcome of such "pantalar" fusions (27); in the studies of ankle joint fusion in RA, the results of these more complex cases are never clearly identified (7, 9, 12, 22).

In a series of tibiotalar fusions for RA, in patients who had previously undergone knee or hip (total joint replacement) surgery, Cracchiolo *et al.* (7) had disappointing results: six patients had poorer function following arthrodesis, five were unchanged, and only one patient was improved. In the light of these results, the authors stated that they would perform fusion in such multiply operated patients only for pain relief, and not as a means of improving mobility. On the other hand, Felix and Kitaoka (12), in a study of 26 ankle arthrodeses, did not find any poor results in patients who had previously undergone total knee replacement (four cases) or total hip replacement (five cases), and would not consider previous joint replacement surgery as a risk factor for a poor outcome of arthrodesis.

Poor skin and bone stock quality

Long-term use of corticosteroids (8, 12, 22, 23), and, in the opinion of some authors (8), treatment with methotrexate, are risk factors for skin complications and delayed fusion. Thus, Cracchiolo *et al.* (7), in a series of 32 fusions in 26 RA patients, found a

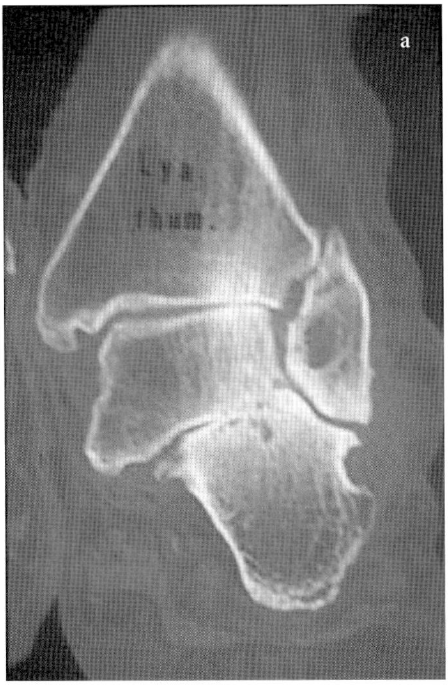

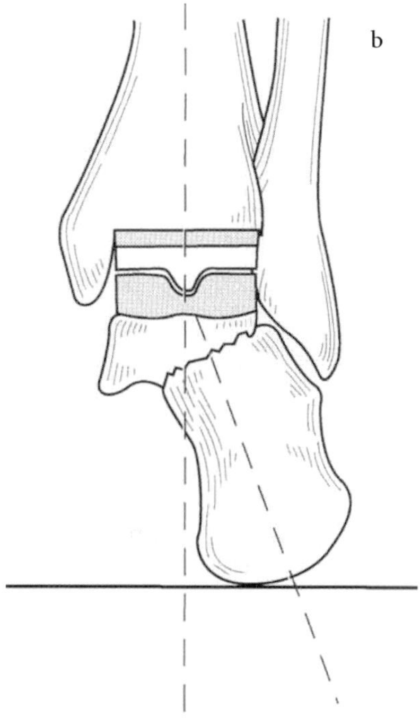

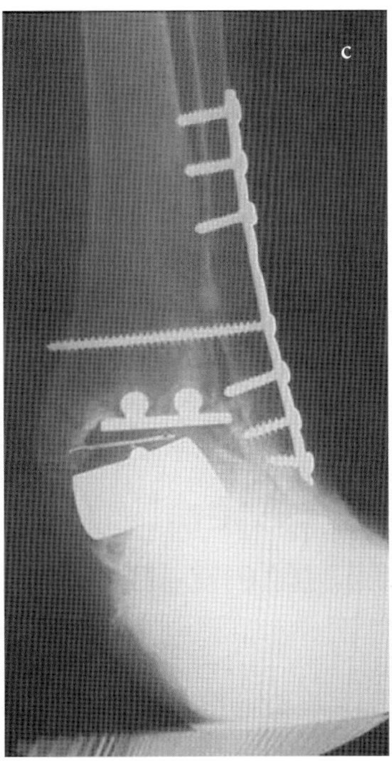

Fig. 1a and b - Associated tibiotalar and subtalar RA, with valgus deformity of mixed aetiology. **a)** Tibiotalar RA with subtalar RA; **b)** If the valgus deformity of the hindfoot is not corrected, the TAR is asymmetrically loaded with early failure (c).

22% rate of nonunion of the arthrodesis and a 33% rate of infection. Moran *et al.* (23) performed 30 fusions in 26 patients, and reported a 40% rate of nonunion and infection. However, Felix and Kitaoka (12) had only one case of nonunion and three cases of superficial skin complications, in a series of 26 fusions in 21 patients. With the advent of arthroscopic techniques, the complication rate has dropped. Nowadays, more than 95% of primary fusion may be obtained, and skin complications have virtually disappeared.

Soft-tissue and bone healing problems may also occur following TAR. Thus, Kofoed and Sørensen (20) had problems in one RA patient out of 23 (4%), while Kitaoka (17) and Kitaoka *et al.* (18) reported soft-tissue complications in 14 out of 204 cases (7%), without, however, specifying whether these problems were encountered in OA or in RA patients (fig. 2).

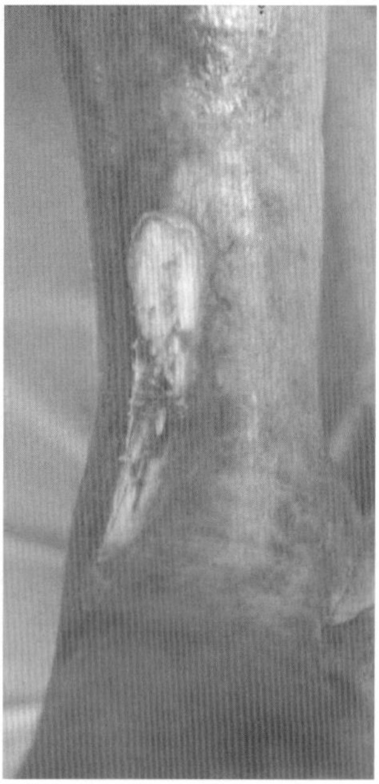

Fig. 2 - Skin necrosis after TAR in a patient with RA.

Consideration of the patient's general condition in planning the treatment strategy

More often than not, surgery of the foot and ankle in RA patients will require the patient to be kept off weight-bearing for long periods of time, and will necessitate lengthy immobilization in casts or splints. RA patients have great difficulty using walking aids, because of associated involvement of upper-extremity joints (elbow, shoulder, wrist, hand). This makes the postoperative period an ordeal for the patient. It follows that the patients should be comprehensively managed, if possible in a rehabilitation facility, following a plan worked out before any surgery is performed. Also, care should be taken to ensure that as many procedures as possible are performed at the same time, rather than addressing each joint separately, in a series of operations.

Treatment strategy

Tibiotalar fusion in RA patients is difficult and may produce a poor outcome. This is why attempts have been made to use TAR in this patient population. The first results were, indeed, encouraging. In 1989, Johnson (15) felt that the best candidates for TAR were "RA patients without hindfoot deformity and with a stable ankle." Since then, this optimism has been somewhat tempered, following the reports of failure rates in major studies: Kitaoka *et al.* (18) reviewed 96 implants at nine years, and reported a failure rate of 32%; while Kofoed and Sørensen (20) had a failure rate of 24% at 14 years, in a study of 27 TARs. These two studies are the largest to date, as well as the ones with the longest follow-up. They would appear to have involved a number of risk factors (1). The implants used were of the cemented type, and Kitaoka *et al.* used only constrained cylindrical devices, with a single degree of freedom (2). In the study by Kofoed and Sørensen, 13 cases were managed with two-component implants, and 14 with three-component (meniscal bearing) devices; however, the results are not broken down by implant type (3). In both series, there was a high rate of secondary subtalar involvement, which means that the implant may have failed as a result of hindfoot valgus deformity. Kofoed and Sørensen found 18% secondary subtalar involvement; Kitaoka *et al.* reported 57%, without, however, distinguishing between OA and RA patients.

Meniscal bearing designs hold great promise, since they place less stress on the implant fixation devices and allow the use of cementless prostheses. The literature on these implants in RA patients is as yet scarce (1, 10, 20), and follow-up to date has been short.

In view of all these factors, some rules have been established to govern ankle surgery in RA patients.

- A global lesional and deformity analysis should be performed, to cover the tibiotalar, subtalar, and midtarsal joints.
- Tibiotalar fusion should be avoided. Such fusion is likely to affect the surrounding joints, and may rapidly lead to a poor outcome, especially if subtalar and midtarsal fusion have to be performed, or if fusion of the first metatarsophalangeal joint has already been performed.
- Whenever possible, surgery of the ankle, the hindfoot, the midfoot and the forefoot should be combined, so as to spare the patient repeated spells of postoperative disability.
- The skin over the ankle should be carefully protected and watched throughout the postoperative period. Discontinuing steroids and methotrexate until healing has been obtained may be a useful precaution (fig. 2).

- Postoperative care should be part of a comprehensive management plan, and should be provided at a specialized facility.

The treatment strategy will need to be guided by the overall alignment of the hindfoot, by the involvement of the subtalar joint, and by the condition of the tibialis posterior tendon. The patient should be checked in meticulous detail, with and without weight-bearing. In addition to the clinical examination, weight-bearing radiographs and, if need be, thin-section coronal CT scans should be obtained, to show the condition of the subtalar joint. In some cases, MR imaging will need to be performed, to study the tibialis posterior tendon. Hindfoot valgus may be due to three anatomical causes, which may be associated (fig. 3): subtalar RA; lateral wear of the tibial pilon, in tibiotalar RA; and/or tibialis posterior tendinopathy with rupture of the tendon. A search for these causative factors should be made preoperatively, so as to enable the surgeon to optimize the procedure.

There are three distinct patterns (fig. 4).

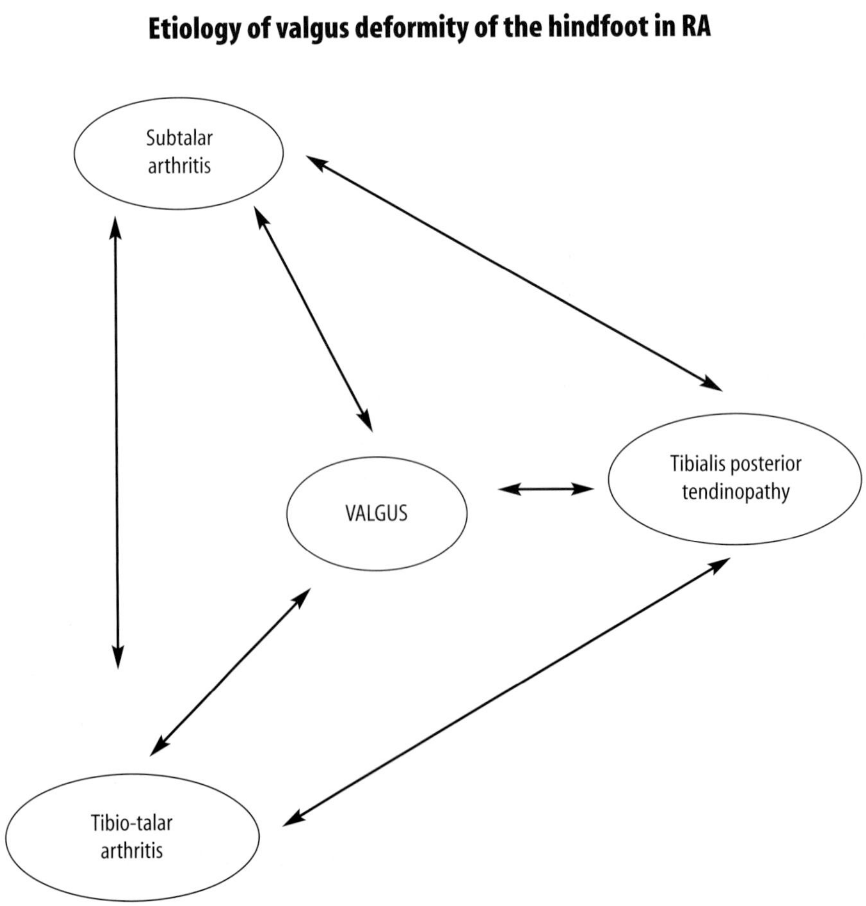

Fig. 3 - Causes of hindfoot valgus deformity in RA.

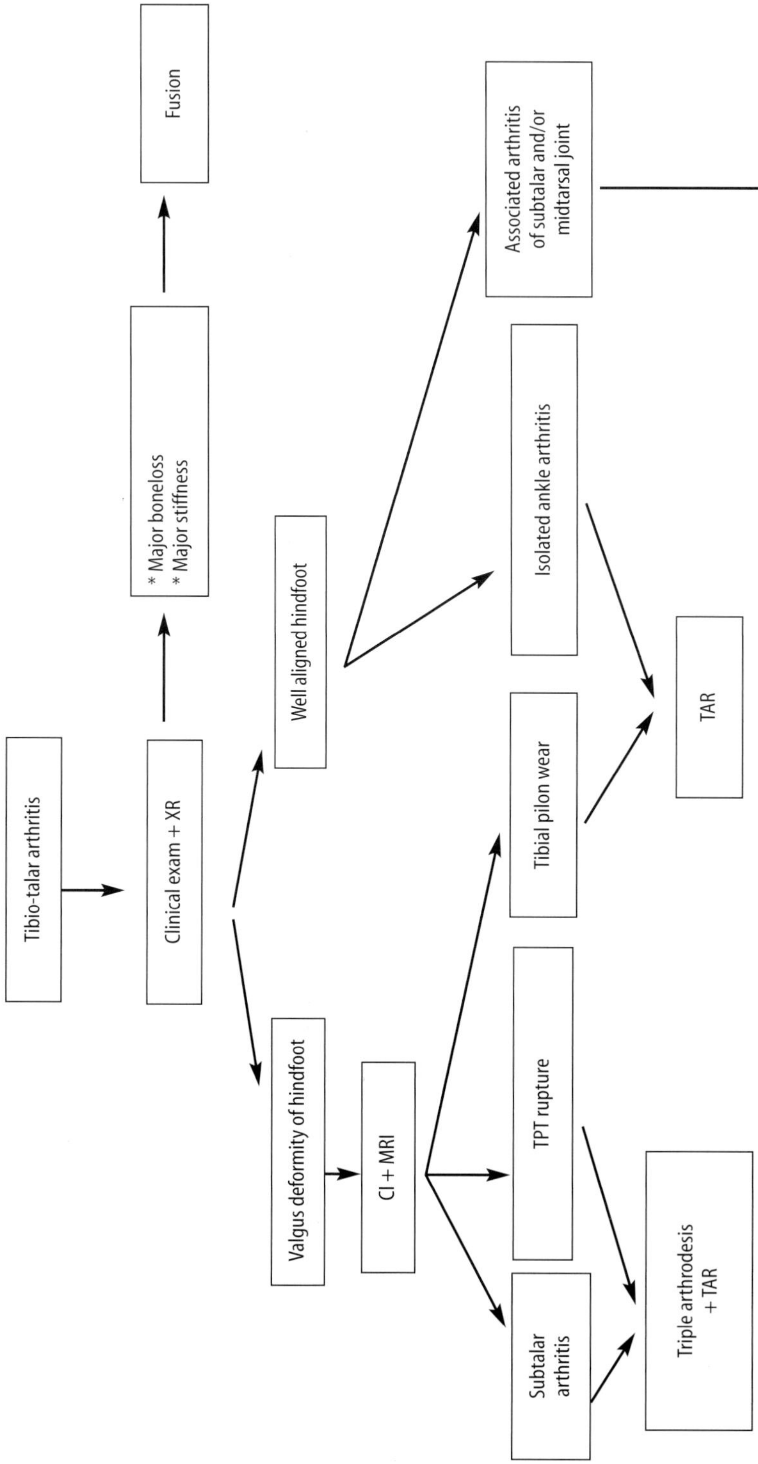

Fig. 4 - Management algorithm in tibiotalar disease.
TPT: Tibialis Posterior Tendon

Isolated involvement of the tibiotalar joint, without any deformity

Where the hindfoot is in correct alignment and the subtalar joint is intact, in correct position or spontaneously fused (cavus deformity), TAR may be performed as an isolated procedure (fig. 5).

Deformity confined to the tibiotalar joint

More often than not, the deformity will be associated with loss of bone stock from the tibial pilon. The deformity may be corrected by the prosthesis, which allows filling in the bone defect (fig. 6).

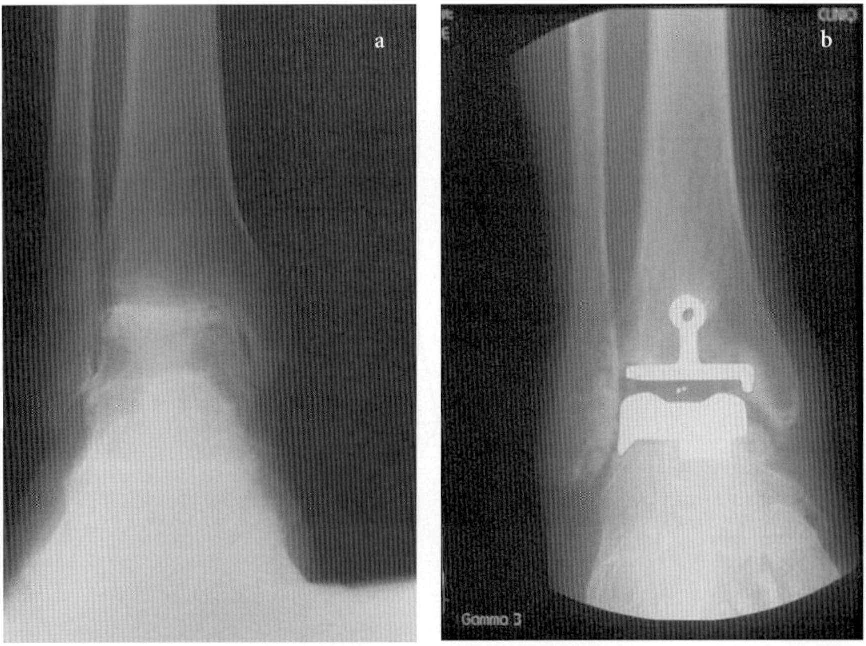

Fig. 5 - Management of isolated tibiotalar disease. **a**) Isolated tibiotalar RA; **b**) Treatment with isolated TAR.

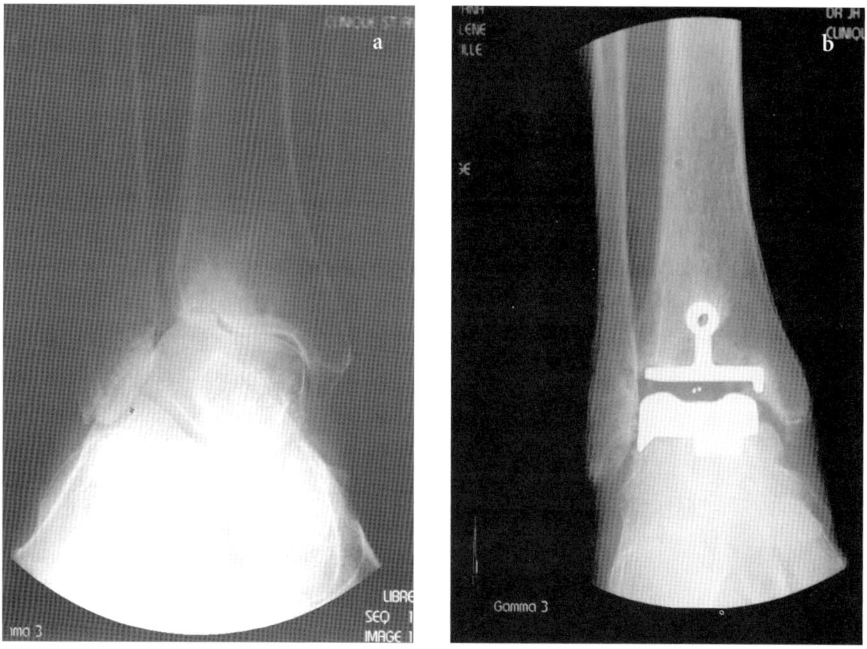

Fig. 6 - Management of isolated tibial pilon wear. **a**) Valgus deformity resulting from isolated tibial pilon wear; **b**) Treatment with isolated TAR.

Deformity affecting the ankle and the hindfoot

If the hindfoot is in valgus, as a result of associated subtalar or midtarsal RA or of advanced tibialis posterior tendinopathy, the outcome of an isolated procedure on the ankle joint is likely to be poor. Tibiotalar fusion may lead to rapid deterioration of the hindfoot joints, while any TAR may be doomed to early loosening in the malaligned ankle. Similarly, where there is associated talonavicular or talocalcaneal RA, albeit without deformity, addressing the tibiotalar joint in isolation may not afford the desired pain relief.

In such cases, two procedures may be considered: pantalar (tibiotalar, subtalar, and midtarsal) arthrodesis, or a combination of subtalar and midtarsal fusion with a TAR.

If there is no major loss of bone stock, it is our policy to avoid "fusion escalation", and to aim for ankle mobility. These complex cases are operated on in two stages. First, subtalar and midtarsal fusion are performed, followed at a later stage by TAR (1, 3). In order to minimize the period of immobilization, the subtalar and midtarsal fusions are performed first. The patient then spends 45 days in a plaster cast, prior to receiving his or her TAR. Following the arthroplasty procedure, a walking cast is worn for another 45 days (fig. 7).

In some cases of subtalar and midtarsal RA, spontaneous fusion in malposition may occur, with calcaneal valgus and forefoot abduction. In such cases, we feel that it would make little sense to implant a TAR above a malaligned hindfoot, and that these patients are better served by an osteotomy of the spontaneous fusion line, to allow correction of hindfoot and midfoot malalignment before TAR is performed. This pattern may also be encountered where subtalar and midtarsal fusions have been carried out previously, with insufficient correction of hindfoot and midfoot malalignment.

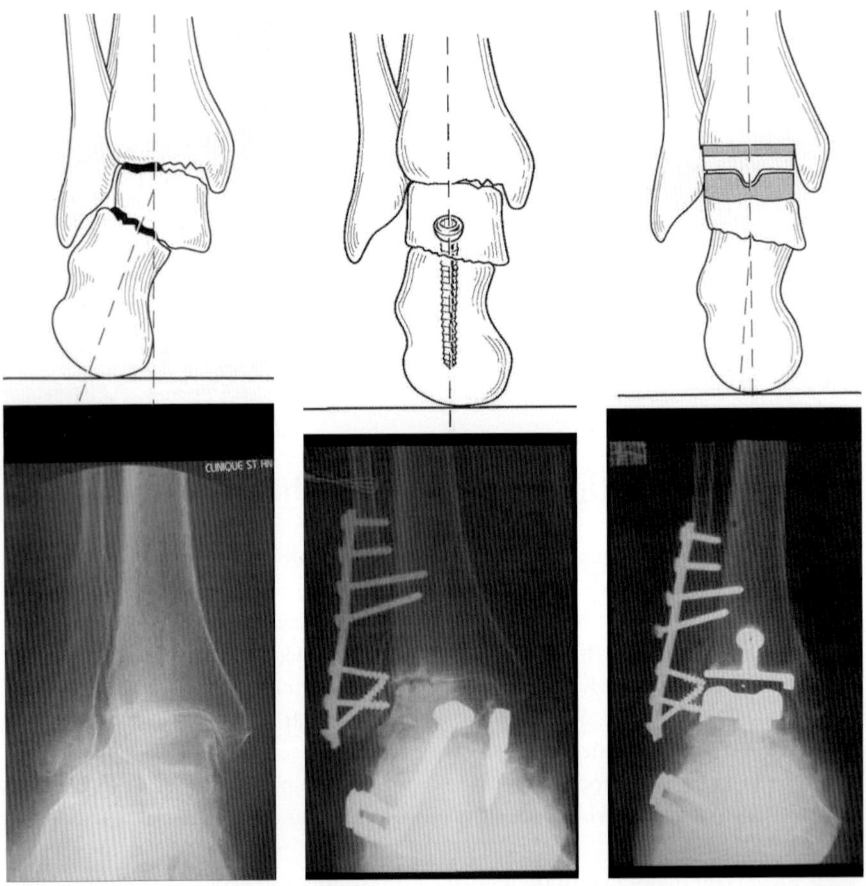

Fig. 7 - Management of multi-joint (tibiotalar and subtalar) disease). **a**) Associated tibiotalar and subtalar RA, with hindfoot valgus and stress fracture of lateral malleolus; **b**) First stage of surgical management: Subtalar and midtarsal fusions, and corrective osteotomy of the lateral malleolus; **c**) 45 days later, second stage of surgical management: TAR in an ankle above a correctly aligned hindfoot.

Where the forefoot is also affected, surgery at this level may be performed under the same anaesthetic as the subtalar and midtarsal fusions; if possible, the first metatarsophalangeal joint should be managed with arthroplasty rather than with fusion, so as to avoid excessive loading of the ankle.

In our opinion, tibiotalar arthrodesis and pantalar fusion should be performed only in patients with very severe loss of bone stock or with major stiffening of the different joints.

Between 1993 and 1999, we operated on 32 ankles in RA patients (3). Of these patients, 26 were female, and six were male. The mean age at surgery was 55 years (range: 32 to 81 years). The mean duration of RA was 17 years (range: two to 35 years). Eighteen patients had been treated with corticosteroids, and 17 with methotrexate. Eleven patients had isolated tibiotalar disease, and were managed with an isolated TAR. In 21 cases, there was multiple-joint involvement, and the protocol described above was applied.

Mean follow-up to date has been 57 months (range: 26 to 100 months). None of the patients were lost to follow-up. The functional results were analyzed using the AOFAS (American Orthopaedic Society of Foot and Ankle Surgery) scoring system. The results are shown in tables I and II.

Table I - Functional outcome of 32 total ankle replacements in RA patients.

AOFAS Score	Pre-op	Post-op	p value
Global score	33 ± 16	82 ± 8.6	<0.05
Pain/40	5 ± 9	35 ± 17	<0.05
Function /50	21 ± 7	35 ± 5.7	<0.05
Alignment/10	3.4 ± 2	7.6 ± 2	<0.05

AOFAS = American Orthopaedic Foot and Ankle Society

Table II - Functional outcome in the two groups (isolated TAR, and TAR plus subtalar and midtarsal fusions).

Procedure (n)	Age (years)	Duration of RA (years)	AOFAS Score
TAR only (11)	52.8	17.8	88.8 ± 6.1
TAR+ST-MT-F (21)	56.5	16.9	80.9 ± 8.6
p value	NS	NS	<0.05

RA = rheumatoid arthritis; AOFAS = American Orthopaedic Foot and Ankle Society; TAR = total ankle replacement; ST-MT-F = subtalar and midtarsal fusions; NS = not significant

References

1. Bonnin M, Bouysset M, Tebib J *et al.* (1999) Triple arthrodesis associated with total ankle arthroplasty in rheumatoid arthritis. American Orthopaedic Foot and Ankle Society, 29th meeting, Anaheim, California
2. Bonnin M, Judet T, Siguier T (2000) La prothèse totale de cheville. In: M. Bouysset Le pied en rhumatologie. 2nd edition. Paris Springer-Verlag
3. Bonnin M, Bouysset M, Tebib J *et al.* (2001) Total ankle arthroplasty in rheumatoid arthritis. ERAS: European Ankle Arthritis Surgery Society, Montpellier
4. Bouysset M, Tebib J, Noel E *et al.* (1992) Le métatarse rhumatoïde: évolution originale du premier métatarsien Rev Rhum Mal Ostéoartic, 59: 408-12
5. Bouysset M, Tavernier T, Tebib J *et al.* (1995) CT and MRI evaluation of tenosynovitis of the rheumatoid hind foot. Clin Rheumatol, 14: 303-7
6. Carlsson ÅS, Henricson A, Linder L, *et al.* (1994) A survival analysis of 52 Bath & Wessex ankle replacements. A clinical and radiographic study in patients with rheumatoid arthritis and a critical review of the literature. The Foot 4: 34-40
7. Cracchiolo A III, Cimino WR, Lian G (1992) Arthrodesis of the ankle in patients who have rheumatoid arthritis. J. Bone Joint Surg 74-A: 903-9
8. Cracchiolo A (1997) Rheumatoid arthritis. Hind foot disease. Clin Orthop 340: 903-9
9. Dereymaeker GP, Van Eygen P, Driesen R, *et al.* (1998) Tibiotalar arthrodesis in the rheumatoid foot. Clin Orthop., 349: 43-7
10. Doets HC (1997) Ankle arthroplasty for rheumatoid arthritis (New Jersey Ankle). First International Congress on Ankle Arthroplasty, Copenhagen, 20-21 June 1997
11. Evanski PM, Waugh TR (1977) Management of arthritis of the ankle. An alternative to arthrodesis. Clin Orthop, 122: 110-5
12. Felix NA, Kitaoka HB (1998) Ankle arthrodesis in patients with rheumatoid arthritis. Clin Orthop, 349: 58-64
13. Gschwend N, Steigen U (1987) Stable fixation in hind foot arthrodesis. A valuable procedure in the complex RA foot. Rheumatology 11: 113-25
14. Jakubowski S, Mohing W, Richter R (1970) Operationen am rheumatischen Fuss Therapiewoche 20: 762-8
15. Johnson K (1989) Replacement arthroplasty of the foot and ankle: total ankle arthroplasty. In Surgery of the foot and ankle arthroplasty. K.A. Johnson, New York Raven Press, 265-80
16. Kirkup J (1990) Rheumatoid arthritis and ankle surgery. Ann Rheum Dis 2: 837-44
17. Kitaoka HB (1989) Rheumatoid hindfoot. Orthop Clin North Am 20: 593-604
18. Kitaoka HB, Patzer GL, Ilstrup DM, *et al.* (1994) Survivorship analysis of the Mayo total ankle arthroplasty. J Bone Joint Surg 76-A: 974-9
19. Kitaoka HB, Patzer GL (1996) Clinical results of the Mayo total ankle arthroplasty. J Bone Joint Surg 78-A: 1658-64
20. Kofoed H, Sørensen TS (1998) Ankle arthroplasty for rheumatoid arthritis and osteoarthritis. Prospective long-term study of cemented replacements. J Bone Joint Surg 80-B: 328-32
21. Lachiewicz PF, Inglis AE, Ranawat CS (1984) Total ankle replacement in rheumatoid arthritis. J Bone Joint Surg 66-A: 340-3
22. Miehlke W, Gschwend N, Rippstein P, *et al.* (1997) Compression arthrodesis of the rheumatoid ankle and hindfoot. Clin Orthop, 340: 75-86

23. Moran CG, Pinder IM, Smith SR (1991) Ankle arthrodesis in rheumatoid arthritis. 30 cases followed for 5 years. Acta Orthop Scand 62: 538-43

24. Tillmann K. (1990) Recent advances in the surgical treatment of rheumatoid arthritis. Clin Orthop 258: 62-72

25. Tillmann K (1997) Point de vue sur la chirurgie du pied rhumatoïde. In Bouysset, Le pied en rhumatologie, Paris Springer-Verlag 151-6

26. Unger AS, Inglis AE, Now CS, *et al.* (1988) Total ankle arthroplasty in rheumatoid arthritis: a long-term follow-up study. Foot Ankle 8: 173-9

27. Vahvanen VAJ (1967) Rheumatoid arthritis in the pantalar joints. A follow-up study of triple arthrodesis on 292 adult feet. Acta Orthop Scand Suppl 107: 3

28. Vainio K (1956) The rheumatoid foot. A clinical study with pathological and roentgenological comments. Ann Chir Gynaecol 45 (1): 1-12

29. Vidigal E, Jacoby RK, Dixon AS, *et al.* (1975) The foot in chronic rheumatoid arthritis. Ann Rheum Dis 34: 292-7

30. Wood P (1997) Total ankle replacement (STAR-Link) for rheumatoid arthritis. First International Congress on Ankle Arthroplasty. Copenhagen, 20-21 June 1997

Respective indications of talo-crural arthrodesis and ankle prosthesis with different situations in rheumatoid arthritis

K. Tillmann and B. Fink

When systemical and local conservative treatment fails in the case of rheumatoid affection of the ankle joint, synovectomy should be the first consideration and option. The functional results of a timely and technically correct synovectomy cannot be equalized by any reconstructive surgery, neither by arthrodesis nor by endoprosthetic replacement. Even late synovectomies (LED-grade 2-3) may render acceptable results, preserving any possibility of retreat in case of failure: this is important especially for young patients (33).

In case of progression to serious painful destruction, the differential indication between arthrodesis and alloarthroplasty has to be considered.

Actual and promising ankle replacement started exactly in 1973 with the first publications of Lord and Marotte (21) and in the first line of Buchholz and Engelbrecht (2). The latter concept, the so-called St. Georg-prothesis, became the prototype of all "two components" endoprostheses: unconstrained, cemented, with a cylindrical concave tibial polyethylene component and a sled-like convex metal part, resurfacing the talar dome.

In close cooperation with the authors we started with this in January 1976. But at the end of the year facing the disavantages of a transfibular approach and of a missing side protection, we changed to the Thompson-Parkridge-Richards (TPR) prosthesis (23, 27), which we used up to 1990.

Since this time we did try different three component (35) designs: LCS (4), S.T.A.R (17) and Alphanorm (36). All these are characterized by metal components for the tibia and for the talar dome: with a flat undersurface on the tibial side and a convex contoured surface on the side of the talus. A mobile polyethylene bearing matches with both of them, permitting free sliding including rotation to the flat tibial component. To the talar side the bearing is semi-constrained and by this protected against luxation. For these implants we prefer a cementless press-fit fixation.

Parallel to alloarthroplasty we continue to indicate and to perform arthrodeses, even somewhat more frequent actually.

In order to preserve as much function as possible for the patient, we try to limit the fusions to only the severly destructed and deformed painful joints of the hindfoot, leaving free intact tarsal joints as far as possible and reasonable (36).

Due to the great variety of single and combined joint affections and of the different character and grade of destruction it would be inadequate to stick to only one technique for any arthrodesis: flexibility is required. Whenever possible, we perform open surgery and internal fixation, often in combination with bone grafting. The post-operative care is less demanding for patients and surgeons as well, compared to external fixation.

More recently, also for rheumatoid patients, arthroscopic (24, 26, 37) and percutaneous (19) techniques have been recommended in case of a well protected form and bone stock of the ankle joint (table II). For just these patients up to now we personally prefer an ankle prosthesis because the local situation is more suitable.

This statement may serve as a transition to the essential item of this chapter: the differential indication of fusion versus arthroplasty with respect to typical situations of the rheumatoid disease.

For this decision in the first line the local situation has to be considered. Serious destructions with major bone loss in the ankle and hindfoot region, especially necrosis of the talar dome, mutilating courses and massive cystic lesions are left for arthrodesis. Even this can be technically very difficult and extremely problematic. The success of the primary surgery can never be guaranteed. A non-union rate of about 20% in the literature (table I) may illustrate the difficulties.

To some degree bone grafting may render or improve the preconditions for the implantation of an endoprosthesis, but performed to a major extent it is too hazardous to rely upon such an "artificial" fixation.

In case of serious painful destruction of the neighboured tarsal joints it depends on the general situation of the patients, if a fusion should preceed an ankle arthroplasty, or if it will be preferable to combine it with an extended arthrodesis including the ankle joint in only one session.

Only exceptionally it is possible to combine tarsal fusions with ankle replacement: the post operative treatment is in general controversial.

In many situations there is no alternative to a fusion, whereas an arthrodesis can always be regarded as a possible alternative to ankle replacement.

So the question may arise: why do we need ankle endoprosthesis? When do we see the justification, facing the general risks of endoprosthetic replacement? Where do we see the inferiority and the superiority of allo-arthroplasty especially of the ankle joint in comparison to its arthrodesis?

The main arguments for the maintenance of the mobility of the ankle joint may arise from biomechanical considerations. By an arthrodesis the spring effect of the ankle gets lost to both directions, proximal and distal. This can cause disadvantages for severely affected or replaced hips and knees as well as for osteo-arthritic or inflamed tarsal and tarso- metatarsal joints and forefoot disorders (34). Especially in the region of the hind-and midfoot, serious pre-existing arthric or degenerative lesions will inevitably deteriorate after ankle arthrodesis (6, 20).

In contrast we did observe marked improvement of related problems after successful replacement of painfully destroyed ankle joints. The tendency of a spontaneous fusion of affected tarsal joints can be accelerated by the improved mobility of the ankle with the consequence of a well-formed "os tarsale" under protection of a suitable insole: a very happy outcome for these patients.

Forefoot problems in rheumatoid patients always become deteriorated by an ankle fusion, with and without forefoot surgery.

The frequently symmetrical rheumatoid affection of both ankles causes particular problems. In the case of bilateral ankle fusion the use of rocker-soles on both sides interferes seriously with the stability of the patients in standing and walking. The older the patients become, the more difficulties they will have to cope with this situation. They may lose a lot of independence and freedom by the limitation of locomotion (32, 34).

In the case of severe osteoporosis stress-fractures of the distal tibia have been observed, not only by ourselves (9, 12, 31). These fractures, if recognized and treated immediately, heal rapidly, but anyhow they cause painful additional problems and a delay of the rehabilitation.

Another very important argument for ankle replacement in our special experience with multiply disabled rheumatoid patients is the much more comfortable and much less demanding postoperative treatment in comparison to arthrodesis. Using suitable light- weight orthoses after the implantation of an ankle endoprosthesis, full weight-bearing can be permitted a few days after surgery already, whereas after arthrodesis disloading for several weeks, plaster cast immobilisation for about three months and usually an immobilizing below-knee custom-made boot will be necessary. This can cause great problems for severely affected rheumatoid patients regarding the general function of the locomotion system and will impair their rehabilitation.

Respecting biomechanical considerations, function, post-operative care and acceptance by the patients there cannot be great discussion regarding the superiority of ankle replacement compared to arthrodesis in suitable cases. But the deciding question of the responsible surgeon as an advocate of his patients interests has to be answered: what is the outlook of both procedures on short and long terms, what are the risks?

High failure rates of some cemented two-component ankle endoprostheses of the "first generation" (11, 15, 22) are certainly the main source of the still existing sepsis and reserve of many surgeons. The implantation is difficult and needs a lot of special experience in ankle surgery.

Moreover, the way of retreat in case of failure to an arthrodesis is risky and not easy. With growing experience and improving technique it may become more successful, but partly due to the need of bone grafting in many cases, the non-union rate will always be higher compared to primary arthrodesis.

In our experience an exchange operation can be easier and safer in suitable cases (34, 36).

Even in primary arthrodeses the main risk in open procedures is non-union (table I). In cases suitable for arthroscopic or percutaneous fusions (table II), we

Table I - Ankle arthrodesis in R.A. (7, 14, 28, 29, 38, 39) - Material/Complications.

	Pseud. -Rate		**Compl.**	
	n		**Skin**	**Inf.**
1969 Vahvanen V	32	19%	0%	0%
1980 Iwatawa H *et al.*	10	0%	./.	10 %
1987 Steiger U, Gschwend N	13	0%	0%	10%
1987 Uuspää V, Raunio P	148	22%	25%	./.
1990 Smith EJ, Wood PRL	11	18%	9%	36%
1992 Cracchiolo A. *et al.*	32	22%	9%	22%
TOTAL	**246**	**19%**	**17%**	**13%**

Table II - Ankle arthrodesis in R.A. (19, 24, 26, 37).

	n	**Pseud. -Rate**	**Compl.**		
			Skin	**Inf**	**Others**
PERCUTANEOUS:					
1998 Lauge-Pedersen H *et al.*	11	0%	0	0	2 (Fr.)
ARTHROSCOPIC:					
1995 Turan I *et al.*	10	0%	0	0	0
1998 Schmidt K, Haaker R	8	0%	0	0	0
2000 De Palma L *et al.*	7	0%	0	0	0

personally have no experience: the majority of just these cases is technically most appropriate for an alloarthroplasty (s. a).

The great advantage of an arthrodesis is that once fused in a good position, the ankle itself will be painfree and, except the above mentioned possible problems, the result will last for ever. But in general this procedure will be irreversible.

The long-term outcome of ankle arthroplasties, especially of the "second generation" (tri-component implants), is up to now scarcely known. Compared to more than one century of experience with ankle arthrodesis, that of "modern" ankle arthroplasty encloses only three decades (including the "first generation").

Some of our own experiences are shown in table III. With cemented two-component implants, type TPR, in rheumatoid joints after 14.6 years we had a failure rate of 24%. This may not be just encouraging, but less disastrous than commonly suggested. Lacking an actual follow-up of uncemented three-component implants, we may present in our opinion the most significant results of the two first designs (New Jersey and STAR) of the second generation, which we also used to a major extent (table IV).

Actually since 1995 we use mainly, due to biomechanical considerations, our own design with new materials ("Alphanorm") with very encouraging results.

Other designs followed later ("Hintegra", "Salto", "Ramses"), but for all of them in our opinion it is still to early too publish results.

Also two-component designs have been made suitable for cementless implantation, "TKN" (30) and "Agility" (1). For both these implants good medium-term results have been published (see table V).

Table III May mirror in some respect our own differential indication for rheumatoid patients by the numbers of different surgical procedures at the ankle joint. The relation has been maintained in the last years, so that it may be considered as current. The predominant role of arthrodesis may result from the typical situation of a well known and highly specialized combined unit for arthritis surgery, which attracts preferably most serious and late cases of inflammatory arthritic diseases. By

Table III: Ankle surgery in R.A. (Bad Bramstedt I/76 – XII/97 (22 Y) (Prim. Op. n = 502 Jts.).

Syn.	Fus.	Ankle joint replacement n = 159 Jts					
n =	n =	Cemented*			Uncem.**		
Jts.	Jts.	Prim. Impl.	Fus.	Exch.	Prim. Impl.	Fus.	Exch.
129	214	67	13	3	92	5	2 Total
				↓ Uncem			1 Bearing
FU (years)		14.6 (6.1-21.2) Y.			3.4 (0.6-7.6) Y.		
Failure Rate:		* 24%			** 8,7%		

Table IV - Ankle endoprotheses, tri component (3, 8, 13, 16, 25, 40).

	n	F.-U.	Surv. -R	ROM		COMPL.
				Prae	*post*	*(radiol.)*
N.J. – LCS						
1992 Buechel FF I	40	10 Y	95%	26°	25°	45%
Pappas MJ II	14	3 Y	100%	27°	28°	7%
1998 Doetz HC	21	6 Y	100%	25°	31°	9.5%
S.T.A.R.						
1998 Schill S, Thabe H	22	6 Y	94%	26°	34°	5%
1998 Wood PRL	19	-	100%	23°	29°	5%
1999 Hintermann B	50	1,5 Y	100%	-	30°	14%
1999 Kofoed H (cem.38, unc.59)	97	8 Y	96%	-	-	-

Table V - Ankle endoprotheses, two component – cementless (10, 30).

	n	F.-U.	Surv-R	ROM		COMPL.
				prae	*post*	*(radiol.)*
CYOCERA						
1990 Takakura Y *et al.*	38	4.1 Y	97%	-	29°	23%
AGILITY						
1998 Hansen ST Jr	56	4.8 Y	-	-	36°	21%

this the number of arthrodeses surpasses somewhat that of endoprotheses and - not to our delight – that of synovectomies.

To summarize, we feel that endoprosthetic replacement of the ankle joint cannot be regarded as an experimental procedure anymore after three decades of experience (18). The number of implantations is increasing on costs of fusions. But arthroplasty of the ankle joint will never edge out arthrodesis in the same way as in hip and knee, notwithstanding further technical progress. Personally I even think that just for rheumatoid patients the relation, as mirrored in our own statistics (see table III), will not change dramatically in the near future.

References

1. Alvine, FG (1991), Total ankle arthroplasty: concepts and approach. Contemporary Orthopaedics 22: 387-403
2. Bucholz, H.W, Engelbrecht E, Siegel A (1973), Total Sprunggelenksendoprothese Modell St Georg. Chirurg 44: 241-4
3. Buechel FF, Pappas MJ (1992), Survivorship and clinical evalution of cementless meniscal bearing total ankle replacement. Sem Arthroplasty 3: 43-50
4. Buechel FF, Pappas M.J, Iorio LJ (1988), New Jersey low contact stress total ankle replacement. Biomechanical rationale and review of 23 cementless cases. Foot & Ankle 44: 279-90
5. Carlsson AS, Henricson A., Lindner L *et al.* (2001), 10 years survival analysis of 69 Bath and Wessex ankle replacements. Foot and Ankle Surg 7: 39-44
6. Coester L.M, Saltzmann CL, Leupold J *et al.* (2001) Long-term results following ankle arthrodesis for posttraumatic arthritis. J Bone Joint Surg 83-A: 219-28
7. Cracciolo III A., Cimino WR, Lian G (1992), Arthrodesis of the ankle in patients who have rheumatoid arthritis. J Bone Joint Surg 74-A: 903-9
8. Doets HC (1998), The low Contact Stress Buechel-Pappas total ankle prothesis. In: Kofoed H (ed): Current status of ankle arthroplasty. Springer-Verlag pp. 29-33
9. Garcia S, Camacho JM, Segur P *et al.* (2001) Stress fractures of the tibia after ankle arthrodesis: a review of three cases. Foot and Ankle Surg 7: 175-80
10. Hansens ST Jr (1998), Cementless ankle arthroplasty in the United States of America: The Alvine Agility Total Ankle Arthroplasty. In: Kofoed H. (ed): Current status of ankle arthroplasty. Springer-Verlag pp. 37-40
11. Hay S.M, Smith TWD (1994), Total ankle arthroplasty: a long term review. The Foot 4: 1-5
12. Hilker A, Miiehlke R (1997), Das rheumatische Sprunggelenk. Med Orth Techn 117: 102-10
13. Hintermann B (1999), Die S.T.A.R.-Sprunggelenkprothese. Kurz- und mittelfristige Erfahrungen. Orthopäde 28: 792-803
14. Iwatawa H, Yashuhara N, Kawashima K *et al.* (1980), Arthrodesis of the ankle joint with rheumatoid arthritis. Clin Orthop 153: 189-93
15. Kirkup J (2002), Personal communication
16. Kofoed H (1999), Die Entwicklung der Sprunggelenksarthroplastik. Orthopäde 28: 804-11
17. Kofoed H., Stürup J (1994), Comparison of ankle arthroplasty and arthrodesis. A prospective series with long term follow-up. The Foot 4: 6-9
18. Kofoed H, Tillmann K (2000), Das obere Sprunggelenk Bemerkung zu einem Beitrag. In: Der Orthopäde (1999) 28: 529-237 und die Erwiderung der Autoren. Orthopäde 29: 171-2
19. Lauge-Pedersen H, Knutson K, Rydholm U (1998), Percutaneous ankle arthrodesis in the rheumatoid patient without debridement of the joint. The Foot 8: 226-9
20. Leicht P, Kofoed H (1992), Subtalar arthrosis following ankle arthrodesis. The Foot 2: 89-92
21. Lord G, Marotte JH (1973), Prothèse totale de cheville. Technique et premiers résultats. À propos de 12 observations. Rev Chir Orthop 59: 139-51
22. Müller EJ, Wick M, Muhr G (1999), Chirurgische Therapie bei Inkongruenzen und Arthrosen am oberen Sprunggelenk. Orthopäde 28: 529-37

23. Pahle JA (1987), Möglichkeiten und Komplikationen der operativen Behandlung am rheumatischen Fuß. Akt Rheumatol 12: 25-31
24. De Palma L, Santucci A, Verdenelli A *et al.* (2000), Arthroscopic arthrodesis of the ankle in rheumatoid patients. Foot an Ankle Surg 6: 261-6
25. Schill S, Thabe H (1998), Ankle arthroplasty: A clinical follow-up. In Kofoed H. (ed), Current status of ankle arthroplasty. Springer-Verlag pp. 90-3
26. Schmidt K, Haaker R (1998), Arthroskopische Behandlung des rheumatischen Sprunggelenks. Arthritis + Rheuma 18: 46-53
27. Sinn W, Tillmann K (1986), Mittelfristige Ergebnisse der TPR-Sprunggelenksendoprothese. Akt Rheumatol 11: 231-6
28. Smith E, Wood PRL, Ankle arthrodesis in rheumatoid patients. Foot & Ankle 10: 252-6
29. Steiger U, Gschwendt N (1987), Die Zugschraubenarthrodese nach Wagner bei Destruktion des Rückfußes. Akt Rheumatol 12: 41-4
30. Takakura Y, Tanaka Y, Sugimoto K *et al.* (1990), Ankle arthroplasty. A comparative study of cemented metal and uncemented ceramic protheses. Clin Orthop 252: 209-16
31. Thodarson DB, Chang D (1999), Stress fractures and tibial cortical hypertrophy after tibiocalcaneal arthrodesis with an intramedullary nail. Foot & Ankle 20: 497-500
32. Tillmann K (1979), The rheumatoid foot. Diagnosis, Pathomechanics and Treatment. Thieme, Stuttgart
33. Tillmann K (1990), Value of synovectomy. In: Revisional surgery in rheumatoid arthritis (eds. Hämäläinen M., Hagena F.-W., Schwägerl, W., Teigland, J. Rheumatology 13: 1-13
34. Tillmann K (1995), Eingriffe am oberen Sprunggelenk In: Wirth, CJ, Kohn, D, Siebert, WE: Rheumaorthopädie - untere Extremität. Springer-Verlag 166-73
35. Tillmann K (1998) Ankle joint replacement. In: Wülker, N, Stephens, M, Cracciolo III, A: An atlas of foot and ankle surgery. London, Dunitz 345-50
36. Tillmann K (2003), Differentialindikation zwischen OSG Arthrodese/Endoprothese beim Rheumatiker In: Imhoff A., Zollinger-Kies H (ed.), Fußchirurgie, Stuttgart
37. Turan I., Wredmark T, Fellender - Tsal L (1995) Arthroskopie ankle arthrodesis in rheumatoid arthritis. Clin Orthop 320: 110-4
38. Uuspää V, Raunio P (1987), Ankle arthrodesis: Rheumatology 11 104-13
39. Vahvanen V (1969) Arthrodesis of the TC or pantalar joints in rheumatoid arthritis. Acta Orthop Scand 40: 642-52
40. Wood, PLR (1998), Total ankle replacement (Link S. T. A. R.) for rheumatoid arthritis. In: Kofoed H (ed.) Current status of ankle arthroplasty. Springer-Verlag 34-6

Surgical strategy in surgery of the lower limb in rheumatoid arthritis

W.A. Souter

One of the great triumphs of orthopaedic surgery in the past half century has been the reconstruction of the multiply affected lower limb in rheumatoid patients. Previously an inexorable deterioration was liable to occur, especially if one or both hips became involved and the end product was all too often a wheelchair or bed-bound patient. Today this should only occur in very few patients since in order to pre-empt such a disastrous outcome a whole armamentarium has now been evolved, comprising forefoot arthroplasty, various forms of hindfoot fusion, ankle arthrodesis and ankle arthroplasty, total knee and hip replacement. Nearly all these operations are of proven and durable efficacy, only ankle arthroplasty being in the relatively experimental development phase and even this operation is now proving much more promising and durable. If, however, programmes of reconstruction are to reach their full potential of success, it is very important for the rheumatoid surgeon to be constantly mindful of the natural history of lower limb involvement and to use this knowledge in the selection of the most appropriate operations. Moreover, their optimal timing is still a major challenge demanding wisdom and experience.

Presentation

Programmes of multiple operations may be required in two different situations:

- as a straight sequence of operations carried out during a single programme of surgical therapy;
- as an intermittent cumulative series of operations which may be spread over many months or years.

The first of these possibilities was encountered fairly frequently in the early years of total joint replacement due to a backlog of extremely disabled untreated patients. At the present time this formidable challenge is much less frequently encountered due to improved ongoing care.

Modern care of the polyarthritic patient tends is follow the second pattern intermittent cumulative operations, the aim being to maintain the patient on a level or improving functional gradient.

It is now generally agreed that rehabilitation is much easier, providing intervention can be carried out before the patient has become too disabled and fallen into a lower functional category. This is not only of importance with regard to the patients coping with his or her own personal rehabilitation, but also carries major implications in terms of cost-effectiveness and manpower requirements. Kolstad and Wigren (1981) showed that with hospitalised patients who were still relatively independent and mobile, the workload assessed as the number of minutes per day provided in personal care from a variety of heath professionals averaged 112 minutes. By comparison the daily workload in caring for the severely disabled patient averaged 292 minutes.

Natural history of multiple joint disease in the lower limbs

The natural history of severe rheumatoid involvement in the lower limbs needs to be considered along several lines of potential deterioration. There is the progressive erosive pathology in the different joints leading to an associated increase in the sites and severity of pain. Inexorable functional deterioration is the inevitable result. What is less frequently realised is that there are accompanying systemic penalties, particularly with regard to the cardio-pulmonary physiology. All the foregoing have adverse implications for the patient's socio-economic welfare and although it is customary to somewhat belittle the importance of cosmesis for some patients, the progressive deformity accompanying severe lower limb pathology may be an important part of social isolation. It is very important for the rheumatoid surgeon to be fully aware of the "knock-on" effect or chain reaction implicit both in these individual lines of deterioration and operating across the lines as interacting adverse influences.

Progressive painful forefoot problems can render walking intolerable for the patient. Moreover, in order to gain some relief, patients are forced to rock back on their heels with resulting abnormal stresses on the hindfoot joints and ankle, so that pre-existing disease in these joints may be greatly exacerbated.

Severe valgus or varus deformity of a knee may result in corresponding valgus or varus deformity of the hindfoot or vice versa, Similarly, a flexion/adduction deformity of the hip can result in major erosive disease of the lateral compartments of the ipsi or contra-lateral knee (the latter having been referred to as long-leg arthroplasty).

A flexion contracture of the hip will induce a compensatory postural flexion deformity in the knee and if the latter joint is itself the site of erosive disease, this deformity will rapidly become a fixed contracture. Obviously the reverse process can occur where the primary joint involved is the knee. The combination of knee and hip deformities will necessitate the patient adopting an exaggerated lumbar lordosis which will inevitably result sooner or later in the development of back pain. As this postural chain reaction intensifies, the patient may in the end only be able to balance satisfactorily and maintain walking ability by resort to cane support or a walking frame. Under these circumstances upper limb joints have themselves to become weight bearing joints, with all the potential this involves for exacerbating upper limb disease, especially in the wrist, elbow and shoulder.

Because of this potential chain reaction it is very important to prevent the development of significant deformity at any joint in the lower limb in order to safeguard the function and architecture integrity of neighbouring joints. Moreover, when one is faced with multiple joint involvement and deformity at several sites and levels in the lower limbs, it is essential that corrective surgery is performed at all sites of deformity if a full erect posture is to be regained. This was very clearly stressed by McElwain and Sheehan in their review of bilateral hip and knee replacement, when they stated that it had been their policy to get patients to agree to a full programme of surgery before the treatment was commenced.

Moreover, there is a further implication, namely, that it may be necessary to persuade the patient to have surgery and perhaps even the initial surgery to a joint which is pain free due to its having become eroded and deformed relatively silently. For example, one may occasionally be presented with a patient with severely symptomatic knee pathology, where one finds that the trigger problem has been silent erosive disease, resulting in contracture and deformity in one or both hips. Clearly, any surgery to the knees in such circumstances would be futile and indeed irresponsible without first of all operating on the causative hip joint pathology.

In the light of the foregoing discussion, we can now define the aims of reconstructive surgery in the lower limb in rheumatoid arthritis as being:

- the relief of pain;
- the maintenance of function;
- the correction of deformity;
- the maintenance of a normally erect posture, particularly as seen in profile;
- the preservation of optimal walking ability;
- preservation of socio-economic independence and high quality of life.

If these aims are to be achieved and if the surgical interventions are to be appropriately timed, efficient and knowledgeable monitoring of the individual patient is essential, and one of the most important questions facing us at the present time is whose responsibility it should be to perform this monitoring.

Monitoring of the rheumatoid patient

In the pioneer days of rheumatoid surgery regular monitoring in the combined clinics was an unquestioned activity of the latter. Three or six monthly or yearly reviews was the order of the day. With the snowballing of clientele, detailed review of this nature within the combined clinic bas become impracticable and the tendency has been for monitoring to be referred back to the primary care team. It is questionable however, whether such monitoring is likely to be satisfactory, or in any way comparable to what was previously provided by the rheumatologist and surgeon within the milieu of the combined clinic. I would suggest that the reverse is likely to be the case. Whereas the surgeon and physician with a life long interest in rheumatoid problems carry a high degree of expertise with regard to their knowledge of the natural history of the disease, the general practitioner may or may not be interested in rheumatoid and with the best will in the world can only be relatively inexperienced in his knowledge of the natural history of these diseases. With monitoring in the combined clinic, radiographs were personally interpreted by experts. In the primary care scene, the X-rays may never be actually reviewed by the practitioner himself who may merely rely on a report given by a non-specialist radiologist who himself may have comparatively limited data on the clinical situation related to the X-rays. In the combined clinic there was personal knowledge of what surgery can provide. In the primary care situation there may be only very limited or indeed sometimes totally erroneous knowledge of what can actually be achieved by a surgical approach.

In practice, monitoring can probably only be undertaken by three groups of people:

- the medical rheumatologist/rheumasurgeon within the combined clinic which now seems to be impractical;
- the general practitioner who, in general, will tend to be insufficiently experienced;
- the paramedical members of the hospital team.

This last approach may well prove to be the most appropriate since it is probably the only way in which all rheumatoid patients who have come under the care of the specialised hospital rheumatoid service can be kept under permanent review by really knowledgeable health professionals. Physiotherapists, by their specialised training and approach to locomotor problems, are particularly suitable for this activity, but experienced senior nursing staff can also fulfil this role extremely efficiently.

Monitoring is an extremely interesting challenge for health professionals of whatever discipline, since their attention must range over a very wide spectrum of assessment parameters. These include the activity of the systemic and local disease, the severity and pattern of joint erosion, and social factors including age, career demands, leisure aspirations and very individual personal responsibilities. Moreover, all decisions must be taken in the light of the observer's own personal experience of the demands of individual surgical operations and the efficacy and durability of these procedures.

Delivery of surgical care

The first principle of management viz., the establishment of a good doctor patient relationship is of vital importance. In many ways the surgical management of rheumatoid disease can be regarded as a battle, or more accurately, a long war between the rheumatoid disease on the one hand and the surgical armamentarium on the other. In this contest the patient, if correctly handled, can be a vital ally in ensuring the success of the surgical procedures. How is this relationship to be established?

- By communicating to the patient the surgeon's sympathetic appreciation of the patient's very natural apprehension regarding the functional problems and deformities which may arise in the future;

- By a frank discussion of the goals to be aimed for and the delineation of what will and will not be practicable;
- By starting with a "winner" operation, by which I mean an operation likely to tax the patient minimally, while offering maximum pain relief and/or restoration of function. This approach can greatly boost the patient's confidence in facing more taxing and formidable operations at a later date and it is, in my opinion, of such importance that it should be regarded as a tactic in its own right.

Sequence of operations

Where only a single or relatively few joints are involved, the nature of the surgical intervention may be largely predetermined. Where, however, the surgeon is faced with multiple pathology in both lower limbs, the planning of the surgical programme becomes of vital importance.

Where there are severe toe deformities, forefoot arthroplasty constitutes an ideal "winner" operation as it places minimal demands on the patient but is virtually guaranteed to give them tremendous relief from pain. Where the forefoot is not requiring attention, total hip replacement can provide a very useful starting point, as again the post-operative rehabilitation is relatively easy and the functional benefits can be inestimable. Once the patient's confidence has been gained through the successful completion of such operations, they are likely to be much better psychologically adjusted to facing the greater rigours of the recovery from total knee replacement or the more prolonged convalescence from hind foot surgery. Moreover, the completion of the reconstructive surgery at hip and knee level allows the surgeon to plan the final stage of hind foot surgery in the light of the alignment which has already been achieved more proximally.

The above-suggested sequence of operations should not be regarded as an immutable blueprint but merely as a guideline which can be altered accordingly to the pattern of the disease and the severity of the various problems of the individual patient. Moreover, different surgeons may prefer alternative sequences of operations and provided the method of attack has been found efficacious in their hands there is no reason why all should conform to a fixed blue-print. The disease itself can be infinitely variable and therapeutic programmes should be similarly malleable.

The use of early minor operations to pre-empt the need for late major surgery

If early intervention using simple operations may delay or prevent further damage, then this is certainly to be advocated. Full implementation of policy might of course necessitate a considerable increase in the amount of early surgery undertaken, and it is clearly necessary to balance the ideal with what is practical in view of the limited resources available. On the other hand, it has been appreciated that a simple surgical procedure applied relatively early in the course of disease before architectural disintegration and malalignment has supervened, may occupy much less theatre time and require much input during the rehabilitation phase. Clearly this opens a whole field of potential research which is urgently required to assess the efficacy of early simple operative intervention relative to more major interventions at a later

date. Randomised controlled trials of the current laissez-faire approach, frequently requiring later major surgery, versus aggressive surgery using minor conservative techniques would be of great value as they should yield answers to the following important questions:
- does early intervention reduce the necessity for later major surgery or does it render the latter more effective when it is finally undertaken?
- is the policy of early intervention likely to be cost-effective?
- can it yield virtually total pain relief at local sites as compared with the mere partial control which can be effected via analgesia? This certainly has major humanitarian implications, but could also yield cost benefits.

There is a real need for units to develop definite strategies for clinical management in relation to the modification which early surgical interventions, can achieve in the natural history of the disease at local sites, and perhaps this can be well illustrated in relation to the hind foot. All too often the rheumatoid hindfoot reaches the surgical clinic when it has become rigid and hopelessly distorted into a valgus position. There may also be marked tightness and contracture of the lateral tissues including the skin. Medical rheumatologists perhaps do not always appreciate the technical difficulties of rectifying this situation. Triple fusion with full correction of the deformity can be a most demanding operative procedure. For the surgeon two choices are available. He may either elect to build up a pillar of bone on the outer aspect of the foot and, in so doing, maintain heel height, in which case he may be faced with grave problems of wound closure, delayed wound healing and later collapse or partial resorption of the graft with recurrence of the disability. Alternatively, he may go for excision of a medially based wedge. This is technically much more difficult but is much safer with regard to skin healing, bone fusion and durability. If the deformity has been severe however the amount of bone which will need to be removed will inevitably condemn the patient to a very low heel and its attendant problems of discomfort from the uppers of shoes pressing on the malleoli. Karl Tillmann, however, has pointed out that the hindfoot problems almost invariably start in the talonavicular joint. Alternatively the subtalar joint may be the site of initial involvement. The simple operation of talonavicular fusion provides the possibility of maintaining a plantigrade foot and perhaps preventing or lessening further active hind foot disease so that the need for triple fusion may be obviated. If this hypothesis is indeed true, there can be no excuse for failing to monitor hindfoot disease so that early referral to the surgeon becomes possible at a time when serious erosion is limited to the talonavicular joint and the foot still remains plantigrade. I would suggest therefore that an appropriate hind foot therapeutic policy would involve early referral for talonavicular fusion (or for fusion of the subtalar joint should this be the joint which had become primarily involved). Likewise, this policy should also be subjected to strictly controlled trials so that the prevailing laissez-faire approach of so many centres can be scientifically compared with the results which are likely to be achieved with early aggressive surgery aimed at ensuring that the foot remains in plantigrade alignment. The questions to which such controlled trials should yield answers are:

- does talonavicular fusion prevent later hindfoot disease activity and deformity?
- does it render the necessity for triple fusion minimal and if it has to be undertaken, is it likely to be less technically difficult?

- does the resulting more rigid hindfoot accelerate ankle involvement?

Such early intervention at the subtalar metatarsal level and the maintenance of a plantigrade foot may also have major implications with regard to the ease with which ankle arthroplasty may be resorted to, should this joint become involved at a later date. It is now generally agreed that a severe valgus deformity of the hindfoot must be corrected prior to embarking on ankle arthroplasty if this latter operation is to prove successful and durable. If the foot has not been kept plantigrade and these operations have to be tackled in sequence, the patient will inevitably have to cope with a considerable period of morbidity. Early appropriate surgery might hopefully abolish this problem.

The combination of operations under one anaesthetic

One of the major problems of surgical treatment for rheumatoid patients is the sheer number of joints that may be involved in severe cases and, in consequence, the sheer number of anaesthetics and operations which may be required in the course of corrective surgery. Consequently, if operations can be combined under a single anaesthetic there may be very considerable advantages. Bilateral forefoot arthroplasty has of course been long established as the routine approach, but there are now numerous studies in the literature which suggest that bilateral hip and bilateral knee replacements can be undertaken under the same anaesthetic without any adverse result. Indeed it is claimed that the overall hospitalisation and period of rehabilitation is considerably reduced. Where severe hip and knee flexion contractures co-exist in the same limb, simultaneous replacement of the hip and knee may also be worth consideration.

Where a patient is requiring corrective surgery in both upper and lower limbs and where facilities exist for two teams operating simultaneously, the combination of appropriate upper and lower limb operations, under the same anaesthetic, has much to recommend it.

As with other aspects of reconstructive rheumasurgery there should be no fixed blueprint with regard to such a policy. There is always the dread that if infection was to occur post-operatively, all the operated sites might become involved which could prove quite disastrous for the patient. Moreover, not all studies have suggested that combined operative procedures may be completely innocuous. The more cautious surgeon may therefore feel happier with a staged approach carrying out individual procedures at fortnightly intervals. Individual patients may also prefer this approach so that their efforts at rehabilitation can be concentrated on a single site. The policy in any single unit should clearly be determined by the inclinations of the surgeon and the wishes and psychological profile of the individual patients. Complete confidence in and approval of the proposed surgery is indeed a vital factor in ensuring surgical success.

Self-awareness and informed consent in the approach to the planning of surgery

Sadly, no single surgical operation and certainly no programme of surgery can be guaranteed to be successful. Moreover, the same operation in the hands of different surgeons can yield very differing results. It is accordingly always important for the surgeon to be mindful of the serious complications which can occur and to render the patient fully aware of these. Moreover, the varying likelihood of these complications relative to the patient's age and potential activity must also be clearly kept in mind and explained to the patient.

While it is necessary for the surgeon to be knowledgeable with regard to the reported results from individual operations in the literature, it is even more important for him to exhibit full self-awareness as to the results which he or she can personally achieve with any given procedure, as it is entirely on this that the outcome will depend. Provided that a good rapport has been established between surgeon and patient from the outset and given that complete openness has been observed in the discussions leading up to surgery, trust and understanding are likely to be maintained between surgeon and patient even in the event of complications arising. Where this rapport and openness is missing, recriminations are all too likely to occur.

In the rheumatoid field with good patient management and a wisely directed strategy of treatment, reconstructive surgery presents a very rewarding challenge. Most rheumatoid patients show exemplary courage and determination to reap the very best they can achieve from the various surgical procedures which they have to undergo and the privilege of helping them to achieve these aims, frequently over a period of many years can be an exciting and humbling experience for the whole therapeutic team.

Surgery of the foot and ankle in patients with rheumatoid arthritis: some reflexions

F.X. Koeck, G. Heers, W. Caro and J. Grifka

Introduction

When treating rheumatoid patients the foot and ankle surgeon may use established surgical procedures or more recent techniques and procedures for this difficult problem. However, careful and critical evaluation is important when considering deviations from the established methods of treatment. Total joint arthroplasty of the ankle joint using the latest generation of uncemented prosthesis and open or arthroscopic synovectomies with concurrent synoviorthesis for early stages of the disease are considered basic established procedures of every surgeon treating rheumatoid patients.

In the early stages of rheumatoid disease the forefoot is afflicted in 16% of patients, progresses to 53% after three years, until finally 90% of cases will have some involvement (7, 14, 31, 37). Joints involved include the tarsal and metatarsal in 40-60% of cases, whereas the involvement of the talocrural and the subtalar joints depends on the duration of the disease, and ranges from 10-52%. In general, the subtalar joint is more often affected than the talocural joint (1, 14, 25, 36, 40).

The complex physiological interconnections of the fore-, mid-, and hind foot should be considered prior to surgical intervention (36). The multifocal pattern of joint affection and corresponding chain like destruction of the joints necessitate careful planning and order of treatment.

Additional involvement of the hip and knee joint may lead to static alterations of the lower limb. Overall, the correct choice of surgical procedure depends on the pattern and the stage of joint destruction as described by Larsen-Dale-Eek (LDE), and the expected spontaneous course of the disease. We differentiate between an ankylotic, a secondary arthrotic, and a mutilating progress of the disease (26, 35, 36).

Given equal stages of destruction of the upper and lower extremity the lower extremity should be operated on first, as the rheumatoid foot is frequently considered the limiting factor for mobility of the patient. Prior to surgery in the rheumatoid patient, conservative treatments such as corrective shoes and insoles should be pursued (12). The surgeon must be aware of the individual functional status and expectations of the patient (35). Patients with rheumatoid arthritis are at a higher risk for complications following surgery. The increased rate of wound healing impairment and postoperative infections can be explained by the systemic disease itself, and the extended use of medications that may affect normal healing processes and immune responses (28).

Special operative procedures

Generally, one has to choose between joint preservation and reconstructive surgical procedures that include total joint replacement or arthrodesis.

Joint preserving surgical procedures are performed at the early stages LDE 0-3. Reconstructive surgeries are necessary at advanced stages LDE 4-5 (41). Procedures to preserve the joint should be performed as early as possible. If conservative treatment fails and joints and tendons are threatened by destruction and disabling deformities a synovectomy of the foot is performed. A synovectomy is called early synovectomy when done during stages 0 to 2 and late synovectomy during stages LDE 2-3.

Tibiotarsal joint and hindfoot

Rheumatoid hind foot is characterized by changes in the subtalar, tibiotarsal, and the talonavicular joints, and synovitis of the peroneal and tibialis posterior tendon (5, 35). The combined destruction of articular and extraarticular structures leads to pes planovalgus (15, 38).

The timing of synovectomy is the key factor that determines the status of the hindfoot and the long term outcome.

Arthroscopic synovectomy is the chosen method to treat early LDE 0-2, in which isolated synovitis of the tibiotarsal joint, especially in its ventral parts, and a low grade tendon destruction is present without accompanying inflammation (fig. 1 and 2).

In addition, radio- (rhenium) or chemosynoviorthesis (sodium-morrhuate) has been advised (31).

Open synovectomy should be performed during stage 2-3, when a distinct villous proliferative synovitis and middle graded destructive changes at the joint are present. The surgical approach is dependent on which additional procedures will be needed. Open synovectomy can be combined, if necessary, with tenosynovectomy of the fibular and tibialis posterior tendons, or with subtalar arthrodesis to correct the anatomical position of the joint.

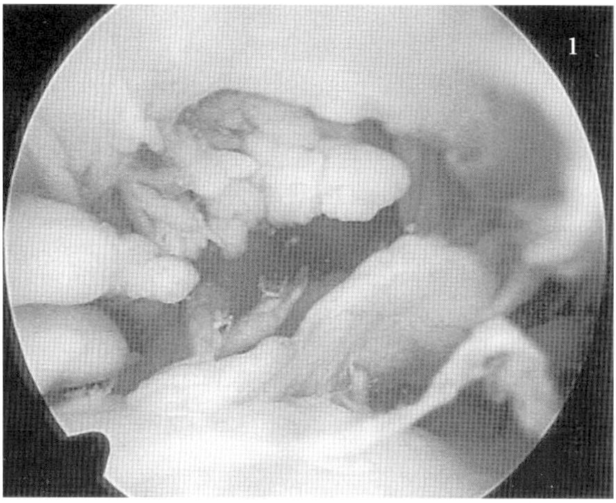

Fig. 1-

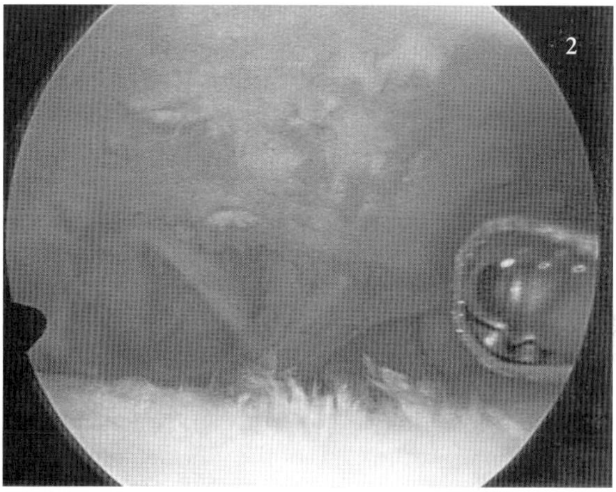

Fig. 2 -

Several studies concerning the combined strategy report good results with reduction of pain and swelling in 70-80% of the cases and satisfactory function (1, 3, 31).

Transfer of the flexor digitorum longus tendon as described by Johnson performed for stage LDE 2 is rarely indicated, as dysfunction of the tibialis posterior tendon in cases of an rigid pes planovalgus may lead to complaints (10, 20).

At the advanced stages LDE 4-5 there is, in addition to arthrodesis of the tibiotarsal joint, the opportunity of total joint replacement after excluding contraindications. Apart from the prosthesis design, surgical technique, and the postoperative treatment regime, it is primarily the correct indication for surgery that decides between success and failure.

Residual function of the tibiotalar joint, intact and stabile ligaments, good bone stock for the prosthesis, and kinematic variations of the hindfoot (varus-/valgus malposition maximum of 15°) must be be considered (17). Necrosis of the talar dome in cases of advanced tibiotarsal joint destruction is considered an absolute contraindication for arthroplasty (33). Newton in 1982 and Bolton-Maggs in 1985 reported rheumatoid arthritis itself as a contraindication for total tibiotarsal joint replacement. At the time of these reports, first generation cemented TAA were very disapointing (4, 29). The improved outcomes of more current, newly designed, uncemented, unconstrained TAA incorporating plastic slide bearings (LCS®, New-Jersey®, STAR®) make them a viable treatment of the rheumatic ankle joint (6, 23, 37). The high satisfaction of patients in up to 94% of the cases does not correlate with the gained range of motion of the ankle joint (17, 33, 37). The survival rate of the latest prothesis designs are reported to be 85-96% with a medium-term follow-up of 8-10 years.

Advanced stages of the disease (LDE 4-5) are considered a contraindication for total joint replacement. In these cases arthrodesis remains the treatment of choice. Arthrodesis leads to higher mechanical stresses on the adjacent joints and a non-physiological gait (8,25). Resulting severe deformities, especially deformities of the hind foot, and instabilities may be corrected (35). Compression-arthrodesis using cannulated cancellous bone screws may be considered is the most common technique. Use of External fixation may lead to infections or diminished blood perfusion and should therefore be limited to revision surgery (8,9). The lateral transfibular approach in patients with limited bone quality has the advantage of a possible fibula grafting (18) as compared to the anterior approach to the talocural joint. Neutral hindfoot position regarding to rotation, flexion/extension and varus/valgus is considered the ideal position for ankle fusion in rheumatoid arthritis. If necessary, a complementary arthrodesis of the subtalar and chopart joint as well as a complete hindfoot arthrodesis may be performed. If further correction of the axis of the hindfoot is unnecessary, one may consider an arthroscopically assisted arthrodesis of the talocural joint (19, 34). Post-operative care should include a cast for 8-12 weeks and no or partial weight bearing 4-8 weeks to ensure osseous healing. Once healing is confirmed radiologically mobilisation using corrective shoes should be performed until the end of the first postoperative year. Good results have been reported in 70-90% in rheumatoid patients (8, 42). However, a rate of 20-44% non-unions has been reported depending on the method of fixation (8,13).

Synovectomies of the subtalar, talonavicular and calcaneocuboidal joint are only rarely performed. Corrective shoes and insoles are absolutely necessary when radiographic changes in these joints are present. We perform arthrodesis in these joints when persistent pain, destruction and malalignment are present. Arthrodesis should be limited to the joints involved due to biomechanical disadvantages (35). An arthrodesis of the talonaviclar joint alone (fig. 3, 4) or a double arthrodesis of the chopart joint can be fixed using Blount staples.

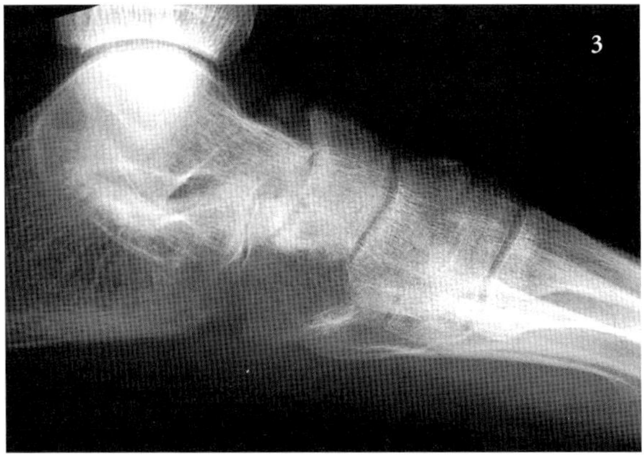

Fig. 3 -

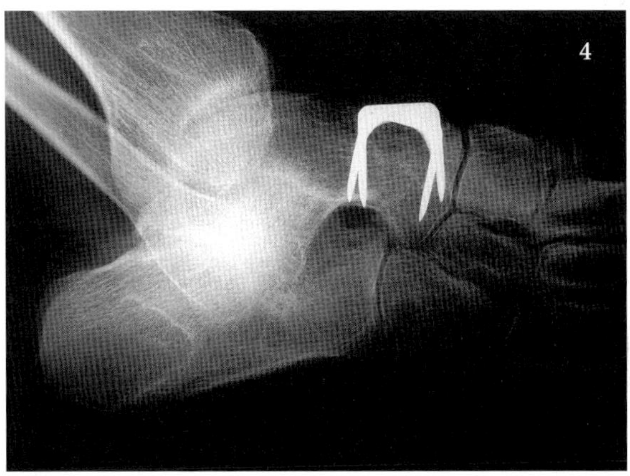

Fig. 4 -

A rigid pes planovalgus often makes a triple arthrodesis necessary. The subtalar joint may be fixed using a cancellous bone screw and concurrent autologous iliac crest bone graft inserted laterally (30). Furthermore, hindfoot arthrodesis sometimes makes cancellous bone grafting necessary to fill bony defects and correct bony alignment. As with arthrodesis of the talocural joint, partial or non-weight bearing periods following the cast immobilisation must be sufficiently long to ensure healing. The lever arm forces present in the subtalar joint are generally less than in the hindfoot, which reduces the risk of complication due to weight-bearing.

Forefoot

Apart from destruction of joint architecture of the forefoot, hindfoot deformities influence forefoot deformities in the rheumatoid patient (10, 36). Understanding this will help avoid multiple surgeries on the forefoot.

Advanced forefoot deformity in rheumatoid arthritis typically consists of extensive hallux valgus with concurrent bursitis at the first metatarsal head, lateral deviation of hammertoes 2-5, digitus quintus varus, plantar subluxation of the metatarsal heads 2-5 with concurrent plantar bursal synovitis, and destruction of the plantar tendinous plate (pes transversoplanus) (fig. 5). If only inflammatory changes of the forefoot are present, surgery may be avoided by proper management of corrective shoes or specific insoles (35, 36).

In cases of persistent pain and evidence of rheumatoid fore-foot deformities, surgery remains a rewarding procedure in the hands of an experienced surgeon.

Synovectomy of the toe joints alone should not be considered a routine operation and is rarely indicated in advanced stages of the disease (LDE 0-2). If surgery is necessary and subluxation in the MTP joint is present an additional lengthening of the extensor tendon may be necessary.

For advanced subluxation of the fifth metatarsophalangeal joint an additional shortening osteotomy according to Weil may be indicated in order to achieve correct

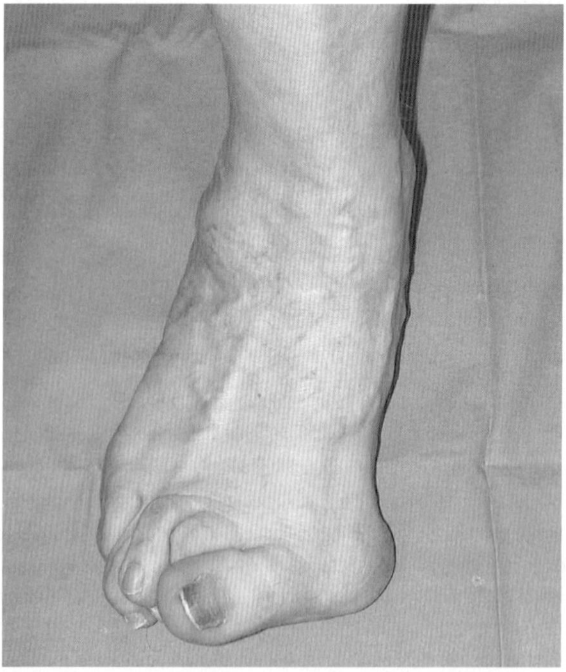

Fig. 5 -

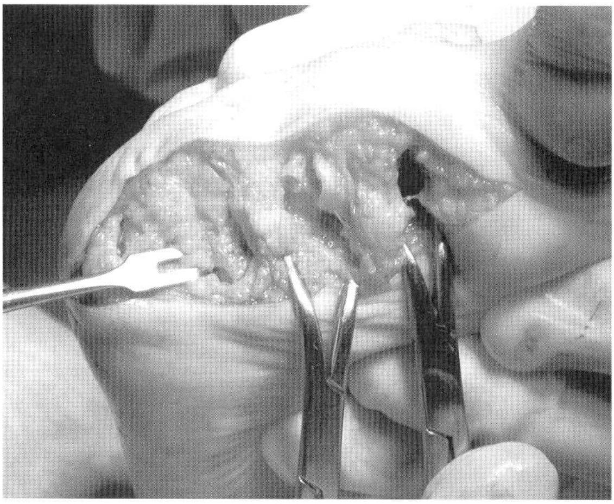

Fig. 6 -

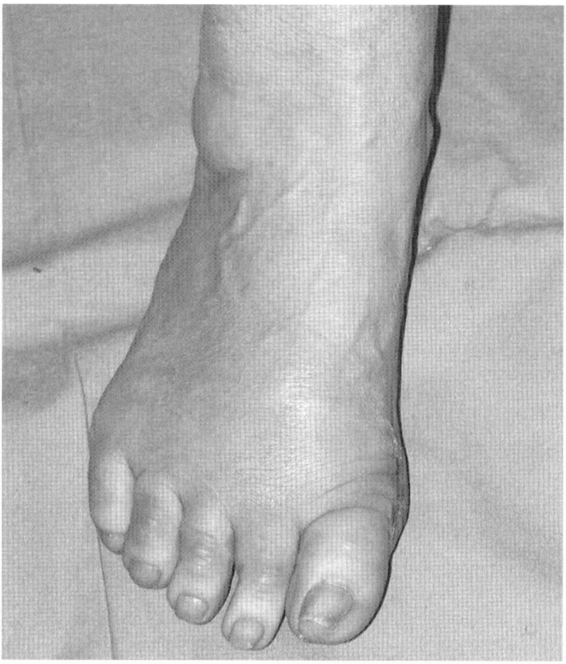

Fig. 7 -

reduction of the joint. Unfortunately, long term results following synovectomy and joint preserving procedures on the toes show significant radiologic progressive changes of the disease (2).

Indications for osseous corrective operations depend both on the level of destruction of the first metatarsophalangeal joint and the functional demands of the patient.

As a general rule joint preserving procedures on the first ray should only be performed in LDE stages 0-3. Similar to therapy of idiopathic hallux valgus, the treatment of choice depends on the degree of malposition, especially the angle between the first and the second metatarsal bone.

If this angle exceeds 15° proximal or diaphyseal corrective osteotomies may be the best procedure (10). The so-called distal and lateral release of the soft-tissues with detachment of adductor tendon combined with medial capsulo- and tenorhaphy should be performed in all surgical cases.

The resection arthroplasty remains the gold standard for complex deformities of the forefoot in advanced stages of joint destruction (LDE 4-5) (figs. 5, 6, 7).

Partial Resection of the first metatarsal head as described by Hueter and Mayo or resection of metatarsal heads 2-5 by plantar approach as described by Hoffmann and Tillmann along with proper after care (adhesive plaster bandage, stable and form protecting insoles and rocker soles) can result in significant long-term pain reduction. Improved walking abilities of the patient should result (11, 21, 22, 36).

Dynamic foot pressure measurements have shown that complete resection of the metatarsal heads, especially the first metatarsal head, is comparable to functional amputation of the forefoot. As such the great toe is not involved in the gait process.

Therefore arthrodesis of the first metatarsal-phalangeal joint is preferred for young and active rheumatoid patients with concurrent resection of metatarsal heads 2-5 as described by Hoffmann/Tillmann (21, 42).

Due to our personal experience of silicon induced synovialitis following implantation of Swanson-Silicast-Spacers in the first metatarsal-phalangeal joint we do not recommend this procedure as a primary treatment. However, good long-term results have been reported using Swanson-Silicast-Spacers with 10year survival rates of over 87% (10, 16, 42).

Conclusion

A pain free, enduring and orthograd foot is the primary aim of surgical intervention in rheumatoid foot deformities. There are several well-established procedures aimed at this goal, which involve either joint-preserving techniques or arthrodesis. Arthroscopic surgery as well as the new generation of total joint replacements should only be performed for the talocrural joint.

References

1. Akagi S, Sugano H, Ogawa R (1997) The long-term results of ankle synovectomy for rheumatoid arthritis. Clin Rheumatol 16: 284-90
2. Belt EA, Kaarela K, Lehto MU (1998) Destruction and arthroplasties at the metatarsophalangeal joints in seropositiv rheumatoid arthritis. A 20-year follow-up study. Scand J Rheumatol 27: 194-6

3. Biehl C, Schill S, Thabe H (2001) Mittel- und langfristige Ergebnisse nach Sprunggelenksynovektomien. Orthopädische Praxis 12: 814-7
4. Bolton-Maggs BG, Sudlow RA, Freeman MA (1985) Total ankle arthroplasty. A long-term review of the London Hospital experience. J Bone Joint Surg B 67: 785-90
5. Bouysset M, Bonvoisin B, Lejeune E *et al.* (1987) Flattening of rheumatoid foot in tarsal arthritis on X-ray. Scand J Rheumatol 16: 127-33
6. Buechel FF, Pappas MJ (1992) Survivorship and clinical evaluation of cementless meniscus bearing total ankle replacements. Sem in Arthroplasty 3: 43-50
7. Clayton ML (1969) Situation of the foot regarding early synovectomy in rheumatoid arthritis. Excerpta Medica (Amsterdam): 146
8. Cracchiolo A, Cimino WR, Lian G (1992) Arthrodesis of the ankle in patients who have rheumatoid arthritis. J Bone Joint Surg A 74: 903-9
9. Dennis DA, Clayton ML, Wong DA *et al.* (1990) Internal fixation compression arthrodesis of the ankle. Clin Orthop 253: 212-20
10. Fuhrmann R (2002) Die Behandlung der rheumatischen Fußdeformität. Orthopäde 31: 1187-97
11. Grifka J, Oest O (1989) Verlaufsbeobachtungen nach Mittelfußköpfchenresektion nach Lelievre. Z Orthop 127: 561-5
12. Grifka J (1997) Shoes and insoles for patients with rheumatoid foot disease. Clin Orthop 340: 18-25
13. Günter U, Zacher J (2000) Die Pseudarthrose nach Arthrodese – Eine Analyse der Indikationen und Methoden bei 64 Sprunggelenken. Orthop Praxis 36 (8): 490-6
14. Gschwend N (1977) Die operative Behandlung der chronischen Polyarthritis. Thieme (Stuttgart) 2nd edition
15. Haas C, Kladny B, Lott G *et al.* (1998) Progression von Fußdeformitäten bei rheumatoider Arthritis – eine radiologische Verlaufsbeobachtung über 5 Jahre. Z Rheumatol 58: 351-7
16. Hanyu T, Yamazaki H, Ishikawa H *et al.* (2001) Flexible hinge toe implant arthroplasty for rheumatoid arthritis of the first metatarsophalangeal joint: long-term results. J Orthop Sci 6: 141-7
17. Hintermann B (1999) Die STAR-Sprunggelenkprothese. Orthopäde 28: 792-803
18. Iwata H, Yasuhara N, Kawashima K *et al.* (1980) Arthrodesis of the ankle joint with RA: experience with transfibular approach. Clin Orthop 152: 189-93
19. Jerosch J (1999) Arthroskopische Operationen am oberen Sprunggelenk. Orthopäde 28: 538-49
20. Johnson KA, Strom DE (1989) Tibialis posterior dysfunktion. Clin Orthop 239: 196-206
21. Jüsten HP, Berger W, Leeb I *et al.* (2000) Langzeitergebnisse nach Metatarsalköpfchen-Resektion bei rheumatoider Arthritis. Z Rheumatol 59: 101-7
22. Köck FX, Fischer M, Schill S (2002) Die Schuhversorgung. Orthopädie-Schuhtechnik. Sonderheft Rheuma: 11-22
23. Kofoed H, Danborg L (1995) Biological fixation of ankle arthroplasty. The Foot 5: 27-31
24. Kofoed H, Lundberg-Jensen A (1999) Ankle arthroplasty in patients younger and older than 50 years: a prospective series with long-term follow-up. Foot Ankle Int (US) 20 (8): 501-6
25. Lachiewicz PF, Inglis AE, Ranawat CS (1984) Total ankle replacement in rheumatoid arthritis. J Bone Joint Surg 66 A: 340-3

26. Larsen A, Dale K, Eek M (1977) Radiographic evaluation of rheumatoid arthritis and releated conditions by standard refernce films. Acta Radiol 18: 481-91
27. Mohing W, Köhler G, Goldewey J (1982) Synovectomy of the ankle joint. Int Orthopedics 6: 117-21
28. Nassar J, Cracchiolo A (2001) Complications in surgery of the foot and ankle in patients with rheumatoid arthritis. Clin Orthop 2001 (1): 142-52
29. Newton SEI (1982) Total ankle arthroplasty. Clinical study of fitfty cases. J Bone Joint Surg A 80: 1410-20
30. Rehart S, Peters A, Kerschbaumer F (1999) Arthrodesen am unteren Sprunggelenk beim Erwachsenen. Orthopäde 28: 770-77
31. Rittmeister M, Böhme T, Rehart S *et al.* (1999) Die Behandlung des rheumatischen oberen Sprunggelenks mit Synovektomie und Synoviorthese. Orthopäde 28: 785-91
32. Schwitalle M, Eckardt A, Rosendahl T *et al.* (1998) Evaluation von Spätergebnissen nach Clayton-Resektions-Arthroplastik bei rheumatischer Vorfußdeformität. Akt Rheumatol 23: 129-33
33. Schill S, Thabe H (1998) Ankle arthroplasty. A clinical follow-up. Current status of ankle arthroplasty. Koefed (Ed.) Springer-Verlag: 90-3
34. Schmidt K, Willburger RE, Miehlke RK (1997) Arthroskopische Behandlung des rheumatischen Sprunggelenks. Arthritis + Rheuma 18: 46-53
35. Schill S, Thabe H, Grifka J (2002) Operative Versorgung des rheumatischen Fußes. Orthopädie-Schuhtechnik. Sonderheft Rheuma: 11-22
36. Tillmann K (1977) Der rheumatische Fuß und seine Behandlung. Bücherei des Orthopäden. Band 18. Enke Verlag (Stuttgart)
37. Tillmann K (2004) Differenzialindikation zwischen OSG-Arthrodese/Endoprothese beim Rheumatiker. In: Imhoff A, Zollinger-Kies H (Ed.) Fußchirurgie. Thieme (Stuttgart, New York): 280-90
38. Vahvanen V (1967) Rheumatoid arthritis in the pantalar joints. Acta orthop Scand 107
39. Vainio K (1956) The rheumatoid foot: A clinical study with pathological and roentgenological comments. Ann Chir Gynaecol Fenn Suppl 1: 5-10
40. Wörner A (1973) Über den prozentualen Anteil der Kiefergelenksbeteiligung beim Krankheitsbild der chronischen Polyarthritis. Dissertation (Mainz)
41. Wolfrum U (1997) Die Sprunggelenke. Praktische Rheumaorthopädie. Thabe H (Ed.) Chapman &Hall: 264-79
42. Wolfrum U (1997) Der Vorfuß. Praktische Rheumaorthopädie. Thabe H (Ed.) Chapman &Hall: 280-308
43. Wülker N, Flamme CH, Müller A *et al.* (1997) 10-Jahresergebnisse nach Arthrodesen der Rückfußgelenke und des oberen Sprunggelenks. Z Orthop 135: 509-513

Mise en page: Déclic Graphique

Achevé d'imprimer en 2005
par EPEL Industrie Graphique
64700 Hendaye